CANCER ETIOLOGY, DIAGNOSIS AND TREATMENTS

LEIOMYOSARCOMA

RISK FACTORS, DIAGNOSIS AND TREATMENT OPTIONS

CANCER ETIOLOGY, DIAGNOSIS AND TREATMENTS

Additional books in this series can be found on Nova's website under the Series tab.

Additional e-books in this series can be found on Nova's website under the e-book tab.

CANCER ETIOLOGY, DIAGNOSIS AND TREATMENTS

LEIOMYOSARCOMA

RISK FACTORS, DIAGNOSIS AND TREATMENT OPTIONS

ROSEMARY H. LEACH
EDITOR

New York

For permission to use material from this book please contact us:
Telephone 631-231-7269; Fax 631-231-8175
Web Site: http://www.novapublishers.com

Library of Congress Cataloging-in-Publication Data

ISBN: 978-1-63117-940-2

LCCN: 2014938748

Published by Nova Science Publishers, Inc. † New York

Contents

Preface

Leiomyosarcomas (LMS) are soft tissue tumors derived from smooth muscles cells, often in the uterus, retroperitoneum, skin, vessels, and bone. They are one of the most common types of sarcoma. Most leiomyosarcomas are sporadic, but may develop in the setting of genetic syndromes such as hereditary retinoblastoma and L-Fraumeni syndrome. Leiomyosarcomas may also be a result of radiation exposure; however, radiation-induced sarcomas are typically undifferentiated, fibrosarcomas or malignant peripheral nerve sheath tumors. Like other sarcomas, prognosis is worse with higher grade tumors. Although chemotherapy and radiation are sometimes used as adjuvant therapy, the mainstay of therapy, and the only chance for cure, is surgery. The management of LMS is especially complex when the tumor involves major blood vessels. This book discusses the diagnosis and treatments most effectively used for Leiomyosarcomas. It also provides insight on the specific areas that LMS is found and how it affects that area.

Chapter 1 – *Introduction*: Leiomyosarcomas (LMS) are soft tissue tumors derived from smooth muscles cells, often in the uterus, retroperitoneum, skin, vessels, and bone. They are one of the most common types of sarcoma. Like other sarcomas, prognosis is worse with higher grade tumors. Although chemotherapy and radiation are sometimes used as adjuvant therapy, the mainstay of therapy, and the only chance for cure, is surgery. Full resection with R0 borders is necessary for cure. The question of management of LMS is especially complex when the tumor involves major blood vessels. To date, there are between 300-400 reported cases of LMS invading the inferior vena cava, about 12 cases of aorta involvement, and 38 cases involving renal vessels, splenic, or mesenteric vessels. In these reports, the management of the vessels is discussed, whether primary or patch repair, simple ligation, or replacement with a tube graft or autologous vein graft. There have been only seven papers reporting *ex vivo* surgical resection for LMS.

Data: In this chapter, the authors conduct the largest review to date of the literature regarding LMS involving each of the vessels above.

The authors identify several factors that correlate with disease-specific mortality, survival time, and recurrence, including grade, tumor location, and negative margins. The authors also provide the largest single-center case series to date of ex vivo surgery for treatment of these tumors.

Discussion: Finally, the authors discuss the major surgical considerations and debates regarding this topic, including the various approaches to managing the resected IVC, the best choice of graft materials, and the roles of anticoagulation, arteriovenous fistula creation, and chemotherapy/radiation. The authors evaluate the options using the perspectives gained from having reviewed the bulk of the world's experience to date as well as their own analysis of the data, which is the world's largest to date. Thus, their chapter both summarizes the experience with aggressive surgical resection of LMS and contributes new knowledge regarding ex vivo surgery for LMS invading major blood vessels.

Chapter 2 – Leiomyosarcomas (LMS) are a common subtype of sarcoma that is frequently characterized by aneuploidy. However, leiomyosarcomas of the genitourinary (GU) tract make up less than 5% of all leiomyosarcomas. Areas of involvement includes bladder, prostate, seminal vesicle, and renal which will be discussed herein. Given rarity of these tumors, no consensus on treatment guidelines are available. However, a common unifying theme suggests that these are highly aggressive tumors that have a high propensity for metastasis even with adequate surgical extirpation. This review will discuss the common presentation, risk factors, treatment and prognosis associated with these GU tumors.

Chapter 3 – Leiomyosarcoma represents a particular subset of malignant connective tissue neoplasms arising from smooth muscle. Soft tissue sarcomas themselves are relatively uncommon, and leiomyosarcomas represent less than 10% of this group of cancers. These tumors are traditionally quite resistant to radiation and chemotherapy, and surgical intervention remains the best option for affected patients. Smooth muscle is located throughout the entire body, including intra-abdominal organs, blood vessel walls and skin. Many of these cancers occur in the gastrointestinal tract and uterus, with extirpation and wound closure performed by the primary surgical team. They can also be found in the abdominal wall, retroperitoneum, thorax, and pelvic viscera which introduces certain reconstructive challenges. As plastic and reconstructive surgeons, we are often called upon to assist our oncologic surgical colleagues to help restore the integrity of the abdominal wall, chest wall, and pelvis following excision. Techniques utilized range in complexity from primary closure and local tissue rearrangement to free microvascular tissue transfer. In this chapter the authors will speak to the basics of leiomyosarcoma tumor biology and then highlight some of the principles of reconstructive surgery as well as challenges specific to defects created by soft tissue sarcoma resection.

Chapter 4 – Leiomyosarcomas are rare and often aggressive forms of sarcoma that arise from various anatomic locations. Leiomyosarcomas commonly originate from the smooth muscle of the soft tissues, gastrointestinal tract and uterus and account for approximately 5% to 10% of all soft tissue sarcomas. Diagnosis and treatment of leiomyosarcomas involves a multimodality approach; however, even with aggressive treatment, survival and prognosis of this disease is relatively poor. This chapter highlights the risk factors, diagnosis, and treatment options for localized and metastatic leiomyosarcomas.

Chapter 5 – Primary intracranial leiomyosarcoma is a malignant intracranial tumor of smooth muscle origin. Limited literature data suggest that it may have unique pathogenesis, which raises the possibility of special treatment and different prognosis from conventional extracranial leiomyosarcomas. This chapter discusses the epidemiology, pathology, and treatment of this tumor.

Chapter 6 – Sarcomas represent a rare class of soft tissue cancers that can occur anywhere in the body. Soft tissue sarcomas represent 0.7% of all malignant tumors. Urologic primary sarcomas are extremely rare. They can arise from the testes, paratesticular tissues, penis, bladder, prostate, kidneys and retroperitoneal tissue. The most common type is a leiomyosarcoma (LMS), but other types of sarcomas can occur including liposarcomas, rhabdomyosarcomas, and fibrosarcomas.

The purpose of this review is to present the epidemiology and possible risk factors in each of the urogenital sites, together with clinical presentation and imaging modalities that can assist in diagnosing LMS. Also presented are histological diagnosis and the immunohistochemical use of myogenic markers (h-caldesmon, desmin and muscle-specific actin) to help define smooth or skeletal muscle differentiation in soft tissue tumors (skeletal alpha actin, myogenin, MyoD1 and myoglobin). Current treatment options for genitourinary tumors are addressed: surgery, radiation therapy, chemotherapy and new targets such as antiangiogenic therapy. This review also examines the systemic approaches currently used, or which are under evaluation, to improve the outcome of patients with this disease.

Chapter 7 – Leiomyosarcoma is an aggressive mesenchymal tumor derived from smooth muscle cells accounting for up to 30% of all sarcomas. Cardiac impairment is often a character of its metastatic involvement or, less likely, the heart can be the only organ targeted by this rare tumor disease. Patients with established diagnosis of cardiac leiomyosarcoma present with various symptoms relating to the tumor disease itself or may have symptoms associated with the location and extent of the tumor mass in the heart. Imaging modalities used in routine practice are of great importance in establishing diagnosis, assessing tumor disease staging and in evaluating the response to the selected therapeutic modality. Unfortunately, the long asymptomatic course of cardiac leiomyosarcoma and the aggressive behavior of this tumor have made available therapeutic interventions at presentation of limited efficacy. While the role of chemotherapy is not well established and considering that leiomyosarcoma is known to have a low radiosensitivity, surgical resection of the tumor mass is the treatment option with proven positive impact on patient's survival, symptoms and quality of life. In general, leiomyosarcoma is difficult to treat and has a poor prognosis.

In this article the authors review cardiac leiomyosarcoma, its prevalence, clinical manifestation, the diagnostic modalities used for establishing the diagnosis of leiomyosarcoma, current treatment options available for the management of this disease and patient prognosis and outcomes.

Chapter 8 – Atypical intradermal smooth muscle neoplasms (AISMN, formerly known as cutaneous leiomyosarcomas) are uncommon neoplasms, which seem to be remarkable for their excellent prognosis in contrast to their deeper counterparts. The authors evaluated the histologic and immunohistochemical features of 4 cases of AISMN.

The immunohistochemical stains such as smooth muscle actin and muscle specific actin, when are used in combination, can identify smooth muscle differentiation in 100% of the cases. With some caveats, CD34, S100, and CK 5/6 are helpful in ruling out other important cutaneous spindle cell neoplasms. Malignancy criteria established by WHO include high cellularity, nuclear atypia significantly and at least one mitosis by 10 high power fields. Actually noted the utility of immunohistochemical marker of mitosis phosphohistone H3 (phH3) in diagnostic leiomyosarcomas with mitotic activity and some degree of atypia nuclear.

AISMN can have significant morphologic variation and overlap with other spindle cell neoplasms of the skin and that a limited panel of key immunohistochemical stains should be used to distinguish this lesion.

Chapter 9 – Uterine leiomyosarcoma, though the most common mesenchymal tumor, yet constitutes only 1-2% of all uterine malignancies. This malignancy is well known for its aggressiveness and confers a poor prognosis, even if diagnosed at an early stage; once disseminated, the overall survival is usually only 2.8 years. The majority of these tumors are only identified at histopathological examination of hysterectomy or myomectomy specimens. An increasing trend towards conservative treatment of leiomyomas such as uterine artery embolization and gonadotropin-releasing-hormone agonists, may further delay the accurate diagnosis of these tumors, posing the risk of an increased incidence of high-grade tumors at presentation.

Chapter 10 – Leiomyosarcoma (LMS), one of the most commonly diagnosed subtypes of sarcoma, is an aggressive malignancy of smooth muscle (SM) origin for which the basis of transformation and mechanisms of progression are mostly unknown. This tumor usually occurs in middle-aged or older adults. Given the variety of anatomical locations of SM tissues, LMS can arise in various regions of the body, and forms a significant percentage of retroperitoneal, vascular, extremity, and uterine sarcomas. Imaging studies often demonstrate LMS as a nonspecific soft tissue mass; the definitive diagnosis relies on histological examination. Following diagnosis of LMS, the first line of defense is surgical resection of the primary tumor, radiotherapy or chemotherapy is also needed due to common involvement of adjacent tissues and high recurrence rates. Although tumors from the various regions are histologically similar, they often have different clinical courses and chemotherapeutic responses. Clinically, LMS of cutaneous origin usually has a favorable outcome than of deep tissue origin, such as the frequent retroperitoneal tumors. This review delineates the risk factors, diagnosis and treatment of LMS in different sites; aim to better manage the care of those diagnosed with LMS.

Chapter 11 – The vast majority of mesenchymal neoplasms of the gastrointestinal (GI) tract are currently identified as GI stromal tumors (GISTs). According to the World Health Organization's classification of the tumors of the digestive system 2010, primary GI leiomyosarcoma (GI-LMS) in the post-GIST era is so rare that there are no significant data on clinicopathological features of this tumor. Because of different treatment options available, it is crucial to distinguish the GI-LMS from the GIST accurately, on the basis of histological criteria combined with smooth muscle antigens as well as GIST-specific molecular markers. In this review, the authors summarize immunohistochemical diagnosis, prognostic factors as well as clinical management of the GI-LMS and the GIST.

Chapter 12 – Primary ovarian sarcoma is a very rare tumor, accounting 1% of all ovarian malignancies. The most common histologic subtypes are: mixed mullerian tumor, stromal cell sarcoma and fibrosarcoma. Primary ovarian leiomyosarcoma is an extremely rare histologic subtype of ovarian sarcomas. Until now, about 66 cases have been reported in English literature. Among them, 43 were primary ovarian leiomyosarcoma without heterologous elements and 23 were primary ovarian leiomyosarcoma with heterologous elements. It is usually occurs in postmenopausal women, although sometimes younger women may be affected. The mean age at diagnosis is 52 years (range 12-84 years). The precise histogenesis of primary ovarian leiomyosarcoma is relative unknown. It is probably originates from smooth muscle present in the walls of the blood vessels in the cortical stroma, in the corpus luteum, in the ovarian ligaments at their point of attachment to the ovary, in remnants of Wolffian ducts and in totipotential cells of ovarian mesenchyme. Most patients with primary ovarian leiomyosarcoma usually have nonspecific symptoms and signs. Also they have pressure symptoms on adjacent organs. Primary ovarian leiomyosarcoma is typically present as a solitary, large, lobular, soft, fleshy, solid mass with hemorrhage and cystic degeneration.

It is usually unilateral and may reach more than 10 cm in diameter. The diagnostic criteria for primary ovarian leiomyosarcoma are: hypercellularity, nuclear atypia, pleomorphism, coagulative necrosis and high mitotic activity. Immunohistochemical staining for primary ovarian leiomyosarcoma is generally positive for muscle specific actin, SMA, desmin, vimentin, p53 and proliferation markers and negative for cytokeratins and S-100. Due to the rarity of primary ovarian leiomyosarcoma, it is very difficult to determine the optimal therapy. Surgery is the baseline therapy and complete resection should be attempted whenever possible. Postoperative adjuvant radiotherapy is used for local disease control. Postoperative adjuvant chemotherapy is used in patients with locally advanced or metastatic disease. The prognosis of primary ovarian leiomyosarcoma is generally unfavorable, depending on mitotic activity and stage at diagnosis. Most patients die with extended local disease and multiple distant metastases.

Chapter 13 – Leiomyosarcoma, a malignant tumor that arises from mesenchymal tissues, is the most common soft-tissue sarcoma. Although rarely found in the female genital tract, leiomyosarcoma is the most malignant tumor that can occur in the female genital tract. Although leiomyosarcomacan occur anywhere through the female genital tract (including the uterine body, uterine cervix, ovary, salpinx, vagina and vulva), it is most commonly found in the uterine body. Uterine leiomyosarcoma is the most common uterine sarcoma, with an incidence of uterine leiomyosarcoma of 0.64 per 100,000 women. It is the single largest site-specific group of leiomyosarcoma. Given the rarity of leiomyosarcoma in the female genital tract, the causes and risk factors are not well known. The pretreatment diagnosis of leiomyosarcoma in the female genital tract is challenging because most cases are diagnosed after inadvertent surgery for presumed fibroids. Surgery is the only curable treatment for leiomyosaroma, with rates of cure of other treatment modalities (including radiation therapy, chemotheprapy, and targeted therapy) remaining uncertain. This review summarizes the most recent findings regarding the risk factors, diagnosis, and treatment options for leiomyosarcoma in the female genital tract.

In: Leiomyosarcoma
Editor: Rosemary H. Leach
ISBN: 978-1-63117-940-2

Chapter 1

Surgical Management of Leiomyosarcoma Involving the Major Abdominal Vessels

Joshua Weiner, Adam Griesemer and Tomoaki Kato*

Columbia University College of Physicians and Surgeons, Center for Liver Disease and Transplantation, New York, NY, US

Abstract

Introduction: Leiomyosarcomas (LMS) are soft tissue tumors derived from smooth muscles cells, often in the uterus, retroperitoneum, skin, vessels, and bone. They are one of the most common types of sarcoma. Like other sarcomas, prognosis is worse with higher grade tumors. Although chemotherapy and radiation are sometimes used as adjuvant therapy, the mainstay of therapy, and the only chance for cure, is surgery. Full resection with R0 borders is necessary for cure. The question of management of LMS is especially complex when the tumor involves major blood vessels. To date, there are between 300-400 reported cases of LMS invading the inferior vena cava, about 12 cases of aorta involvement, and 38 cases involving renal vessels, splenic, or mesenteric vessels. In these reports, the management of the vessels is discussed, whether primary or patch repair, simple ligation, or replacement with a tube graft or autologous vein graft. There have been only sever papers reporting *ex vivo* surgical resection for LMS.

Data: In this chapter, we conduct the largest review to date of the literature regarding LMS involving each of the vessels above.

We identify several factors that correlate with disease-specific mortality, survival time, and recurrence, including grade, tumor location, and negative margins. We also provide the largest single-center case series to date of ex vivo surgery for treatment of these tumors.

Discussion: Finally, we discuss the major surgical considerations and debates regarding this topic, including the various approaches to managing the resected IVC, the

* Corresponding author: Tomoaki Kato. E-mail address: tk2388@cumc.columbia.edu.

best choice of graft materials, and the roles of anticoagulation, arterio-venous fistula creation, and chemothera-py/radiation. We evaluate the options using the perspectives gained from having reviewed the bulk of the world's experience to date as well as our own analysis of the data, which is the world's largest to date.

Thus, our chapter both summarizes the experience with aggressive surgical resection of LMS and contributes new knowledge regarding ex vivo surgery for LMS invading major blood vessels.

Introduction

Some topics in medicine, as is popular culture, disproportionately seem to influence those involved those whom they engage. It was once said of an iconic album, "The first Velvet Underground album sold only 10,000 copies, but everyone who bought it formed a band."

So it is with leiomyosarcoma (LMS) cases involving large abdominal vessels. The widely repeated shibboleth is that there have been roughly 300 known cases of this presentation, but it seems that every one of these cases has spawned a case report, if not more than one. One speculates that this topic is so frequently reported when it occurs because of its relative rarity, the uniqueness and often heroic nature of each patient's surgical treatment, and finally because of the way the evolution in treatments has reflected the most recent technical advances in surgical oncology.

In this chapter, we consolidate what is known about surgical treatment of LMS involving major abdominal vessels by synthesizing the disparate case reports. This is also the first manuscript that will present data from all major abdominal vessels side by side.

Finally, we present the world's largest case series of *ex vivo* surgeries for LMS involving major abdominal vessels.

General Background

LMS is a malignancy involving mesenchymal cells of smooth muscle origin.

The first reported involvement of LMS in a major abdominal vessel was an IVC tumor described by Perl in 1871 (Perl 1871), and the first resection of such a tumor was performed by Melchior in 1928 (Melchior 1928). LMS makes up 0.5-1% of all malignant tumors (Tan 2009, Dull 2013), between 5-7% of all sarcomas (Kulayat 1997, Gage 2012), and 45% of retroperitoneal malignancies (Tan 2009). LMS has a strong female predilection, with a reported overall 2:1 or greater sex ratio (Gage 2012). Most LMS occurs in the uterus, subcutaneous soft tissue, and retroperitoneal soft tissue, with only about 2% or fewer involving blood vessel walls (Gage 2012, Kwon 2003, Tan 2009). However, this is enough to make it the most common type of sarcoma involving vessel walls (Mayer 2007). When these tumors do involve blood vessels, the inferior vena cava (IVC) is the most common location making up 50-75% of vascular LMS cases (Aguilar 2005, Dzinich, Tan 2009), followed by the thoracic aorta and pulmonary arteries (Kevorkian 1973, Kulayat 1997, Kwon 2003). In fact, LMS is the most common tumor involving the IVC (Cacoub 1991).

Among abdominal vessels, LMS next most commonly involves the renal vessels followed by the superior mesenteric vein (SMV) (Gage 2012). Overall, venous location of LMS is 5 times more common than arterial (Kevorkian 1973).

Other features of LMS are either unique to their location or have not been shown to be universally true of all LMS locations. However, a few basic tenets are common to all LMS tumors. One is that chemotherapy and radiation, while possibly having a palliative effect, have never been definitively shown to improve survival with LMS of any kind (Bathan 2013). It follows that the second basic tenet is that the only potentially curative treatment is full resection (Bathan 2013). 95% of cases are treated surgically, with advanced disease, inoperable tumor, and preoperative death being the most common reasons for not operating (Gage 2012). For retroperitoneal sarcomas as a whole, decreased local recurrence is seen with radical en bloc resection (Zaenkert 2013). En bloc resection is successful since the tumor is usually confined by its capsule (Illuminati 2006, Kulayat 1997). Therefore, aggressive resection is recommended, even if the tumor invades a major vessel requiring replacement. Full resection is the standard of care and the only chance for cure of vascular LMS (Keiffer 2006, Hollenbeck 2003, Hines 1999).

Given that full en bloc resections are complex and difficult procedures, with each one requiring unique approaches to removing the tumor and all associated organs and structures, a high level of skill and experience is necessary.

It makes sense that survival and functional outcomes after resections of retroperitoneal sarcomas as a whole are therefore also generally better at high-volume centers, especially if the tumors are large or high grade (Gutierrez 2007, Zaenkert 2013). In fact, one study showed that inadequate resection at a non-specialized center could later be corrected with good outcomes by repeat resection at a high-volume center. In contrast, the survival of patients not treated by resection or treated with inadequate resection is dismal (Mann 2012, Hollenbeck 2003).

Another basic tenet about all vascular LMS is poor prognosis. In one study of 143 patients with LMS in various locations, 1 and 3-year survival was 87% and 58% with too few remaining patients to calculate 5-year survival (Gage 2012). In comparing vascular LMS to LMS at other locations, Bathan et al. speculate that vascular LMS have very poor prognosis in particular due to its unchecked local spread and frequent hematogenous metastates (Bathan 2013). There is no existing literature comparing the prognosis between LMS affecting different vessels, mostly because the reports of LMS in vessels besides the IVC are so limited.

Beyond the facts above, which are applicable to LMS located in any vessel, almost the entirety of the remainder of knowledge about vascular LMS in the abdomen is limited to the IVC. The overwhelming majority of vascular LMS literature concerns the IVC, literally hundreds of reports and case series. Consequently, there is a great deal known about IVC LMS, and this makes up the bulk of our knowledge and our discussion below. LMS cases involving other vessels are described in only a handful of reports, too few to make any definitive conclusions or even to debate conflicting findings or approaches. However, it is possible that much of what we know about LMS of the IVC can apply to LMS of the other vessels. We will present and analyze these cases to the extent that they are available in the literature.

IVC

General Background

As previously noted, 50-60% of vascular LMS are found in the IVC, and LMS is the most common tumor of the IVC.

LMS of the IVC, like LMS as a whole, has a strong female predilection, with a reported 4:1 to 6:1 sex ratio (Tan 2009, Cacoub 1991, Mingoli 1991, Kulayat 1997). Some authors speculate that the female predominance might represent occult spread from the uterus, which is a frequent LMS location (Laskin 2010). Certainly there have been confirmed cases of IVC spread from uterine tumors (Moorjani 2005). Although these tumors can affect patients at any age, they most frequently affect women in their sixth decade and men in their seventh (Cacoub 1991). The overall mean age at presentation is reported as 54.4-58 years for IVC LMS tumors (Tan 2009, Kulayat 1997).

Mean reported size of IVC LMS is 11 +/- 5.3 cm (range 2-30) with grade evenly split between low (25.7%), moderate (27.1%), and high (25%) (Mingoli 1991). For the purpose of identifying tumor location, the IVC is commonly divided into three regions: infra-renal (I), between renal and hepatic vessels (II), and superior to the hepatic vessels (III) (Figure 1).

In previous large IVC LMS case series, region II is almost always the most common location followed by region I then region III (Mingoli 1991, Cacoub 1991, Laskin 2010).

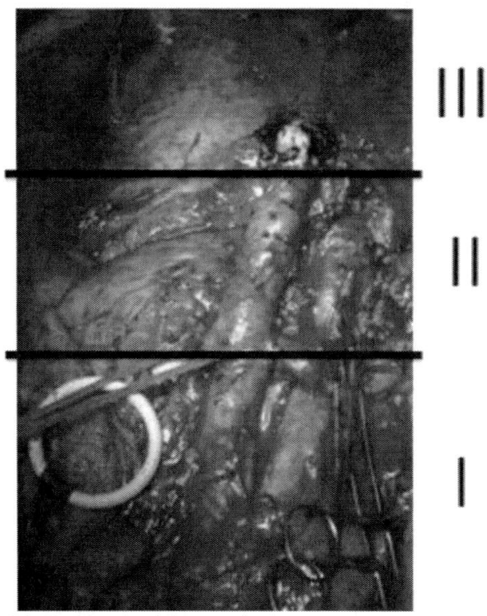

Photo by Yojiro Kato, M.D., Ph.D. Used with permission.

Figure 1. Regions of the IVC. Region I is inferior to the renal vessels. Region II lies between the renal vessels and hepatic veins (here shown as a Dacron patch where the hepatic veins have been resected). Region III lies superior to the hepatic veins.

Specifically, Mingoli et al. in their International Registry of IVC Leio-myosarcoma, which analyzed 144 previous patients with IVC LMS through a combination of literature review and personal correspondence, found the distribution to be 41.7% region II, 34% region I, and 24.3% region III (Mingoli 1991). Only very few smaller case series found region I to be the most common (Dew 2005, Dzsinich 1992, Kualayat 1997). The largest of these, Kulayat et al., in their review of 133 cases found the distribution to be 27.8% region I, 27% region II, 4.5% region III, and 21.5% mixed (Kulayat 1997). Within the IVC, as in other vessels, LMS originates in the smooth muscle of the media. In a review of 211 patients with IVC LMS by Hilliard et al., the tumor was found to grow murally in 5%, extraluminally in 23%, intraluminally in 23%, bidirectionally in 19%, and not specified in 30% (Hilliard 2005). In the large series in Kulayat et al., the growth was found to be mural in 6.8%, extraluminal in 29.3%, intraluminal in 24%, bidirectional in 27.8%, and unspecified in 12% (Kulayat 1997). One study found extraluminal growth to be as high as 60% (Laskin 2010).

Diagnosis

IVC LMS may be difficult to diagnose since it often presents with no symptoms or signs (Kulayat 1997). In fact, 50% of cases are diagnosed at autopsy (Mingoli 1991). Lab values are almost always normal, unless tumor-related hepatic vein obstruction causes elevated liver function test values (Kulayat 1997).

LMS tumors can be seen well on various imaging modalities, where they are often found incidentally. CT, MRI and ultrasound are all useful for showing both tumor and tumor thrombus, and venography can also show intraluminal thrombus as well as collaterals (Dull 2013, Bonura 2006, Bathan 2013, Luigi 2011).

When LMS symptoms are present, they are often non-specific, and LMS is rarely suspected due to its rarity (Kulayat 1997). In one study, the average duration of symptoms prior to diagnosis was 8 months with a range of 2 weeks to 12 months (Hilliard 2005).

The International Registry of IVC Leiomyosarcoma lists the most common presenting symptoms and signs of IVC leiomyosarcoma as follows: abdominal pain (66%), abdominal mass (47.9%), LE edema (38.9%), Budd-Chiari as a result of tumor in region III (22.2%), weight loss (30.6%), increased abdominal girth (30.6%), weakness (14.6%), nausea (14.6%), anorexia (13.2%), dyspnea (13.2%), vomiting (10.4%), fever (9%), jaundice (4.2%), nocturnal sweating (4.2%) (Mingoli 1991).

Other studies present similar findings (Kieffer 2006, Kim JT 2012, Kulayat 1997, Laskin 2010, Lovisetto 2013, Luigi 2011, Ito 2007). When the tumors occlude the renal ostia, they can occasionally contribute to acute renal failure (Hilliard 2005). Abdominal pain is especially common in region II, likely because of the many vital organs and nervous structures in this area (Laskin 2010). Although abdominal mass is listed as the second most common symptom or sign in the International Registry, IVC LMS is not detected on exam in 2/3 of cases (Kulayat 1997). It is possible that the proportion with palpable mass in the 1991 report of the Registry study was higher than it would be today due to more delayed diagnosis resulting from less frequent and less reliable imaging in 1991. IVC LMS presents earlier if intraluminal (Lovisetto 2013), likely because of effects on the circulation, such as edema, cardiac disease, hepatic and renal congestion, and pulmonary embolism (Kulayat 1997). 12% of all LMS tumors are metastatic at the time of diagnosis (Gage 2012).

Prognosis

The prognosis for IVC LMS, like that for other LMS, is poor. Part of the reason for the poor prognosis is advanced disease at diagnosis (Mayer 2007). In various literature reviews with large numbers of patients after tumor resection, Hollenbeck et al. put 3 and 5-year survival rates at 76% and 33% with no 3-year survivors among those with incomplete resections (Hollenbeck 2003); Ramponi et al. put 5 and 10-year survival rates at 30-54% and 7.4% (Ramponi 2012); and Mann et al. estimate 5-year disease-free survival at 30-53% and 5-year overall survival at 56%. In the 1991 report of the International Registry, 3 and 5-year survival rates were 76% and 33% with up to 50% recurrence, mostly within 30 months of resection (Mingoli 1991).

Of note, IVC LMS has a worse prognosis compared to other retroperito-neal sarcomas (Hines 1999, Hollenbeck 2003). On the other hand, its prognosis compares favorably to other tumors invading the IVC (Illuminati 2006) and to LMS in other locations (Hines 1999).

Prognostic Features

There is highly variable evidence regarding which factors affect prognosis of IVC LMS. Some of the potential factors that have been suggested include grade, location of IVC tumor, size of tumor, intraluminal versus extraluminal position, presence of liver failure, and Budd-Chiari, which correlates with tumor location in region III.

Margins are frequently listed as a prognostic feature as well.

For the purposes of this chapter, we will consider margins not as a prognostic factor but instead as a factor that is an important surgical considera-tion that affects operative planning, which we will present in greater detail in our discussion section.

Tumor grade affects prognosis in some study but not others. Kulayat et al. found a weak correlation between grade based on mitotic activity and distant recurrence, with 31% recurrence rate for grades 1 and 2 but 43% for grade 3 (Kulayat 1997). Poorly differentiated tumors, meaning higher grade, were also found to be a poor prognostic sign in the International Registry (Mingoli 1991).

Other studies found that higher grade was not a poor prognostic sign. While Kim et al. say grade is important, some of their longest survivors were high grade (Kim JT 2012). Dzsinich et al. found no correlation between grade and survival, and Laskin et al. found that necrosis (indicating high grade) does not decrease survival and that higher grade tumors were not more common in short-term survivors compared to long-term survivors (Dzsinich 1992, Laskin 2010). It is the rare study that finds that tumor location does not affect survival, especially location in the upper regions of the IVC. Two studies have shown tumor location not to be important for survival, but these results are directly challenged by Mingoli et al. using the data from the much larger International Registry (Dzsinich 1992, Hines 1999, Mingoli 1991, Mingoli 1993). Almost all other studies find that location matters and that more cephaled tumors in particular have worse prognosis (Lotze 2012, Laskin 2010, Mingoli 1991, Lovisetto 2013, Kulayat 1997, Monig 1995). This prognosis grows even worse if tumor invades the right atrium (RA), possibly even causing right-sided heart failure (Laskin 2010, Monig 1995). This is most likely because of the increased propensity of more cephaled tumors to grow intraluminally, which has worse prognosis, to block blood flow to the heart, and to make resection more technically difficult (Laskin 2010). The most superiorly located tumors are also associated with Budd-Chairi syndrome, which conveys even greater morbidity (Lovisetto 2013). It is worth noting, however, that the poor region III outcomes historically might be changing since many of these tumors used to be considered inoperable (only 3/35 were resected in the 1991 International Registry report), but that would likely not be the case today with more experience with these procedures (Mingoli 1991).

Most studies also found that level II tumors have better prognosis than level I tumors. The International Registry is an important exception. In that study, 5 and 10-year survival of those with segment I tumors was 9.3% and 0% versus 48.3% and 34.4% for those with segment II tumors (Mingoli 1991).

One possibility for the poor prognosis observed in LMS tumors of region I is that the relatively unconfined anatomical area allows a large amount of growth before detection or containment by surrounding structures (Mingoli 1991).

Relatively little is found in the literature regarding size as a prognostic factor. The most prominent example is a study by Ito et al. finding that smaller tumors correlated with better disease-free survival (Ito 2007).

A few studies attempt to analyze several prognostic factors. Perhaps the best is a study by Laskin et al. employing regression analysis of different factors. Poor prognostic features for long term survival in their findings included location in region III, intra-atrial invasion, positive margins, and intraluminal location, but not grade.

They also found several other factors with non-significant trend towards worse prognosis. Factors that correlated with worse survival on univariate analysis were intraluminal location, Budd-Chiari, liver failure of any cause, and moderate to poor tumor differentiation.

However, only liver failure correlated with worse survival on multivariate analysis (Laskin 2010).

In a separate analysis of 14 patients, Hines et al. found that factors that did not affect survival included age, gender, tumor size, tumor grade, and lymph node status. Tumor location (especially a beneficial location in region II) and negative margins did improve survival (Hines 1999).

Finally, the International Registry sheds light on several prognostic factors. Those associated with longer survival included radical resection, presentation with abdominal pain (perhaps because of earlier detection), and absence of palpable abdominal mass (perhaps indicating smaller size).

Factors that did not affect survival included age, gender, tumor size (maybe because resected tissues are sometimes included in the tumor size), presence of metastases, and use of adjuvant therapies. Nor did type of IVC management (ligation, graft, etc.) affect metastasis occurrence (Mingoli 1991).

Treatment

Radical curative resection is the only effective therapy for LMS (Mingoli 1991). Full resection is the standard of care and the only chance for cure (Keiffer 2006, Hollenbeck 2003, Hines 1999), even if it necessitates maxima-lly invasive surgery with multiple specialists doing their part (Wang 2007).

One of the reasons for the poor prognosis of LMS of the IVC is that complete resection of retroperitoneal tumor is technically difficult (Zaenkert 2013).

In one relatively but very thorough review of previous cases, only 66.7% of tumors could be resected: 56.9% with curative resection and 9.8% with palliative resection.

When resection is performed, there are many possibilities for addressing the vessel defect. The major categories of options include primary repair, patch repair, ligation without reconstruction, and graft replacement (Tan 2009, Fiore 2008). Again, most of these options, and the vast majority of the literature, are based on surgery of the IVC. It makes sense that primary repair is best if possible (Hollenbeck 2003). Advantages include shorter operative time, less lower extremity edema, less hemodynamic and coagulation complications, and less use of foreign material (Tan 2009, Fiore 2008).

Often, however, primary repair is not consistent with either full resection or the ability to maintain adequate blood flow (Spinelli 2008). In this case, autologous vein patch (saphenous or otherwise) is the next best option (Tan 2009, Fiore 2008). Another potential option is using a peritoneofascial (or fascio-peritoneal) patch, in which a flap of posterior rectus sheath is brought down to patch the defect (Fiore 2008).

Segmental resection of the vessel without reconstruction is one option if primary or patch repair are not possible. In this case, the vessel is simply ligated. In general, this option is quicker and less technically demanding than reconstruction and tends to have low morbidity if collaterals are well-developed (as they tend to be if the vessel is obstructed by tumor). It also avoids complications associated with later graft thrombosis, including major embolic events. However, without good collaterals, and sometimes even *with* good collaterals, the venous congestion can cause morbidity in regions proximal to the ligation (Tan 2009, Fiore 2008). As the outcomes after ligation and the surgical decision-making are complex and nuanced, a more extended consideration of vascular ligation can be found in the Discussion section.

When ligation is judged not to be appropriate, the vascular defect can be repaired with various types of grafts (Figure 2). The first description of IVC replacement with graft after resection for neoplasm in Starzl 1980 (Madariaga 2000).

Possible graft replacement materials include both natural and artificial materials. Natural materials consist of banked vena cava or aortic homograft (DiBenedetto 2012, Fiore 2008, Praseedom 2007, Zaenkert 2013), bovine pericardium (Mondragon-Sanchez 1998), or tube cavoplasty using autologous vessels, such as Soejima et al.'s use of internal jugular and external iliac veins sutured together into a tube (Soejima 2013). Graft materials consist of PTFE, Dacron, and Gore-Tex.

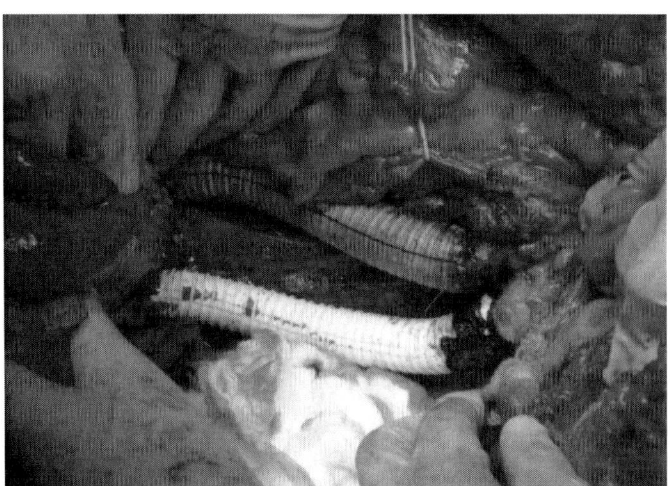

Photo by Yojiro Kato, M.D., Ph.D. Used with permission.

Figure 2. Example of graft replacement of major abdominal vessels after resection for sarcoma. At the top of the picture, the aorta is replaced with a Dacron graft, and the IVC is replaced with a Gore-Tex graft at the bottom of the picture.

The two most important complications of graft replacement are thrombosis and infection, and the risk of both is increased with synthetic grafts (Tan 2009). On the other hand, synthetic grafts have some advantages, such as the ability to resist compression and ready availability (Fiore 2008).

Once again, the choice of grafts is nuanced and will be addressed in greater detail in the Discussion section.

Regarding incision options, the choices differ depending on the level of IVC requiring resection. Tumors in IVC region I are usually approached via lower midline laparotomy (Kieffer 2006, Tan 2009).

If the pelvic space is too limited to permit access to the entirety of the tumor for mobilization, particularly the posterior aspect, a pelvic osteotomy can be performed to open the pelvic brim.

We employed that technique together with our orthopedic colleagues on one patient at our center with LMS in the pelvis involving the iliac vessels (Tomoaki Kato and Francis Lee, personal communication, unpublished report). Tumors in region II are approached via laparotomy or, even better, right subcostal incision if the top of the tumor does not extend above the lower edge of the liver, perhaps with the patient slightly in lateral decubitus to better expose the retrohepatic IVC (Kieffer 2006, Tan 2009).

A thoracoabdominal approach is mandatory for region III. Authors tend to prefer midline laparotomy and sternotomy to thoracophrenotomy (Kieffer 2006, Spinelli 2008).

This also provides a better position for establishing cardiopulmonary bypass if intracardiac surgery becomes necessary and is also better from a postoperative respiratory standpoint. A transdiaphragmatic pericardial window for intrapericardial IVC isolation has been described as an alternative to sternotomy (Chen 2007).

When the tumor is inferior to the renal vessels, resection of the IVC can be carried out prior to resection of the remaining tumor. This is not the case if the tumor is in regions II or III, in which vein clamping and resection must be performed last (Shindo 2002).

Venovenous bypass is an adjunct technique used for some cases of IVC LMS. It is used when surgeons cannot clamp proximally enough to prevent tumor embolus with very proximal tumors or if deep hypothermic circulatory arrest (DHCA) is required (Spinelli 2008) or to avoid massive bleeding or avoid low cardiac return and hemodynamic instability, but it should be avoided if possible due to requirement for anticoagulation and resulting risk of bleeding (Spinelli 2008).

Otherwise, IVC clamping without venovenous bypass is an acceptable option. The question is when is bypass necessary? Tan et al. write that venovenous bypass should be instituted if systolic blood pressure cannot be maintained at or above 100 mmHg and should be adjusted to keep the blood pressure at that level and central venous pressure at 10-12 mmHg (Tan 2009). It appears that venovenous bypass was used more in the earlier years of IVC reconstruction (a byproduct of experience with liver transplantation) and has become less favored as surgeons have gained experience without it and as data have shown that it is not necessary in most cases unless there is hemodynamic instability (Mingoli 1994).

For otherwise unresectable tumors, *ex vivo* resection remains an option. *Ex vivo* advantages include bloodless resection field, reduced time pressure, improved ability to perform R0 resection, providing better access to hepatic tumor and hepatic vasculature without risking warm hepatic ischemia and jeopardizing liver function, and decreased risk of iatrogenic tumor perforation or hematological dissemination of the malignant cells (Gruttadauria 2005, Brekke 2003).

Despite these advantages, *ex vivo* is not yet considered standard of care, however, and applies in only a few select cases. It should be performed only at a referral center for liver resection/transplantation. (Gruttadauria 2005).

The surgical techniques described above have developed over time, and therefore the ability to resect IVC LMS has improved with time. In particular, it is experience with liver transplantation and organ preservation that have fostered the evolution in these techniques, especially those necessary for IVC replacement, venovenous bypass, and ex vivo surgery (Brekke 2003).

Table 1 contains a partial list of the important milestones in surgery for LMS involving the IVC.

Table 1. IVS LMS Milestones

Perl 1871	First reported case of IVC LMS
Melchior 1928	First resection of IVC LMS
Cope 1954	First re-resection of IVC LMS for recurrence
Demers 1992	First failed resection followed later by definitive resection
Fabre 1995	First case report of leimyosarcoma of the middle and upper part of the vena cava successfully treated by surgical resection, complete vena cava replacement and disobliteration of the hepatic veins under veno-venous bypass and liver hypothermic perfusion using "ex-situ, in-vivo approach."
Mondragon-Sanchez 1998	First use of bovine pericarium graft
Chin 1999	First use of peritoneofascial flap
Kaushik 2002	First report of banked homograft use
Wong 2005	First report of emergent resection of IVC LMS, due to PE in this case
Kleisli 2006	First report of cavoatrial tumor resection without sternotomy
Chen 2007	First transdiaphragmatic pericardial window for intrapericardial IVC isolation
Guerrero 2007	First use of fresh allograft
Lygidakis 2007	First case of tumor involving all IVC segments resected by ligation alone
Fiore 2008	First case of banked iliac vein homograft use for IVC replacement
Tranchart 2008	First description of restoring right renal vein drainage in IVC resection by reimplanting into portal vein
Tan 2009	First description of IVC LMS with double IVC
Nayyar 2010	First description of left renal vein reconstruction after IVC resection by using saphenous vein jump graft to infratumoral IVC
Angiletta 2011	First use of Adams-DeWeese clip inferio to reval veins to prevent pulmonary embolism in case with known iliac thrombus
DiBenedetto 2012	First use of banked depopulated cryopreserved IVC homograft for IVC replacement
Liu 2013	First reported case of both renal veins reanastomosed directly to inferior caval segment
Soejima 2013	First reported case of tube cavoplasty

Surgical Outcomes

Due to the rarity of these surgical interventions, the surgical outcomes are best represented in reviews of large numbers of cases. The most often cited collection of cases is the International Registry of IVC Leiomyosarcoma, with publications by Mingoli et al.

In their 1991 report, surgical interventions included direct suture or patch in 27 patients, segmental caval resection with or without reconstruction in 51 patients, and unknown in 4 patients (Mingoli 1991). A 1994 update clarified that 7 of these cases replaced the IVC with prosthetic graft and 2 with autolo-gous vessel (Mingoli 1994).

There were 2 perioperative deaths, and the only early complication was lower extremity edema (27.5%). 22.9% of patients received chemotherapy 22.9%, 18% radiation, and 0.7% immunotherapy, although it is difficult to know how many of these were in patients who underwent resection as 16 of the 49 patients receiving any kind of adjuvant therapy were not operated upon, and 22 instances of adjuvant therapy were initiated after disease recurrence and not after the initial surgery.

Long-term follow up was available for 107 patients (74.3%). All without tumor resection died at a mean of 3 +/- 4.8 months. Of 8 patients with palliative resection, 2 were lost to follow up at 50 and 60 months, and the remaining 6 died at a mean of 21.11 +/- 19.8 months. Of 82 patients who underwent curative resection, 11 (13.4%) recurred locally (mean 24.5 +/- 20.2 months); 25 (30.5%) recurred distantly (mean 30.5 +/- 17.8 months); and 7 (8.5%) had local and distant recurrence (mean 30.5 +/- 17.8 months).

Of these recurrences, 26 died of recurrent disease (mean 36.8 +/- 13.9 months). 19 remained alive: 12 without recurrence (survival mean 63.1 +/- 56.9 months) and 7 with recurrence (mean 84 +/- 36.3 months). 5 of 7 of that remained alive with recurrence were reresected. 31 were lost to follow up, but it is known that 10 of these recurred, and 2 with recurrence were reresected. Total 5 and 10-year survival for those with curative resection was 27.9% and 14.2% (Mingoli 1991).

Perioperative mortality rates in the literature range between 0-20% (Hollenbeck 2003, Mann 2012). Local recurrence rates have been quoted at 26.5-33% at median 20-21 months in one review of the literature (Munene 2011), while another puts the overall recurrence rate at 1/3 to ½ within 30 months (Praseedom 2007).

Table 2 presents the outcomes and demographics in several of the largest series in the literature to date.

Introduction to Other Major Vessels

Most cases of vascular LMS in the literature pertain to the IVC, as do all large case series and reviews involving vascular LMS. In addition, all major points of discussion regarding vascular LMS (i.e., debates regarding various therapies and surgical decisions) pertain to the IVC. However, there is an important set of patients affected by LMS of the other major abdominal vessels. Therefore, while these other tumors contribute little to the interesting questions about this topic, their history is worth considering, and this chapter will serve as the largest and most complete review of these cases to date.

Aorta

The first case report of aortic sarcoma was described by Brodowsky in 1873 (Freyrie 2008). By the time Chiche et al. reviewed the topic in 2003, there were 132 documented cases of aortic sarcoma (not limited to LMS), almost all malignant (Chiche 2003). According to this excellent review, aortic sarcomas most often affected men (63.7%) with a mean age of 59.7 +/- 1.13 years (range 3.5 months to 85 years). Of all aortic sarcomas, the abdominal aorta was affected in 27.3% of cases. Tumors were classified into those that that grew from the intima into the lumen versus those that grew from the adventitia outwards, and it was rare to invade neighboring structures (Chiche 2003). Symptoms are highly variable, depending on which portion of the artery is occluded, and therefore which distal regions become ischemic or experience embolic events (Testini 1996). Intimal tumors usually present with severe hypertension caused by renal artery obstruction, ischemia caused by mesenteric artery obstruction, or embolic events. Medial or adventitial tumors most often present with back pain, anorexia, and mass effect, mimicking aneurysms (Malone 1996). There is also high risk from occluding intercostal vessels or even the artery of Adamkawiecz (paralysis) (Chiche 2003).

The first case of aortic LMS was described by Hernandez et al. in 1979. It was a 12 cm tumor associated with a pseudoaneurysm found during surgery in a 42-year-old man. The tumor was not resected and progressed despite chemotherapy and radiation. The patient died 2 years later (Hernandez 1979). Malone et al. described the first successful resection of aortic LMS in 1996 (Malone 1996). Other notable milestones include the first descriptions of survival after surgery for rupture of aortic LMS tumors (Testini 1996, Szekely 2000) and the first intravascular approach to graft replacement with aortic LMS resection (Presti 2012).

Of the 132 cases of aortic sarcoma in Chiche's review, 90 were resected, 44 with graft replacement, and 46 (52.1%) of these resections were complete. Since the margin of safety is not known, intraoperative negative histologic margins were used. There were 15 perioperative deaths (16.7%), usually due to embolic events, and mean survival was 16 +/- 2.4 months (range 0 – 168 months). Only 9 patients lived longer than 3 years after diagnosis. For those operated upon, 3 and 5-year survival was 16.5% and 11.8%, and both survival and metastases rates were better in those with mural versus intimal tumors. In contrast 1 and 3-year survival rates for those treated non-operatively were 13.4 % and 0 %.

The authors were unable to evaluate the benefit of chemotherapy and/or radiation due to small numbers and lack of randomized control study (Chiche 2003). In this chapter, we will review cases of aortic resection specifically for LMS.

Renal Vessels

LMS of the renal vessels was first reported by Lopez Varela et al. in 1967. In this case, a 40-year-old woman had an 8cm LMS of her right renal vein resected. No further details about her outcome are reported (Lopez Varela 1967). Just as there is a female-predominance in tumors in other vessels, 67-87% of cases are found in women (Aguilar 2005, Brandes 1996), and the average age is a mean of 57 (range 27-88) (Aguilar 2005). 60-64% of cases occur on the left side. Presenting symptoms include abdominal pain in 49-63%, flank mass in 15-18%, and weight loss in 13-26% (Aguilar 2005, Brandes 1996). After the first report, other notable milestones include the first report of prolonged survival (2.5 years) after resection of recurrence (Radhakrishnan 1978), the first report of multiple re-resections for recurrent metastases (Herman 1981), the first reported resection of renal LMS with a large tumor thrombus (Lipton 1995), and the first case of renal vein anastomo-sis to the IMV due to venous congestion (Arkadopoulos 2012).

Superior Mesenteric Vein

There are very few documented cases of LMS of the superior mesenteric vein (SMV), and no documented reports involving the superior mesenteric artery primarily. The first case of LMS arising primarily from the IMV was reported by Goldin et al. in 2002, and only 3 other reports have followed (Goldin 2002). Patients tend to present with epigastric discomfort or pain radiating to back and bloating and discomfort exacerbated with food intake (Goldin 2002) as well as abdominal fullness and appetite loss (Kuma 2008).

Symptoms can often be similar to those found with tumors of the portal vein, and the distinction lies primarily in the portal hypertension additionally seen with portal vein tumors (Madariaga 1995). In this chapter, we will present the largest series of SMV LMS to date and will review the surgical approaches and outcomes.

Inferior Mesenteric Vein

There are only 3 cases of LMS of the inferior mesenteric vein (IMV) and none of the artery. The first report was by Choquart et al. in 1976 (Choquart 1976). In this chapter, we will present the largest series of IMV LMS to date and will review the surgical approaches and outcomes.

Portal Vein

There are only 2 reported cases of LMS arising primarily from the portal vein, the first by Sundaresan et al. in 1990 (Sundaresan 1990). In this chapter, we will present the largest series of portal vein LMS to date and will review the surgical approaches and outcomes.

Splenic Vein

There is similarly very limited history of LMS of the splenic vein, and no reports of LMS in the splenic artery. The first reported case was in 1950 and appeared to have a good outcome, although the details are not specified (NEJM 1950). Presentation depends on the specific site of the tumor but tends to involve a palpable abdominal mass with abdominal pain, nausea, and fever associated with splenic vein occlusion (Aguilar 2005). Occasionally, tumor thrombus can extend into the portal vein (Gage 2012). In this chapter, we will present the largest series of splenic vein LMS to date and will review the surgical approaches and outcomes.

Ex Vivo

Typically, resectability is limited by involvement of hepatic veins (Spinelli Eur J Surg Onc 2008, Cacoub 1991, Delaunay 1991). *Ex vivo* was the next step to solve this problem. There are only 5 cases in the literature of *ex vivo* resections for LMS involving major abdominal blood vessels. In 1995, Fabre et al. described the first "*ex situ in vivo*" resection of LMS (Fabre 1995), but the first true *ex vivo* resection for LMS was described by Kraybill et al. in 1997 (Kraybill 1997). The surgical approaches and outcomes are highly variable from case to case. In this chapter, we will present the largest series of *ex vivo* resection for LMS to date and will review the surgical approaches and outcomes. In addition, we will present our own series of 5 cases of *ex vivo* resections for LMS involving major abdominal blood vessels, which is the world's largest single institution case series.

Data

Our inclusion criteria for articles included all publications in English available through the Columbia University library system concerning LMS involving major abdominal vessels. We further limited to selection to full articles (not abstracts) describing surgical management of these tumors unless used for background sections. Given the large number of articles concerning LMS of the IVC, these were further limited to the previous 10 years unless they involved three or more patients or were important landmark articles for any reason (novel technique, early cases, etc.). The tumors were categorized by vessel based on where the tumor initiated. To be considered renal vessel tumors, they must have been limited to the renal vessels.

For outcomes analysis, margins for tumors with multiple resections were only described for the first resection since the main goal of this chapter is analysis of the surgical approach to de novo disease rather than every recurrence. Tumors were graded as recurrent not if margins were microscopi-cally positive (R1) but if the patient developed clinically apparent disease. We did not differentiate retroperitoneal tumors invading the IVC from those arising from IVC because only rarely is this distinguished in the literature and the distinction does not affect management.

If information was not given for a particular variable (e.g., whether or not chemotherapy was used), we coded the answer as unknown rather than no. If a patient received adjuvant therapy after surgery due to recurrence, they were not coded as having received adjuvant therapy. This is because our aim was to see whether outcome depended on use of adjuvant therapy, not whether adjuvant therapy was used at all. For the purpose of analyzing complications, lower extremity edema was not in itself counted as a complication as it was not universally considered a complication throughout the literature and would have been difficult to compare. It was also an expected and usually transitory outcome of IVC resection. The vessels that we considered "major" were: IVC, aorta, splenic artery, splenic vein, SMA, SMV, hepatic veins, IMA, IMV, renal artery, renal vein, and portal vein.

Before showing the data, it is important for us to note that the information provided by the various papers we reviewed is highly heterogeneous.

Therefore, the numbers, ratios, and percentages differ from variable to variable based upon the sum of information that is provided by the pooled literature for each variable.

IVC

Overall, 111 papers meeting the inclusion criteria pertained to LMS tumors of the IVC. These papers described 363 total cases. There are many more cases if one considers those that fall outside the inclusion criteria, especially all the case reports before 2003. There were 247 female patients and 89 male patients (64% female) for an overall female-to-male ratio of 2.8:1, which is slightly lower than that previously described (Tan 2009, Cacoub 1991,

Mingoli 1991, Kulayat 1997). Mean age was 54.7 +/- 13.3 years (range 22-85). This lies in the same range previous reported in smaller series (Cacoub 1991, Tan 2009, Kulayat 1997).

Location of IVC tumors is shown in Figure 3. As in previous studies, we found the most common location to be region II. The locations were as follows: I 23% (n = 74), I/II 9% (n = 29), II 51% (n = 165), II/III 7% (n = 22), III 4% (n = 12), and I/II/III 6% (n = 18). Mean size of largest dimension was 10.0 +/- 5.4 cm (range 0.75-20). Of the 243 patients for whom tumor grade is provided, 34 (14.0%) were low grade, 76 (31.3%) were moderate grade, and 133 (54.7%) were high grade. For the purposes of our grading, low grade is defined as those identified as either low grade or grade 1, moderate grade is defined as those identified as moderate grade or 2, and high grade is defined as those identified as either high grade or 3-4. See Table 3 for summary of demographic information for IVC LMS tumors.

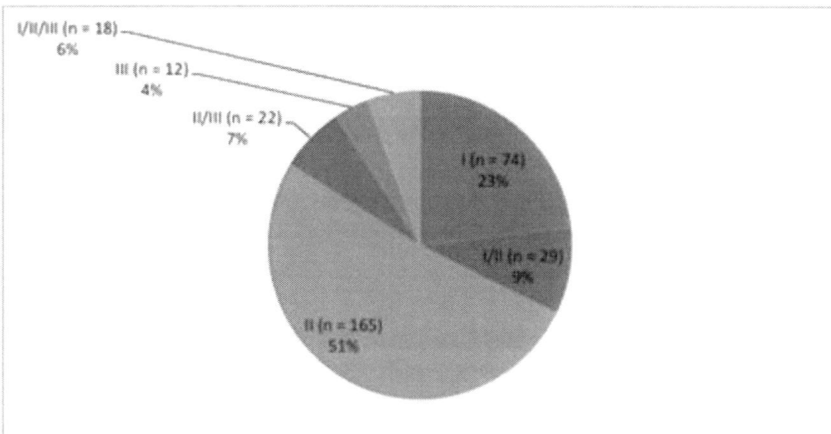

Figure 3. Location of IVC LMS by Region.

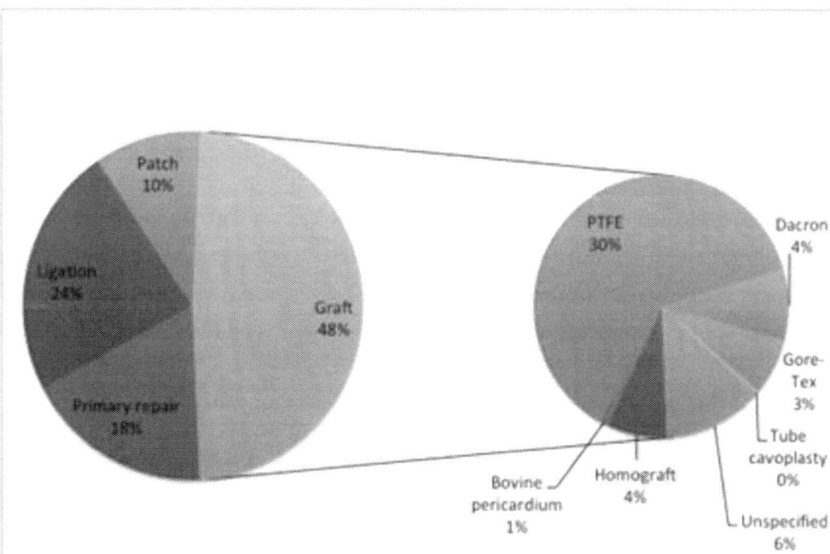

Figure 4. Management of IVC by Percentage.

Choice of approach to the surgical management of the IVC is shown in Figure 4. The IVC defect was able to be repaired by simple primary closure or patch in 18% and 10% of cases respectively. In 24% of cases, the IVC was ligated after resection, and the IVC was replaced by a graft after resection in 48% of cases. When a graft was used, PTFE was chosen 62.3% of the time (30% of all cases) followed by Dacron at 8.8%, homograft at 7.5%, and Gore-Tex at 6.9%. The choice of graft material was unspecified 12.6% of the time. In addition to surgery, neoadjuvant chemoradiation was used in 38 cases (10.5%), and any kind of chemotherapy or radiation was used in 97 cases (26.7%). The overall death rate from data that are available is 118/293 (40.3%). The overall disease-specific death rate is 111/293 (37.9%). The mean follow up is 37.6 +/- 39 months (range 0-216) with mean survival of 69 months and 3, 5, and 10-year survivals of 69.2%, 54.4%, and 28.2% (see Figure 5 and Table 4). These long-range survival values are in roughly the same range as those previously reported in smaller case-series (Hollenbeck 2003, Ramponi 2012, Mingoli 1991).

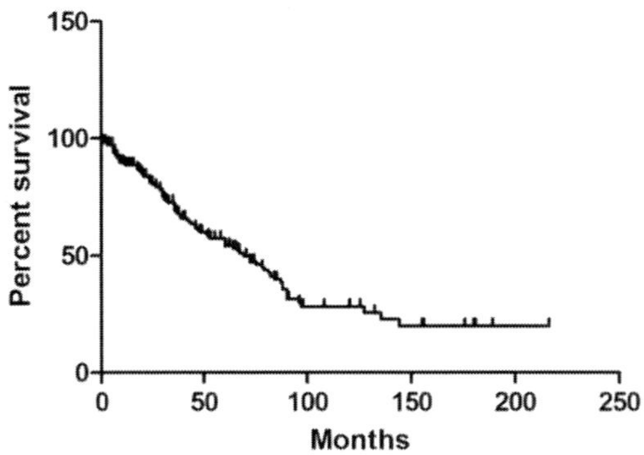

Figure 5. Overall Postoperative Survival After Surgery for IVC LMS.

Out of 287 patients for whom recurrence data are provided, 160 (55.7%) recurred, and mean time to recurrence was 20.6 +/- 23.3 months (range 1-156), although for earlier recurrence times it is not clear if these represent recurrences or failure to resect fully. Of the 167 patients for whom margin data are provided, 43 (25.7%) had positive surgical margins.

Table 5 reviews the relationship between several variables and survival, and Table 6 reviews the relationship of these same variables and recurrence. Table 7 evaluates the correlation between tumor location and size, which was significant, and the correlation between positive/negative margins and tumor size, tumor location, and the use of neoadjuvant therapy, none of which were significant.

Age does not appear to affect the rate of recurrence but may affect the time to recurrence. The mean recurrence rate in those younger than 50 was 53.7 % compared to a 58.8% rate in those older than 50 (p = 0.488). However, there was a non-significant trend towards shorter time to recurrence in those younger than 50 (16.71 +/- 19.03 months versus 23.37 +/- 25.64 months, p = 0.0635). This might indicate more aggressive tumors in younger patients. There was no significant difference in disease-specific survival rates or length of survival based on age. Gender did not affect the overall recurrence or disease-specific survival rates, but there were non-significant trends towards longer time to recurrence (23.19 +/- 26.11 months versus 14.81 +/- 13.02 months, p = 0.122) and longer survival (39.60 +/- 41.07 versus 30.86 +/- 30.20 months, p = 0.092) in women versus men.

Table 2. IVC LMS Large Case Series to Date

	Operative Patients (#)	M/F	Surgeries	Recurrence (#, %)	Mortality	Tumor grade	Tumor locations	Postoperative mortality	Postoperatve morbidity
Kulayat	132	75-80% female	Not resected: 30%; Resected: 70% (6.7% partial, 93.3% complete); Graft replacement in 11 (12.4%)	30 of 78 surgical survivors (38.5%)		High grade in 39% of specified case	I: 6, 45; II: 36, 27; III: 37, 27.8	5 (5.6%)	15% (mostly phlebitis)
Mingoli 1991	144	26/118	No resection: 51 patients; Partial resection: 11 patients; Complete resection: 82 patients (primary repair: 27, ligation: 42, prosthetic graft: 7, autologous graft: 2)	43 (52.4%)	5-year: 27.9%, 10-year: 14.2%	Low grade: 33%, Moderate grade: 35%, High grade: 32%	I: 49, 34, II: 59, 41.7; III: 34, 24.3	2 (2.4%)	27.5% with self-limited lower extremity edema
Mann 2012	233	unknown	Ligation: 29 patients (total number unclear); Cavoplasty: 87 patients; Prosthetic graft: 105 (total number unclear)				I: 15.2%%; II: 50.1%; III: 34.7%		
Hilliard 2005	211	54/157	Complete resection in 151 (71%), IVC handling not specified	56%	42% disease-specific mortality		I: 12% II; 51%; III: 33%; Unknown: 23%	4%	unknown
Daylami 2010	111	unknown	Ligation: 41/111 (37%); Reconstruction: 70/111 (63%)	47/111 (42.3%), some data missing	5-year survival: 35/111 (31.5%), some data missing	unknown	unknown	unknown	unknown

Table 3. Demographics of Patients with IVC LMS Tumors

	Number	%
Patient #	363	
Female: Male	247:89 (2.8:1)	64% Female
Mean Age	54.7 +/- 13.3 (range 22-85)	
Mean Size (cm)	10.0 +/- 5.4 (range 0.75-20)	
Low	34	14
Moderate	76	31.3
High	133	54.7
I	74	23
I/II	29	9
II	165	51
II/III	22	7
III	12	4
I/II/III	18	6

Table 4. Analysis of Outcomes

	Number	%
Overall Survival	118/293	40.3
Overall Disease-Specific Survival	111/293	37.9
Mean Survival (Months)	37.6 +/- 39.0	
Survival Range (Months)	0 - 216	
3-Year Survival		69.2
5-Year Survival		54.4
10-Year Survival		28.2
Patients with Recurrence	160/287	55.7
Mean Time to Recurrence (Months)	20.6 +/- 23.3	

Table 5. Relationship Between Variables and Survival

		Died of Disease	Survived	P	Mean Survival (Months)	P
Age	< 50 years	30 (34.1%)	58 (65.9%)	1	40.12 +/- 40.55	0.488
	≥ 50 years	59 (34.9%)	110 (65.1%		36.57 +/- 39.11	
Gender	Male	22 (34.4%)	42 (65.6%)	1	30.86 +/- 30.20	0.092
	Female	67 (35.1%)	124 (64.9%)		39.60 +/- 41.07	
Region	I	11 (22.4%)	38 (77.6%)	0.017	40.23 +/- 36.78	0.148
	I/II	9 (42.9%)	12 (57.1%)		39.59 +/- 41.38	
	II	28 (25.9%)	80 (74.1%)		39.66 +/- 42.03	
	II/III	4 (28.6%)	10 (71.4%)		33.31 +/- 49.37	
	III	7 (77.8%)	2 (22.2%)		22.56 +/- 18.35	
	I/II/III	4 (26.7%)	11 (73.3%)		16.43 +/- 13.56	
Tumor Size	0-5 cm	4 (19.0%)	17 (81.0%)	0.444	43.16 +/- 51.21	0.045
	5-10 cm	20 (28.6%)	50 (71.4%)		42.05 +/- 36.90	
	10-15 cm	9 (36.0%)	16 (64.0%)		39.50 +/- 47.44	
	15-20 cm	2 (25.0%)	6 (75.0%)		16.14 +/- 10.29	
	> 20 cm	2 (66.7%)	1 (33.3%)		19.33 +/- 20.68	
Grade	Low	7 (22.6%)	24 (77.4%)	0.33	44.62 +/- 43.10	0.77
	Moderate	24 (36.4%)	42 (63.6%)		43.05 +/- 41.84	
	High	29 (36.7%)	50 (63.3%)		40.59 +/- 42.78	
Margins	Positive	22 (53.7%)	19 (46.3%)	<0.0001	40.22 +/- 38.54	0.725
	Negative	23 (19.8%)	93 (80.2%)		34.79 +/- 36.90	
Any chemotherapy or radiation	Yes	29 (31.5%)	63 (68.5%)	0.346	40.80 +/- 38.37	0.126
	No	64 (37.6%)	106 (62.4%)		36.11 +/- 39.27	

Table 5. (Continued)

		Died of Disease	Survived	P	Mean Survival (Months)	P
Neoadjuvant chemoradiation	Yes	10 (27.0%)	27 (73.0%)	0.272	30.42 +/- 24.21	0.684
	No	83 (36.9%)	142 (63.1%)		38.68 +/- 40.65	
Recurrence	Yes	78 (60.0%)	52 (40.0%)	<0.0001	44.45 +/- 38.95	0.0001
	No	5 (4.5%)	105 (95.5%)		32.33 +/- 39.16	
Reresection for Recurrence	Yes	17 (50.0%)	17 (50.0%)	0.135	59.61 +/- 37.52	0.0005
	No	48 (66.7%)	24 (33.3%)		38.72 +/- 38.13	
Graft type	Allograft	0 (0%)	12 (100%)	0.308	24.46 +/- 20.79	0.085
	Bovine pericardium	0 (0%)	2 (100%)		54.00 +/- 59.40	
	PTFE	19 (29.7%)	45 (70.3%)		31.14 +/- 28.21	
	Dacron	2 (18.2%)	9 (81.8%)		60.20 +/- 64.44	
	Gore-Tex	2 (18.2%)	9 (81.8%)		12.55 +/- 12.72	
	Peritoneofascial flap	1 (50%)	1 (50%)		6	
	Tube Cavoplasty	0	1 (100%)		8	
IVC Treatment After Resection	Ligation	15 (27.3%)	40 (72.7%)	0.284	33.82 +/- 35.95	0.572
	Graft (Any)	35 (36.5%)	61 (63.5%)		35.02 +/- 33.94	

Note: Bold P values are significant ($p < 0.05$). Chi-squared test used for analysis of survival. ANOVA (multiple variables) or student's t test (2 variables) used for analysis of survival time.

Table 6. Relationship between Variables and Recurrence

		Recurrence	No Recurrence	P	Mean Time to Recurrence (Months)	P
Age	< 50 years	80 (53.7%)	69 (46.3%)	0.488	16.71 +/- 19.03	0.0635
	≥ 50 years	47 (58.8%)	33 (41.2%)		23.37 +/- 25.64	
Gender	Male	33 (55.0%)	27 (45.0%)	1	14.81 +/- 13.02	0.122
	Female	95 (55.9%)	75 (44.1%)		23.19 +/- 26.11	
Region	I	21 (51.2%)	20 (48.8%)	0.079	25.04 +/- 19.85	0.019
	I/II	9 (45.0%)	11 (55.0%)		6.75 +/- 3.40	
	II	63 (69.2%)	28 (30.8%)		20.11 +/- 17.91	
	II/III	7 (50.0%)	7 (50.0%)		8.80 +/- 5.93	
	III	7 (77.8%)	2 (22.2%)		8.08 +/- 2.76	
	I/II/III	6 (42.9%)	8 (57.1%)		6.67 +/- 3.22	
Tumor Size	0-5 cm	11 (47.8%)	12 (52.2%)	0.737	25.58 +/- 24.94	0.082
	5-10 cm	45 (58.4%)	32 (41.6%		20.60 +/- 18.25	
	10-15 cm	17 (58.6%)	12 (41.4%)		15.80 +/- 10.76	
	15-20 cm	10 (66.7%)	5 (33.3%)		7.23 +/- 3.88	
	> 20 cm	4 (57.1%)	3 (42.9%)		20.13 +/- 16.90	
Grade	Low	11 (37.9%)	18 (62.1%)	0.016	29.00 +/- 10.10	0.07
	Moderate	31 (50.8%)	30 (49.2%)		16.38 +/- 11.12	
	High	46 (67.6%)	22 (32.4%)		18.78 +/- 20.23	
Margins	Positive	27 (75.0%)	9 (25.0%)	0.001	24.77 +/- 22.48	0.23
	Negative	46 (43.4%)	60 (56.6%)		17.25 +/- 16.71	
Any chemotherapy or radiation	Yes	44 (55.7%)	35 (44.3%)	1	21.18 +/- 19.61	0.249
	No	85 (56.3%)	66 (43.7%)		20.32 +/- 25.12	
Neoadjuvant chemoradiation	Yes	16 (48.5%)	17 (51.5%)	0.352	19.48 +/- 13.18	0.439
	No	114 (57.3%)	85 (42.7%)		20.73 +/- 24.49	

Table 6. (Continued)

		Recurrence	No Recurrence	P	Mean Time to Recurrence (Months)	P
IVC Treatment After Resection	Ligation	25 (50%)	25 (50%)	0.863	14.63 +/- 18.60	0.127
	Graft (Any)	47 (48.0%)	51 (52.0%)		25.01 +/- 29.93	

Note: Bold P values are significant ($p < 0.05$). Chi-squared test used for analysis of recurrence. ANOVA (multiple variables) or student's t test (2 variables) used for analysis of time to recurrence.

Table 7. Other Correlations with LMS of the IVC

		Mean Size (cm)		P
Region	I	7.64 +/- 3.21		0.009
	I/II	10.33 +/- 5.07		
	II	10.19 +/- 5.22		
	II/III	9.95 +/- 5.64		
	III	10.97 +/- 5.26		
	I/II/III	14.95 +/- 8.88		
		Positive Margins	Negative Margins	P
Tumor Size	0-10 cm	24 (26.4%)	67 (73.6%)	0.287
	>10 cm	13 (36.1%)	23 (63.9%)	
Neoadjuvant chemoradiation	Yes	9 (27.3%)	24 (72.7%)	0.96
	No	34 (28.1%)	87 (71.9%)	
Region	I	7 (25.9%)	20 (74.1%)	0.935
	I/II	5 (29.4%)	12 (70.6%)	
	II	23 (31.1%)	51 (68.9%)	
	II/III	2 (20.0%)	8 (80.0%)	
	III	1 (33.3%)	2 (66.7%)	
	I/II/III	2 (22.2%)	9 (77.8%)	

Note: Bold P values are significant ($p < 0.05$). Chi-squared test used for analysis of margins. ANOVA used for analysis of mean size.

It has previously been suggested that tumors located more superiorly in the IVC, particularly region III, have worse prognosis due to the difficulty of the surgery and the increased complications associated with tumors in this region. We find evidence that this might be true to some extent. There is a nearly-significant trend towards higher recurrence rates with more superiorly-located tumors, with the highest recurrence rate in region III (77.8%, $p = 0.079$), and the time to recurrence is shorter in region II tumors as well as with tumors involving the entire IVC ($p = 0.019$). The time to recurrence is also shorter in tumors that straddle regions I and II, but this may be to a very low sample number. The increased recurrence rate in these regions appears to affect survival as well. The disease-specific death rate is significantly higher in region III tumors (77.8, $p = 0.017$), and there is a non-significant trend towards shorter survival times in more superiorly-located tumors ($p = 0.148$).

It is not clear whether the size of tumor affects recurrence. There is no significant difference in overall recurrence rate based on size ($p = 0.737$), although there is a nearly-significant trend towards shorter time to recurrence in tumors larger than 15 cm ($p = 0.082$). On the other hand, size does seem to affect survival time, although not the overall disease-specific survival rate. While the recurrence rate of the smallest sized tumors (0-5 cm) appears to be much lower than larger tumors (19% versus rates in the 20-60% range), this is not statistically significant ($p = 0.444$). However, the survival times are significantly shorter in those with tumors larger than 15 cm ($p = 0.045$).

Since prognosis seems to be somewhat worse in those with larger tumors and those with more superiorly-located tumors, it is worth asking if size and region correlate. Our data confirm that mean size of tumors increases in tumors located more superiorly ($p = 0.009$).

It has been suggested that higher grade tumors convey a worse prognosis (Kulayat 1997, Mingoli 1991), and we find evidence that this may be true. In our data, higher grade tumors correlate significantly with increased recurrence rates ($p = 0.016$), with a strong trend towards shorter time to recurrence ($p = 0.07$), with significance likely limited by small numbers (lack of adequate power).

It is not clear if these differences in recurrence translate into differences in survival, however. The percentage of disease-specific deaths increases in patients with higher grade tumors, but this is not statistically significant ($p = 0.330$), and there are no significant differences in survival times based on grade ($p = 0.770$).

Recurrence and survival rates are frequently thought to be strongly related to the presence of negative margins, and we find that this is correct.

The recurrence rate is significantly higher in those with positive margins versus those with negative margins (75.0% versus 43.4%, $p = 0.001$), and the disease-specific death rate is significantly higher (53.7% versus 19.8%, $p < 0.0001$) (see also Figure 6, a Kaplan-Meier curve showing the significant difference in survival time based on recurrence, $p < 0.0001$ by log-rank test).

Strangely, however, the presence of negative margins does not significantly decrease the time to recurrence ($p = 0.230$) or the survival time ($p = 0.725$). This is probably a product of the way in which authors report and evaluate their margins. Negative margins are subjective because they depend on the number of margins sampled and the locations from which the samples are taken. In addition, margins are often not reported in the literature.

Finally, our review is the largest correlation to date of radiation and chemotherapy to recurrence in survival after surgery for LMS if the IVC.

Unfortunately, our review is highly imperfect due to the sparse data regarding these adjunct therapies, the lack of details about the way in which they are used and when/why they are selected for use, and the heterogeneity of the adjunct therapy regimens. This makes comparison highly difficult, if not impossible.

Likely for those reasons, we find no significant differences in recurrence rates ($p = 0.352$ and 1), time to recurrence ($p = 0.439$ and 0.249), overall disease-specific survival ($p = 0.272$ and 0.346), or survival time ($p = 0.684$ and 0.126) between those with or without neoadjuvant or adjuvant chemotherapy or radiation.

Since margins are an important predictor of both recurrence and disease-specific mortality, we analyzed factors that could affect the ability to achieve negative margins, including larger tumor size, the use of neoadjuvant therapy, or the region of IVC involvement.

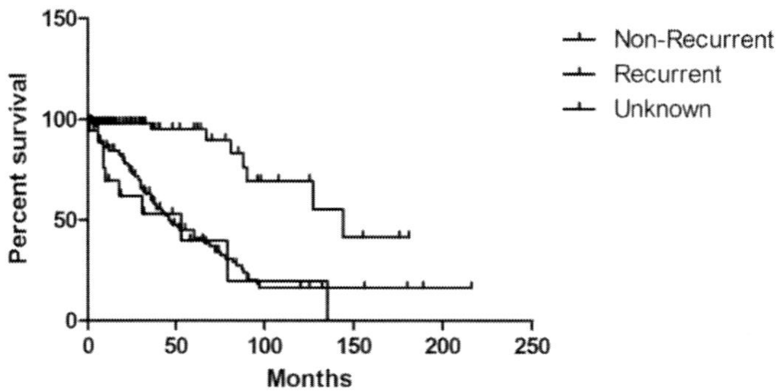

Figure 6. Survival as Function of Recurrence, $p < 0.0001$ (log-rank test).

Neoadjuvant therapy, in particular, has been advocated due to the hypothesis that it might contribute to negative margins (see discussion below).

We find no significant correlation between any of these factors and the achievement of negative margins ($p = 0.287$ for tumor size, $p = 0.96$ for neoadjuvant therapy, and $p = 0.935$ for IVC region).

Until now, we have considered recurrence and survival in parallel, but we also examined the correlation of tumor recurrence with changes in survival.

The disease-specific mortality rate is significantly higher in those with recurrence versus those without (60.0% versus 4.5%, $p < 0.0001$). Strangely, however, survival time is significantly longer in those who recur versus those who do not (44.45 +/- 38.95 versus 32.33 +/- 39.16 months, $p < 0.0001$). This could mean that those with recurrence tend to live longer, although they are much more likely to die of the disease when death finally occurs. More likely, this discrepancy reflects the lack of completeness in the follow up of patients without recurrence. Follow up times for those who do not recur are often shorter since they are either lost to follow up or their ongoing survival is not constantly updated in the literature as they age. On the other hand, those who recur by definition come back into contact with the health care system at whatever length of time that they recur after their original surgery.

Moreover, there is more reason to record their recurrence in the literature than there would be to record another year of survival for a patient who does not recur. Therefore, it makes sense that those who recur might have longer follow up times in the literature.

Finally, the role of reresection of recurrent tumors is debated in the literature (see discussion below). We therefore analyzed the effect of reresection on survival after recurrence. We found a non-significant trend towards lower disease-specific death rates with reresection (50.0% versus 66.7%, p = 0.135) but a very highly significant correlation of reresection and increased survival time (59.61 +/- 37.52 versus 38.72 +/- 38.13 months, p = 0.0005).

We note that one confounding factor might be that a selection bias, since surgeons preferentially resect those who healthy enough to undergo surgery and who have tumors that are considered resectable, meaning less extensive involvement of neighboring structures and less complicated surgery.

We attempted to analyze the effect of anticoagulation on thrombosis rate in our dataset, but the use of anticoagulation is so infrequently recorded in the literature that we are unable to make any conclusions.

Either most surgeons do not anticoagulate, or they chose not to record the use of anticoagulation in their case reports.

We did not compare the outcomes of patients with primary repair of the aorta versus others since those that could be repaired primarily were by definition smaller and almost certainly less morbid. Nor is there an interesting therapeutic question involved since any surgeon would repair primarily or patch if possible preferentially to ligating the IVC or replacing it with a graft. However, when a substantial portion of the IVC must be resected, there is an option between ligation and grafting. We found no significant difference in overall disease-specific survival or length of survival between ligation or grafting (p = 0.284 and 0.572), nor was there any more recurrence in either group (p = 0.863), although there was a very slight and non-significant trend towards shorter time to recurrence in those ligated versus grafted (14.63 +/- 18.60 versus 25.01 +/- 29.93 months, p = 0.127). While this might mean that recurrence occurs more quickly with ligation, there were very few data points for this analysis, and the standard deviation is very wide. Therefore, it is unclear if this trend has any meaning. Nor are we sure if comparing ligation and grafting is even a valid question since ligation might be chosen over grafting for a number of reasons that might affect the outcome. For example, there might be more IVC thrombosis, the surgery might be more emergent, there might be less hemodynamic compromise, or the surgeon might be less comfortable with vascular anastomoses in the ligation group.

Regarding the different types of graft material, comparison is very difficult since the numbers of data points for most graft types is very small, and the reason each graft is chosen over others for a given case is almost never explained. Nonetheless, we present our data regarding the difference between graft choices. We find that there is no significant difference between overall disease-specific mortality between different graft choices (p = 0.308), but there is a nearly significant difference in length of survival after different grafts are used (p = 0.085), with longest survival after Dacron (60.20 +/- 64.44 months, n = 11), then bovine pericardium (54.00 +/- 59.40 months, n = 2), PTFE (31.14 +/- 28.21 months, n = 64), and then allografts of any kind (24.46 +/- 20.79 months, n = 12). Again, we stress both that the number of subjects in most groups is so small and that the reasons for choosing each type of graft are not explained, meaning that comparing these outcomes is probably not valid, even though this is the largest collection of data to date.

Regarding perioperative complications, very few were described. The total list is as follows: acute renal failure (12), respiratory failure (5), intraabdominal hemorrhage (5), pneumonia (4), atrial fibrillation or other arrhythmia (3), wound infection (3), chronic renal failure (2), chylous leak (2), gastro-intestinal bleed (2), sepsis (2), pancreatitis (2), fistula (1), cerebrovascular accident (1), transient hepatic encephalopathy (1), intraabdominal abscess (1), symptomatic graft thrombosis (1), pleural effusion (1), dehiscence (1), psycho-sis (1), temporary liver failure (1), hernia (1), ileus (1), duodenalcaval fistula (1), pulmonary embolism (1), seizure (1), C. difficile infection (1), gastric obstruction by large lymph node (1), duodenal leak (1), and graft infection (1).

Note that most of these complications tended to cluster in a few case reports, indicating that most authors did not fully present the complications or that complications concentrated in a few sick patients.

The full data regarding LMS cases involving the IVC can be found in Table 8.

Aorta

In the largest case series to date, we have identified 12 papers concerning LMS of the aorta including a total of 12 patients. The history of aortic LMS is detailed above. In our series of patient reviewed, the mean age was 55 +/- 10.7 (range 41-71). Of the 11 patients for whom gender is described, 7 (63.6%) were women. The largest size of the tumors ranged between 4-20 cm with an average of 8 +/- 6 cm. Three tumors were described as low grade and 4 as high. Of the 9 patients whose outcome is known, 7 patients died, 5 (55.5%) of them from the disease.

Mean follow up was 32.05 +/- 41.1 months (range 4-127). Margins were negative in 3 and positive in 1. Of the 8 patients whose long-term outcomes are known, 7 recurred (87.5%) and a mean of 7.75 +/- 6.45 months (range 2-17). Two received adjuvant chemotherapy, and 3 received adjuvant radiation. The only reported postop complication was postop ileus. The management of the aorta was as follows: Dacron graft 5/12 (41.7%), unspecified graft 3/12 (25%), ligation 1/12 (8.3%), endovascular stenting prior to resection 1/12 (8.3%), endovascular stenting without resection 1/12 (8.3%), unspecified 1/12 (8.3%). There were no reported complications. The full data regarding aortic cases is found in Table 7.

There are a few noteworthy details from the case reports. One is that, as with the IVC, the aorta can sometimes be ligated instead of replaced with a graft if it is thrombosed with development of adequate collaterals. This is especially useful in those in whom there is a concern about anastomotic healing in the setting of radiation therapy (Malone 1996). Second, we note that, if the tumor causes aortic rupture it can be successfully treated (although disease not cured) by an endovascular stent graft (Stambo 2008, Presti 2012).

Perhaps the aorta should be stented if there is danger of rupture even if there no plans for resection. This could be part of a palliative approach. The endovascular approach to grafting has the advantage of not requiring clamping (Presti 2012). The graft is size-matched to the aorta. Finally, even tumors that cause aortic rupture can be successfully resected emergently with good long-term survival, in one case up to 50.4 months (Szekely 2000, Testini 1996).

Renal Vessels

The history of LMS cases involving the renal vessels is detailed above. We have assembled the most complete series to date in our review of the literature. We have identified 24 papers that met our inclusion criteria including a total of 26 patients. The mean age was 53.9 +/- 15.6 years (range 27-88). There were 21 (80.8%) females for a 4.2:1 F:M ratio. The mean size of the primary renal vessel tumors was 8.5 +/- 4.3 cm (range 5-23) in the greatest dimension. In the 5 tumors whose grade is described, 2 were moderate, and 3 were high grade. Of the tumors whose side was specified, 16/24 (66.7%) affected the left renal vein. This is likely because the left is longer than the right, and it is also possible that primary tumors of the right renal vein might be mistaken for IVC tumors due to the short length of the right renal vein. One of the tumors presented with tumor thrombus of the renal vein. In all cases, the renal vein was resected with the tumor without replacement.

Of the 19 patients whose outcome is described, there were 6 deaths, 5 of them disease-related (26.3% disease-specific mortality). Mean follow up was 35.7 +/- 22.9 months (range 6-90). Where margins are described, they were negative in 2 cases and positive in 1. There was recurrence in 9/18 (50%) patients documented in a mean of 22 +/- 21 months (range 3-60). Four of these recurrences were reresected with survival of up to 60 months. Seven patients received some form of chemotherapy or radiation.

There were no reported complications. The full data regarding renal vein LMS cases can be found in Table 10.

Superior Mesenteric Vein

The history of LMS tumors involving the superior mesenteric vein is detailed above. There are no previous reports of tumors of the superior mesenteric artery.

We have identified 4 papers that met our inclusion criteria involving a total of 4 patients. The mean age was 54.5 +/- 11.8 years (range 40-66). Three of the four patients (75%) were female. The mean tumor size was 6.6 +/- 4.5 cm (range 3-13) in the greatest dimension. All 4 patients remained alive at time of reporting, although one was very close to death at 33 months from her disease process. Two of 4 (50%) recurred, one at an unknown time and one at 6 months postoperatively. The latter had her tumor reresected and remained alive without clinical evidence of disease at 1 year after the original surgery.

One patient received chemotherapy, and one received radiation. In 2 patients, saphenous vein was used to construct a graft, and Gore-Tex was used in a third patient. The SMV was managed with primary anastomosis in the final patient. The only reported complication was an intraabodminal abscess requiring drainage, which, of note, occurred in the one patient with a synthetic graft. The full data regarding SMV LMS cases can be found in Table 11.

Inferior Mesenteric Vein

The history of LMS tumors involving the inferior mesenteric vein is detailed above. There are no reported cases involving the artery. There are only three papers that met our inclusion criteria with a total of three patients, one male and two females. The ages were 64, 66, and 83. Size was not described. The grade of only one of the tumors was described, and it was low.

The vessel was oversewn without replacement in two cases, and the management was not described in the third. Two patients remained alive at time of reporting: one at 13 months after recurring at 6 months and the other at 24 months without recurrence. The third patients recurred at 12 months, but it is not known what happened to him after this. One patient received adjuvant radiation, and this was the only patient who did not recur. There were no reported complications, although it seems that at least one patient had initial congestion of the portal system that was relieved by large gastroepiloic shunts (Cimino 2013). The full data regarding IMV LMS cases can be found in Table 12.

Portal Vein

The history of LMS tumors involving the inferior mesenteric vein is detailed above.

There are only three papers that met our inclusion criteria with a total of two patients (two papers concerning the same patient), both females.

The ages were 28 and 67. The first patient's tumor was 7 cm and low grade, and the other was not specified. The first underwent resection and tumor thrombectomy extending from the portal vein deep to the intrahepatic portal system with unspecified vascular reconstruction.

During a previous laparotomy, portal hypertension was so high and there were so many collaterals around the tumor that she initially required side-to-side mesocaval shunting, followed by the delayed resection 6 months later. Her perioperative course was complicated by bile leak. Margins were R1, and she was given adjuvant radiation, but she had clinical evidence of recurrence at 48 months. She remained alive at 72 months.

The second case was a palliative left hemihepatectomy and was not a definitive resection. Her outcome is unknown. The full data regarding portal vein LMS cases can be found in Table 13.

Splenic Vein

The history of LMS tumors involving the splenic vein is detailed above. There are no reported cases involving the artery. There are only four papers that met our inclusion criteria with a total of three patients (two papers concerning the same patient). There were two females and one male. Ages were 33, 58, and 66. One tumor measured 12 cm, and the vessel was resected as part of a distal pancreatectomy/splenectomy with R0 margins. Adjuvant chemotherapy was given, and she was living without recurrence at 12 months. The second was 3.5 cm, located at the confluence of the splenic vein and SMV with tumor thrombus extending into the portal vein. This tumor was resected with a distal pancreatectomy/splenectomy, the vessel was replaced with a saphenous vein graft, and the tumor thrombus was resected out of the portal vein as it was for the tumor thrombus found in a portal vein LMS (Madariaga 1995, Gage 2012, Niver 2011). Margins were R0, and there was no recurrence. She as still alive at 15 months. The third case lacked most follow up information. All that is known is that distal panreatectomy/splenectomy was performed for this 20cm tumor and that the patient did well with the recovery from surgery. It appears that resection of tumors of the IMV and splenic vein (unlike the portal vein and superior mesenteric vein) are often less technically demanding since the vessels can be resected often without reconstruction.

This also helps to achieve negative margins. The full data regarding splenic vein LMS cases can be found in Table 14.

Ex Vivo

We herein also present our 5 cases of *ex vivo* surgery for resection of LMS tumors invading major abdominal vessels.

This represents the largest single-center case series to date. This will be followed by a complete consideration of the literature to date.

Case 1

A 45-year-old gentleman with a prior history of transient ischemic attack without residual symptoms presented in November 2012 with an large tumor involving the liver (left lobe and caudate), IVC, and hepatoduodenal ligament. The tumor was discovered at an outside institution and deemed unresectable.

He was transferred to our center for surgery.

We performed a left hepatectomy with back-table reconstruction and reimplantation as well as pancreaticoduodenectomy.

Details of the procedure are as follows. We entered the abdomen through a bilateral subcostal incision with midline extension. The tumor was found at the hilum of the liver extensively involving the hepatic hilum. First we dissected the splenic vein below the transverse mesentery. This dissection as done for the purpose of creating a temporary portosystemic shunt for decompression of the venous drainage from the bowel.

We found the splenic vein and the left renal vein relatively close to each other and performed side-to-side anastomosis between the two. We then divided the hepatogastric ligament and mobilized the duodenum. The SMV was exposed, and a few venous branches to the colon and the pancreas head were ligated. Then we divided the stomach and pancreas. The pancreatic duct was identified, and a 7 French tube was inserted and sutured with a 6-0 Maxon stitch. Then we dissected the uncinate process of the pancreas off the SMA as in a routine Whipple procedure. After this was done, we dissected the SMV to the splenic vein confluence and divided the coronary vein. The common hepatic artery was found and was encircled and dissected off the tumor at the GDA junction. Then we mobilized the back of the vena cava. The tumor was infiltrating the left side of the vena cava and the hepatoduodinal ligament. Complete mobilization of the tumor from the left side was not possible. We therefore decided to clamp the portal vein at the splenic junction as well as the common hepatic artery, infrahepatic vena cava, and the supraheptic vena cava, and we divided the portal vein and hepatic artery, exposing the left side of the tumor. After mobilizing the tumor from the retroperitoneum, we divided the vena cava just above the left renal vein inferiorly and at the major hepatic vein orifice superiorly, and the liver and the pancreas head were moved to the back table and flushed. We placed a 19mm ringed tube Gore-Tex to replace the vena cava, after which the clamps were released and the vena cava flow with portocaval shunt was restored. At the back table, we dissected the tumor from the liver. The hepatic artery was divided at the level of the right hepatic artery, and an extension arterial graft was anastomosed at the back table using a piece of proximal hepatic artery that was not involved in the tumor. The left portal vein was divided and the right and the main portal vein were dissected off the tumor. The left hepatic duct was resected, and the gall bladder was removed. The right hepatic vein was preserved. The left and caudate lobes were removed with the vena cava. As soon as the graft was prepared at the back table, we autotransplanted the liver. We made separate large venotomies on the Gore-Tex graft for the right hepatic veins (main plus two accessary veins) and anastomosed the veins to the graft. We then anastomosed the portal vein. Finally, we anastomosed the hepatic artery. Then the liver was reperfused. Significant bleeding from the cut surface was seen, but the patient tolerated reperfusion well. After achieving hemostasis, we decided to redo the hepatic artery anastomosis due to weak pulse. We found an intimal dissection at the common hepatic artery. We therefore decided to mobilize the distal splenic artery, divide it, and flip it to connect to the hepatic artery. This time, the anastomosis was satisfactory. After hemostasis was completed, we performed pacreaticoduodenectomy in the usual fashion. All anastomoses appeared satisfactory. We performed a complete doppler ultrasound of the liver to ensure vessel patency and placed two JP drains. The abdomen was closed. Estimated blood loss was 10 liters.

Pathology showed a grade 3 (high grade) leiomyosarcoma measuring 18 x 12.9 x 6.5 cm arising from the IVC. There were 22 mitoses per 10 high-powered fields (HPF). No lymph nodes were involved, but there was vascular invasion present. The tumor stained positive for smooth muscle actin (SMA), HHF-35, and desmin and negative for CD34 and S-100. All margins were negative.

The patient left the ICU on postoperative day (POD) 7 and was recovering well until the night of POD 10, when he had gross hematemesis, respiratory distress and loss of consciousness. He was intubated and brought emergently to the operating room.

Cardiopulmonary resuscitation was started when he reached the operating room in cardiac arrest. Meanwhile, the abdomen was quickly entered. As massive amount of blood was found in the abdomen, and the amount of blood made it difficult to identify the source.

Therefore, the supraceliac aorta was clamped. The heart was restarted. We found that the surgical margin of the pancreas had become necrotic causing a large hole to form in the hepatic artery anastomosis. This hole was repaired, however hemostasis was extremely difficult due to coagulopathy.

Despite massive amounts of blood products, including over 120 units of packed red blood cells, 92 units of fresh frozen plasma as well as platelets and cryoprecipitate, we could not achieve hemostasis or catch up with blood loss.

The patient's abdomen was packed, and he was brought to the surgical intensive care unit. He continued to hemorrhage and eventually experienced cardiac arrest. Resuscitation was unsuccessful.

Case 2

A 45-year-old woman with history of Wolf-Parkinson-White syndrome was diagnosed with leiomyosarcoma in June 2011 and received a 6 month course of adjuvant chemotherapy. In November 2011, she underwent *ex vivo* resection of the tumor staged over 2 days.

A right subcostal incision was made with a midline extension. The liver was soft, but we found a large tumor occupying most of segments 2 and 3, a relatively large tumor of segment

5, a tumor of segment 7 abutting the IVC, and 2 small tumors in segment 4 in addition to a large abdominal tumor filling the lower abdomen. The liver was completely mobilized and the hilum dissected. An end-to-side anastomosis of the portal vein to IVC was created to maintain portal drainage during the *ex vivo* phase, and the liver was then removed and brought to the back table, where it was perfused with cold solution and kept on ice. During the time, a ringed 19mm Gore-Tex graft was used to replace the resected IVC. On the back table, the liver tumors were resected using a Cavitron Ultrasonic Surgical Aspirator (CUSA). Approaching the liver posteriorly, the segment 7 tumor was resected with 2cm margins. The tumor were separated from the IVC and hepatic veins, and all vascular branches were oversewn. A defect was created in the right hepatic vein at this point and was repaired primarily. The liver was then flipped and approached anteriorly. The segment 4 and 5 tumors were resected in a single pie-shaped incision. All vessel branches were controlled with clips or fine sutures. The liver was then returned to the patient. Cold ischemic time was 2 hours and 10 minutes.

The Gore-Tex graft was removed, and the upper and lower ends of the native IVC were then anastomosed to the portion that remained in the body. The portocaval shunt was then disconnected. The hepatic artery, portal, and biliary anastomoses were completed, and the liver was making bile. Warm ischemic time was 56 minutes. During this time, however, there was massive bleeding, and the patient was hemodynamically unstable, so we packed her abdomen and brought her to the ICU. Total blood loss was 10 L.

The patient was stabilized in the ICU overnight and returned to the OR the next day. The liver was well-perfused, and the bleeding had stopped. We mobilized the retroperitoneal tumor.

The tumor was at the root of IMA involving the IMA and the ureter. We dissected the tumor off the retroperitoneum and iliapsoas muscle fascia. The IMA was divided. The tumor was near the sigmoid colon, however we were able to separate the tumor from the marginal vessels. An excellent pulse was observed at the margin of the sigmoid colon after the tumor resection. The ureter was divided, and a previously-inserted ureteral stent was removed. Uretero-ureterostomy and TAH-BSO were then performed.

The wound was closed temporarily with Gore-Tex mesh and definitively closed on postoperative day 3. Her postop course was complicated by transient delirium, pleural effusions, requiring ventilator support and diuresis, large blood volume loss requiring hemodynamic support and blood products, and an intraabdominal abscess requiring antibiotics and drainage. She recovered well and was discharged home 1 month after surgery.

Unfortunately, she was found to have multiple abdominal recurrences 6 months after surgery causing ascites, abdominal fullness, dyspnea, and lower extremity edema. She underwent debulking 10 months after the original surgery and restarted on chemotherapy.

Unfortunately, she died of her disease soon after. Her exact date of death is not known since she returned to her home country.

Histology showed high-grade leiomyosarcoma. The largest lesion measured 10.1 x 7.5 x 4 cm with multiple smaller lesions.

The margin was microscopically positive in segment 7, and was within 5 mm of the tumor in other segments. The margin was within 1mm of the tumor in a neighboring lymph node. The tumor had spindle cells arranged in fascicles and nests with marked pleomorphism, high mitotic rate (18/ 10 HPF), atypia, confluent necrosis, and vascular invasion.

Case 3

A 53-year old woman presented in August 2013 with abdominal distension, nausea, emesis, and anorexia and was found on CT and subsequent biopsy to have a 16.1cm high grade sarcoma located in the right hepatic/ caudate lobe. There was no evidence of cirrhosis, hepatitis panel was negative, and AFP was not elevated.

While she was being prepared for surgery, she bled from grade II esophageal varices and an ulcerated duodenal lesion and developed a Mallory-Weiss tear associated with vomiting. After being resuscitated and treated with proton pump inhibitors, she was taken to the OR in September 2013.

When her abdomen was opened with a long midline incision with bilateral subcostal extensions, the tumor was found at the hepatic hilum and was exten-sively involving the hilum and the inferior aspect of the liver. The tumor also involved the vena cava just above the right renal vein level. The tumor was not involving the SMA, celiac trunk or abdominal aorta. There was a necrotic area of the tumor between the inferior aspect of the left lateral lobe and the tumor.

The surgical procedure began as a standard pancreaticoduodenectomy, mobilizing the right colon and duodenum, dissecting the SMV, and dividing the stomach and pancreas. A jejunal loop was created as a Roux limb. We then anastomosed a 16mm Dacron graft to the side of the portal vein and the side of the vena cava to create H-graft portocaval shunt. We then dissected the superior aspect of the pancreas off the tumor. The tumor was mobilized from the right side of the retroperutoneum. It was noticed that the tumor was infiltrating to the right kidney. The right kidney needed to be removed together with the tumor. We then mobilized the plane behind the right kidney. The right side of the adrenal gland was included in the specimen. The dissection was further continued at the right of the abdominal aorta. The right renal artery and ureter were divided. The liver was mobilized and its inflow clamped distal to the H-graft. We removed the pancreaticoduodenal complex together with the liver and brought the specimen to the back table, where it was flushed and placed on ice. A right trisegmentectomy was performed at the back table. During that time, the IVC was replaced with a 19mm ringed Gore-Tex graft, and caval flow (with portal flow from the H-graft) was restored. As soon as the graft was prepared at the back table, we autotransplanted the liver. We made separate large venotomies on the Goretex graft for each of the hepatic veins. Then we anastomosed the portal vein. Finally we anastomosed the hepatic artery to the hepatic artery and ligated and divided the H-graft portocaval shunt. The liver was reperfused. There was major bleeding, and significant time was spent achieving hemostasis.

Then we performed the remainder of the Whiple procedure GI reconstruction. We also performed appendectomy in the usual fashion. We then performed complete doppler ultrasound of the liver to ensure vessels patency. Two JP drains were place, one anterior to the pancreaticojejunostomy and the other at the cut surface of the liver. The wound was closed with Goretex mesh since the organ was swollen and was too tight for regular closure. Estimated blood loss was 7000 cc. Cold ischemic time was 1 hour 33 minutes, and warm ischemic time was 42 minutes. The patient was brought to the ICU.

She was returned to the OR on postoperative day 2 because of bleeding, which was found to be coming from the pancreaticojejunal anastomosis. This was repaired. Her abdomen was closed in the OR 12 days after the original surgery. Her postoperative course was otherwise complicated by abdominal abscess requiring drainage and antibiotics, pneumonia, and non-occlusive IVC thrombus. She was discharged to a rehabilitation facility 43 days after surgery.

At her most recent follow up 3 months postoperatively, she has been steadily increasing in strength but continues to experience anorexia and nausea. She has no known recurrence.

Histology showed a soft tissue mass of the right lobe of liver, pancreatic head, right kidney, and portion of duodenum with high grade sarcoma, with features of leiomyosarcoma, pleomorphic undifferentiated high-grade sarco-ma, high grade osteosarcoma and chondrosarcoma, probably originating from the wall of the inferior vena cava. The sarcoma invaded the liver and extended to, but did not invade, the right kidney, the stomach and duodenum, and the gallbladder. The tumor approached, but did not directly involve, the inked surgical margins. At it's largest, the tumor measured 30.5 x 20.2 x 11 cm.

Microscopically, the tumor cells were spindle shaped to pleomorphic, with abundant fibrillary cytoplasm. The tumor cells stained for desmin, SMA, HHF35 and vimentin and were negative for pancytokeratin, EMA, S100 protein and CD34, in keepin with leiomyosarcoma. Margins were negative.

Case 4

A 46-year-old woman with a history of migraines presented with worsening back pain over the previous year and a noticeable abdominal protrusion, which was diagnosed as a large spindle tumor involving the hepatic hilum in close proximity to the hepatic vasculature. The tumor was felt to be unresectable at an outside institution, but we agreed to attempt *ex* vivo resection. She underwent four cycles of neoadjuvant chemotherapy (gemcita-bine/docetaxel) and was taken to the OR for resection in May 2011.

The abdomen was entered through long midline incision with bilateral subcostal extensions. The tumor was at the hilum of the liver extensively involving the hepatic hilum and compressing the liver. First we divided the hepatogastric ligament. The surgical procedure then proceeded as a standard pancreaticoduodenectomy, mobilizing the right colon and duodenum, dissecting the SMV, and dividing the stomach and pancreas. A jejunal loop was created as a Roux limb. An end-to-side anastomosis of the portal vein to IVC was created to maintain portal drainage during the *ex vivo* phase. We then dissected the body of the pancreas off the tumor. Dissection was further continued to the right of the abdominal aorta. The right renal artery was carefully preserved. Then we mobilized the back of the vena cava. We then temporarily disconnected the right renal vein and reimplanted it to the IVC below the area of tumor infiltration. The left renal vein was involved in the tumor. We then clamped the hepatic artery, vena cava below the tumor (above the newly implanted right renal vein) and above the liver, and left renal vein and removed the pancreaticoduodenal complex together with the liver. The specimen was then moved to the back table and flushed on ice. During this time, we replaced the IVC with a 19mm ringed Gore-Tex graft and reimplanted the left renal vein to the Goretex graft. Caval flow was then restored as well as portal flow due to the portocaval shunt. On the back table, we dissected the tumor from the liver parenchyma using CUSA. We exposed the right and left hepatic vein in their entirety and followed the tumor, leaving a thin margin of normal liver without violating the tumor. We divided the liver completely in its superior border and removed segment 8 en bloc with the mass. We developed separate patch orifices for the right and left hepatic veins. All frozen section margins were negative. The liver was then returned to the body. We made separate large venotomies on the Gore-Tex graft for both the right and left hepatic veins and anastomosed them to the graft. Then we dismantled the portocaval shunt and anastomosed the portal vein to the main portal vein, which was separated from the tumor. Finally we anastomosed the hepatic artery to the hepatic artery. Then the liver was reperfused. Significant bleeding from the cut surface was seen but the patient tolerated the reperfusion well. After achieving hemostasis, we completed the Whiple procedure GI reconstruction. Doppler ultrasound of the liver ensured vessels patency. The wound was then closed. Estimated blood loss was 9000 cc.

Her postoperative course was complicated by bile leak, requiring washout and repair, and pleural effusions, and she was discharged on postoperative day 21. Histology showed a semi-soft tan mass measuring 21.5 x 14 x 8.5 cm. Microscopically, the tumor was a high grade leiomyosarcoma.

It had spindle cells arranged in a fascicular pattern with tumor fascicles. There was marked atypia and up to 20 mitoses per 10 HPF. Tumor necrosis was extensive.

The tumor cells stained positively for desmin, SMA and HHF35, with patchy positivity for CD34. Pankeratin and S-100 protein were negative. All the lymph nodes identified and all margins were negative for tumor. The patient was given adjuvant chemotherapy with gemcitabine and docetaxol.

Unfortunately, she was found to have liver recurrence and lung metastases 10 months after her surgery. 14 months after her original surgery, we reresected the tumor, performing partial hepatectomy, removing masses of 10 and 8 cm, and partial lobectomy of her right lung. Histology showed recurrent leiomyosarcoma. At last follow up, the patient had a new tumor nodule in her right breast and had been placed on immunotherapy. She is alive with disease 21 months after her initial surgery.

Case 5

A 65-year-old man with a history of sarcoidosis on steroid therapy, seizure disorder, and gastric reflux was diagnosed at an outside institution with a large tumor at the root of his mesentery that was felt to be unresectable. He was given neoadjuvant chemotherapy and radiation, which did not shrink the tumor, and was referred to our center. We performed *ex vivo* resection of the tumor in January 2009.

The abdomen was entered with a midline incision with right subcostal extension. The liver appeared normal. There was no tumor contamination of the intraabdominal cavity. The tumor was felt at the root of the mesentery. Radiation effect was seen around the tumor that made our dissection very difficult. We dissected the transverse mesentery, dividing the middle colic vessels. We then mobilized the retroperitoneal tumor, separating it from the superior mesenteric vessels. We next mobilized the duodenum and colon in an extensive Kocherization maneuver. This required very tedious dissection as separation of the plane between the vena cava and duodenum was difficult. After this was done, the tumor was separated from the uncinate process of the pancreas. Then we divided the transverse colon and started to separate the tumor completely from the surrounding tissue. Once the tumor was only hanging from the superior mesenteric vein and superior mesenteric artery, we clamped both vessels, and the tumor and entire small bowel together with the right half of the colon was moved to the back table, flushed, and placed on ice. The tumor was relatively densely adhesed to the superior mesenteric vein through its tertiary branches.

The SMA, however, was easy to separate from the tumor. On the other hand, the SMV had to be divided at three major branches, and these branches were reconstructed together using 2 Dacron Y-grafts (22mm and 11mm). The bowel was then brought back to the patient.

The artery was anastomosed first end-to-end. Then the Dacron graft of the resected SMV was anastomosed to the remaining superior mesenteric vein.

The orifice of the superior mesenteric vein was extended to the splenic vein to ensure enough size for the anastomosis. The intestine was then reperfused. Hemostasis was performed, and then we completed reconstruction of the gastrointestinal tract, anastomosing the second portion of the duodenum to the proximal jejunum proximally and the transverse colon to the remaining colon distally. A loop ileostomy was brought out in the usual fashion. The wound was closed, and the patient was brought to the ICU. Estimated blood loss was 2500 cc.

His postoperative course was complicated by self-limited pancreatic ascites, non-ST elevation myocardial infarction, seizures of unknown etiology, atrial fibrillation, and high-output stoma requiring gastrostomy feeding tube. He was discharged 64 days after his surgery. His ileostomy was reversed 4 months after his initial surgery. The patient remains alive with no evidence of recurrence 61 months after his surgery.

Histology showed a rubbery white mass measuring 7.5 x 7.5 x 4.5 cm.

Microscopically, the tumor was a pleomorphic high grade sarcoma with extensive tumor necrosis composed of pleomorphic spindle cells with abundant fibrillary eosinophilic cytoplasm. There was marked atypia but sparse mitotic activity. This was consistent with high grade leiomyosarcoma.

The tumor cells stained positive for desmin, SMA and heavy-caldesmon, in keeping with leiomyosarcoma. Lymph nodes and margins were negative for tumor.

Overall Ex Vivo Review

The history of *ex vivo* resection for LMS involving major abdominal vessels is detailed above. In addition to the 5 patients included in our single-center experience, Dr. Kato also performed another *ex vivo* resection at another institution (Kato 2012). In this case, a 63-year-old woman presented with a 7.6 x 6.4 cm LMS involving the root of her celiac artery and SMA. Her entire intestinal tract from stomach to distal transverse colon was resected together with liver, spleen, pancreas, aorta, and IVC. The aorta and IVC were replaced with PTFE and ringed PTFE grafts respectively, and the kidneys were reimplanted onto the new grafts.

The common hepatic artery and SMA were reconstructed using a bifurcated thin-walled Gore-Tex graft. Margins were negative. The patient was discharged 21 days after surgery and was alive and disease-free 38 months later.

Counting our experience, there are 8 publications describing these cases, which altogether involve 12 patients. The mean age was 53.25 +/- 12.2 years (range 30-75). Of the 12 patients, 7 (58.3%) were female. Tumor size, when provided, ranged from 7-30.5 cm in largest diameter with a mean of 14.67 +/- 8.5 cm. All but one were high grade. The vessels involved were IVC (n = 9), aorta (n = 3), SMA/SMV (n = 2), and celiac/common hepatic arteries (n = 1). Follow up ranged from 4-61 months with a mean of 26.9 +/- 16.7 months. At time of reporting, three patients had died of their disease, 3 were alive with disease, and 5 had no evidence of disease. For IVC replacement, PTFE was used in 2 patients, Dacron in 1, and Gore-Tex in 5. In 1 patient, a Gore-Tex graft was temporarily used until the native IVC was reanastomosed with the autotransplanted liver. For the aorta, Dacron was used in one patient, Gore-Tex in a second, and an unspecified graft in the other. In our ex vivo intestine patient (Patient 5), Dacron was used for the SMV graft, while the SMA was primarily anastomosed.

In the other *ex vivo* intestine patient, PTFE was used for the aorta, ringed PTFE was used for the IVC, and thin-walled Gore-Tex was used for the SMA and hepatic arteries. Margins were negative in all but 2 cases. Of the 10 patients for whom data are provided, recurrence occurred in 5 patients at 3, 6, 10, and 23 months.

Two of these were reresected at 6 and 10 months postoperatively. The first died of her disease, and the second remained alive 21 months after her initial surgery. Chemotherapy or radiation were given in 6 cases, 4 of them neo-adjuvantly in unsuccessful attempts to make the tumors more traditionally resectable.

Reported complications included: intraabdominal abscess (2), acute renal failure (1), paraplegia (1), chylothorax (1), sepsis (1), prolonged ileus (1), chronic diarrhea (1), hemorrhage (1), transient delirium (1), pleural effusions (1), pneumonia (1), bile leak (1), myocardial infarction (1), seizures (1), atrial fibrillation (1), and pancreatic ascites (1).

Postoperative hospitalization times ranged from 10-64 days with a mean of 25.3 +/- 18. The full data regarding *ex vivo* resection for LMS cases can be found in Table 15.

Discussion

Brief Summary of Data

The case reports above are typically snapshots in time, brief descriptions with often little follow up. It is hard to take many conclusions from the individual reports in the literature. Aggregated, however, they point to several important trends regarding the significance of the tumor's location and grade (the two factors most significantly associated with survival and recurrence) as well the detrimental effects of positive margins and recurrence. They also show the value of reresection for recurrence.

Finally, they fail to show a significant advantage to any type of graft choice or even to any particular approach to the IVC resection (ligation versus grafting), although the data are so sparse and heterogeneous that it difficult to conclude much.

The articles above also raise several questions and debates.

These are herein discussed below.

Vessel Management

The most important and widely discussed consideration in resection of LMS of the major abdominal vessels is the question of how to manage the resected vessel. In the literature, this question is almost exclusively limited to the IVC due to the extremely small number of case affecting other vessels. To some extent, the handling of renal vein drainage is also addressed. Other questions addressed under vessel management include the role of arterio-venous fistula when using artificial grafts and the role of venovenous bypass. As discussed above, the best case scenario for vessel management is to be able to repair the vessel primarily without compromising tumor resection or blood flow. If that is not possible, there are several available options, and the choice is often influenced by experience, custom, and availability of collaterals.

Table 8. Leiomyosarcoma of the IVC

Paper	# Patients	Patient age (years)	Patient gender	Tumor size (cm)	Tumor grade (numerical or descriptive)	Region of IVC	Follow up (months)	Outcome	Vessel management	Margins	Recurrence/Time to recurrence (months)	Reresected	Any chemotherapy or radiation (Neo = neoadjuvant)	Notable Features
Abisi 2006	3	60	F	8 x 7	High	II	30	Y/+	PTFE graft		Y/24		Y	
		57	M	10 x 10.5	High	III	7	Y/+	Primary repair		Y/5			
		61	F	9.5 x 7	High	II	16	N (NED)	Vein patch		N		Y	
Al-Saif 2011	1	66	F	6.3 x 5.1 x 4.8	Moderate	I	12	N (NED)	Ligation	R0	N			
Alexander 2009	2	34	M	7	High	II		N (AWD)	Primary repair	R0	Y/6		Y	
		58	F	4	Moderate	II	12	N	PTFE graft	R0	N			
Ameeri 2006	1	73	F	9.5 x 4 x 3.5	High	I/II			PTFE graft	R0	?			
Angiletta 2011	1	39	F	10	3	I	36	N (NED)	Dacron graft		Y/6			Used Adams-DeWeese clip below renal veins due to known iliac thrombus
Arii 2003	1	43	F	15 x 10 x 9		II	11	N (NED)	PTFE graft	R0	N			
Arkadopoulos 2012	1	58	F	5 x 6		I	72	N	PTFE patch	R0	Y/72	Y		
Bertini 2008	1	40	F	12.5	3	II	8	N (NED)	PTFE graft	R0	N			Pregnant, waited until after delivery to treat
Bieliuniene 2010	1	42	F	7 x 5 x 4		II		N (AWD)	Unspecified graft		Y/2			
Bonamigo 2003	1	56	F	8		II	96	N (NED)	Bovine pericardium graft	R0	N			Common femoral artery to greater saphenous vein AVF created to increase caval flow and decrease thrombosis risk, ligated after graft occluded at 3 years
Bonura 2006	1	67	M	1.6 x 1.05 x 0.95	High	I/II			Dacron graft	R0				
Brewster 1976	1	51	M			I								
Cacoub 1991	7	42	F	25		II	38	Y/+	PTFE graft		Y/18		Y Neo	
		73	M			II/III	1	Y/+	Ligation	R2 (lung mets at time of resection)	Y			Had lung mets at time of resection
		63	F	20 x 12		II	10	N (NED)	PTFE graft		N		Y	
		43	F	10		I/II	24	Y/+	Ligation		Y/10	Y	Y	
		63	F			II	72	Y/+	Vein patch		Y/22		Y	
		27	F	18		II	27	Y/+	PTFE graft		Y/14		Y	
		54	F			II	120	N (AWD)			Y/57			
Caso 2009	2	58	F			I/II	38	N (AWD)	Ligation	R0	Y/7			
		63	F			I/II	6	Y/+	PTFE graft	R1	Y/2			
Chan 2012	1	41	F	7.8 x 10 x 19.3		I/II/III			Ligation					
Chen 2007	1						6	Y/+	PTFE graft		Y/3			Transdiaphragmatic pericardial window for intrapericardial IVC isolation
Chiarugi 2009	1	70	F	7.5 x 3.7 x 3.5	High	I			Primary repair	R0			N	
Chin 1999	2						6	Y/+	Peritoneofascial flap		Y/6			
								N (AWD)	Peritoneofascial flap		Y			
Cho 2008	9	55	M	7.5	2	II	73	N (AWD)	Ligation	R0	Y/20	Y	N	
		40	M	9	3	I/II	52	N (AWD)	Ligation	R0	Y/8		N	
		66	F	10	2 to 3	II	47	Y/+	Gore-Tex graft	R0	Y/25	Y	N	
		42	F	12	2	I/II	155	N (NED)	Ligation	R0	N		N	
		76	F	10	3	II/III	12	Y/+	Dacron graft	R1	Y/3		N	
		65	M	22	2	I/II	1	Y periop	Ligation	R1	N		N	
		51	F	6	3	II	181	N (NED)	Dacron graft	R0	N		Y	

Table 8. (Continued)

Paper	# Patients	Patient age (years)	Patient gender	Tumor size (cm)	Tumor grade (numerical or descriptive)	Region of IVC	Follow up (months)	Outcome	Vessel management	Margins	Recurrence/Time to recurrence (months)	Reresected	Any chemotherapy or radiation (Neo = neoadjuvant)	Notable Features
Cho 2008		60	M	30	3	II	8	N (NED)	Ligation	R0	N		N	
		53	M	11.5	3	II	1	N (NED)	Ligation	R0	N		N	
Cina 2013	1	65	F			I	36	N (NED)	Ligation		N			
Cope 1954	1	33	F	6 x 3 x 3		I	35	N (AWD)	Ligation		Y/16	Y x 2		First reported case on IVC LMS resected three times
Daylami 2010	6	60	F	12.5	High	II	9	Y/-	Ligation	R0				
		82	F	9	High	II		N (AWD)	Ligation	R0	Y	Y		
		49	F	7	High	II		N (NED)	Ligation	R0				
		85	F	8	High	II		N (NED)	Ligation	R0				
		79	M	20	High	II		N (NED)	Ligation	R1				
		81	F	8	High	I		N (NED)	Ligation	R1				
Delis 2008	1	65	M	4.8 x 4 x 3.8	Moderate	I	12	N (NED)	Primary repair		N			
Demers 1992	4	42	F		3	I	23	Y/+	Ligation	R1	Y/17	Y	Y Neo	First attempted resection elsewhere followed by good survival after surgery at specialized center.
		73	F		High	II/III	18	Y/+	Ligation		Y/7		Y Neo	
		71	F		High	II	36	Y/-	Primary repair		N		Y Neo	
		24	F	5 x 8 x 4	High		72	Y/+	Primary repair		Y/30	Y	Y Neo	
Dew 2005	8	48	M		Moderate	II	30	Y/+	Primary repair		Y/9			
		66	F		Low	I	127	Y/-	Ligation		N			
		29	F		High	III	39	Y/+	Primary repair		Y/5			
		55	F		High	I	60	Y/+	Primary repair		Y/10			
		62	M		Moderate	II	41	N (AWD)	Ligation		Y/14			
		63	M		Mod	I	38	N (NED)	PTFE graft		N			
		48	M		High	I	7	N (NED)	PTFE graft		N			
		41	F		Moderate	II	1	N (NED)	PTFE graft		N			
DiBenedetto 2012	1	67	F	5.2 x 6.4	High	I	48	N (NED)	Banked homograft	R0	N		Y	
Drucker 2012	1	50	F	6.5 x 3.8	2	I	22	N (NED)	Ligation	R0	N			
Dull 2013	1	62	F	5.5 x 3.3 x 3.4		I	14	N (AWD)	Gore-Tex graft	R0	Y/14		Y Neo	First case report of region II/III resected "ex situ in vivo" approach, reimplantation of hepatic veins of graft
Dzsinich 1992	8	75	F				0	Y periop						First case of banked homograft
		60	F				60	Y	Ligation	R2	Y	Y		
		63	F				24	Y/+	Ligation	R0	Y			
		55	F				3	Y	PTFE graft	R0	N			
		70	F				42	Y/+	Ligation	R0	Y			
		36	F				84	Y/+	Primary repair	R0	Y			
		30	F				90	N (NED)	Primary repair	R0	N			
		74	F				36	N (AWD)	Primary repair	R0	Y			
		42	F				6	N (NED)	Dacron graft	R0	N			
Eder 2008	6	54	F	5 x 4 x 4	Moderate	II/III	15	N (AWD)	PTFE graft	R0	Y/11	Y	Y	
		57	F	5	Moderate	II/III	36	Y/+	PTFE patch	R0	Y/18	Y		
		62	M	5	Moderate	II/III	12	N (NED)	PTFE patch	R0	N			
		61	F	6.5	Low	II	18	N (NED)	PTFE patch	R1	N		Y	
		59	F	5	Low	II	32	N (AWD)	PTFE patch	R0	Y/18			

Paper	# Patients	Patient age (years)	Patient gender	Tumor size (cm)	Tumor grade (numerical or descriptive)	Region of IVC	Follow up (months)	Outcome	Vessel management	Margins	Recurrence/Time to recurrence (months)	Reresected	Any chemotherapy or radiation (Neo = neoadjuvant)	Notable Features
Eder 2008		70	F	6	Moderate	II	58	N (NED)	PTFE patch	R0			Y	
Fabre 1995	1	75	F	20 x 15	High	II/III	15	N (NED)	Gore-Tex graft		N			
Fiore 2008	1	39	F	5	2	II	12	N (NED)	Banked homograft	R0	N		Y Neo	
Fiore 2012	12	42	F	7	3	I	46	Y/+	Ligation	R0	Y		Y Neo	
		39	F	16	2	I/II	62	N (NED)	Banked homograft	R0	N		Y Neo	
		69	F	7	3	I	49	N (AWD)	Banked homograft	R0	Y		Y Neo	
		29	F	15	3	I/II/III	33	Y/+	Ligation	R0	Y		Y Neo	
		52	F	11	2	I/II/III	37	N (NED)	Banked homograft	R0	N		Y Neo	
		57	F	7	1	I/II/III	32	N (NED)	Banked homograft	R1	N		Y Neo	
		47	M	13	1	I/II/III	31	N (NED)	PTFE graft	R0	N		Y Neo	
		35	M	6	3	I/II	20	N (AWD)	PTFE graft	R0	Y		Y Neo	
		57	M	8	3	III	13	N (NED)	Patch	R0	N		Y Neo	
		51	M	5	2	I/II/III	7	N (NED)	Banked homograft	R0	N		Y Neo	
		64	M	10	2	I/II/III	2	N (NED)	Banked homograft	R0	N		Y Neo	
		64	F	5	3	I/II	3	N (NED)	Banked homograft	R0	N		Y Neo	
Goto 2008	1	73	F			II	10	N (NED)	Graft (unspecified)		N			Tumor produced NSE in adrenal
Guerrero 2007	1	56	F			II	14	N (AWD)	Fresh allograft	R0	Y/14			Unique use of fresh allograft.
Hardwigsen 2005	5	55	F	12	3	II	20	Y/+	PTFE graft		Y/17	N		
		50	M	22	1	II	52	Y/+	PTFE graft		Y/38	N		
		60	F	7 x 5	2	II	46	N (AWD)	PTFE graft		Y/33	N		
		54	F	19	2	II	9	Y/+	Ligation		Y/9	N		
		60	M	7	2	II	36	N (NED)	PTFE graft		N		Y	
Hashimoto 2012	1	60	F	20 x 7.4		II	5	N (AWD)	Ligation		Y/5	Y		
Hasan 2010	1	54	F	10	High	III	3	N (NED)	Gore-Tex graft		N			
Hilliard 2005	3	51	F	17.5 x 11 x 10.5	High	II/III	36	N		R0	Y/5		Y Neo	
		66	F	15.8 x 12.2 x 10.1	High	III	24	Y/+		R1	Y/12			
		61	F	12.5 x 6.2 x 5.7	High	II	66	Y/+		R0	Y/36	Y		
Hines 1999	14	Median 54 (34-75)	1:3.66 M:F	Mean 9.38 (3-19)	1	II			PTFE graft	2/14 with R1	Y x 4		Y x 12	
Aggregated data (not specified for each patient)					1	II			PTFE graft					
					2	II			PTFE graft					
					2	II			PTFE graft					
					2	II			PTFE graft					
					2	II			PTFE graft					
					3	II			PTFE graft					
					3	II			Primary repair					
					3	II			Primary repair					
					3	II			Primary repair					
					3	II			Primary repair					
					3	II			Primary repair					
					3	II			Ligation					
					3	II			Ligation					
Hollenbeck 2003	25		F x 17	Median 12 (3-31)	High x 25	II x 15		Y periop x 2	Ligation x 11	R0 x 14	Y x 14/Median 12 (3-43)		Y x 15	

Table 8. (Continued)

Paper	# Patients	Patient age (years)	Patient gender	Tumor size (cm)	Tumor grade (numerical or descriptive)	Region of IVC	Follow up (months)	Outcome	Vessel management	Margins	Recurrence/Time to recurrence (months)	Reresected	Any chemotherapy or radiation (Neo = neoadjuvant)	Notable Features
Aggregated data (not specified for each patient)			M x 8			III x 3	3 and 5-year survival of 21 patient grossly resected: 76% and 33%		Primary repair x 7	R1 x 7	N x 8			
						I x 7			PTFE graft x 2	R2 x 4				
									Vein patch x 1					
Hopson 1968		72	F	4 x 7 x 7	Low	I	9	N	Ligation		N			
Illuminati 2006	11			Mean 15 (7-22)		I	19	Y/+	PTFE graft	R0	Y			
Aggregated data (not specified for each patient)						I	26	Y/+	PTFE graft	R0	Y			
						I	20	Y/+	PTFE graft	R0	Y			
						I	67	Y/-	PTFE graft	R0	N			
						I	48	N (NED)	PTFE graft	R0	N			
						I	108	N (NED)	PTFE graft	R0	N			
						I	62	N (NED)	PTFE graft	R0	N			
						I	40	N (NED)	PTFE graft	R0	N			
						II/III	27	N (AWD)	PTFE graft	R0	Y			
						II/III	18	N (NED)	PTFE graft	R0	N			
						II/III	12	N (NED)	PTFE graft	R0	N			
Ito 2007	20	60	F	8.5	3	II	90.5	Y/+	Primary repair	R1	Y/29.5	Y		
		41	M	17	1	I	6.9	N (NED)	Primary repair	R0	N			
		54	F	7	3	II	175.8	N (NED)	Primary repair	R1	N			
		61	F	6	2	II	44.9	Y/+	Graft (unspecified)	R1	Y/29.4			
		48	M	4	2	I	82.5	Y/+	Graft (unspecified)	R0	Y/26.4	Y		
		57	M	23	3	II	5.5	Y/+	Primary repair	R2	Y/4.4		Y	
		58	F	4.7	2	I	69.4	Y/+	Graft (unspecified)	R1	Y/19.8	Y	Y Neo	
		67	M	6.5		I	21.2	Y/+	Primary repair	R0	Y/6.9		Y Neo	
		68	M	8.8	3	II	78.3	Y/+	Graft (unspecified)	R1	Y/31.2		Y Neo	
		39	F	8.5	2	II	73.9	N (AWD)	Primary repair	R1	Y/49.7	Y	Y Neo	
		75	F	5.2	1	II	5.7	N (NED)	Ligation	R1	N		Y Neo	
		65	F	11.5	2	II	3.5	N (NED)	Ligation	R1	N		Y Neo	
		60	F	10.5	3	II	2	N (NED)	Ligation	R1	N		Y Neo	
		54	F	13	3	II	43.6	Y/+	Primary repair	R1	Y/18.7		Y	
		24	M	14	3	II	75.3	Y/+	Graft (unspecified)	R0	Y/15.7		Y Neo	
		40	F	18	3	III	31	Y/+	Primary repair	R0	Y/8.5		Y	
		76	M	19	2	II	9.4	Y/+	Primary repair	R0	Y/6.1		N	
		64	M	8.6	3	I	66.8	N (AWD)	Primary repair	R1	Y/35.6		N	
		53	F	9.8	2	I	11	N (AWD)	Primary repair	R0	Y/7		N	
		44	F	10	3	II	10.9	N (NED)	Primary repair	R0	N		Y Neo	
Kato 2004	1	59	M	10 x 6.5 x 5.5		II	6	Y/+	Primary repair		Y/1			Arrises from adrenal
Kato 2013	1	65	M			I/II/III	9	N (AWD)	Dacron patch	R0	Y/9			
Kaushik 2002	1	49	F	8.5	High		3.5	N	Banked homograft					
Kawahara	1	74	F	4 x 4.5 x 7	1	I	5	N (NED)		R0	N			
Kieffer 2006	20	Mean 59.5 (28-80)	15F/5M			I x 3	0 x 3, 1 x 1	Y periop x 4	Ligation x 5		Y x 12		Y x 15	
Aggregated data (not specified for each patient)						I/II x 3			PTFE graft x 13					
						II x 11	Mean 43.7 (10-132)	Y/+ x 11	Primary repair x 1					
						II/III x 4	18 +/- 11.3	N x 5						
						I/II/III x 1								
Kim JT 2012	6	55	F	7.3	High	II	132	N (AWD)	PTFE graft	R0	Y/67	Y	Y	

Paper	# Patients	Patient age (years)	Patient gender	Tumor size (cm)	Tumor grade (numerical or descriptive)	Region of IVC	Follow up (months)	Outcome	Vessel management	Margins	Recurrence/Time to recurrence (months)	Reresected	Any chemotherapy or radiation (Neo = neoadjuvant)	Notable Features
Kim JT 2012		25	F	8.9	Low	II	36	Y/+	PTFE graft	R0	Y/18	Y	Y	
		63	F	8	High	II	97	Y/+	PTFE graft		Y/47	Y	Y	
		57	F	5	High	II	97	N (AWD)	PTFE graft	R1	Y/91	Y	Y	
		36	M	8	High	II	91	N (AWD)	Ligation (occluded)	R1	Y/5	Y	Y	
		30	F	20	High	I/II/III	25	N (AWD)	PTFE graft	R0	Y/3		N	
Kleisli 2006	1	37	F			II/III		N (NED)	Ligation (occluded)		N			Cavoatrial tumor removal without sternotomy under circulatory arrest
Kraybill 1997	2	70	F			II	8	Y/+	Ligation		Y/8			
		81	F			II	1	Y periop	Gore-Tex graft					
Kruger 2010	1	49	M		2	II/III	6	N (NED)	Paricardial patch	R0	N			Deep hypothermic circulatory arrest for removal of tumor thrombus to left pulmonary artery.
Kulayat 1997	3	73	F	11 x 9 x 9		II		Y/+	Primary repair		Y/23			
		48	F	11	1 to 2	II	70	N (NED)	Ligation		N		Y	
		77	M		1	II	15	N (NED)	Primary repair		N			
Kwon 2003	4	56	F	7.3 x 4 x 3.5	Low	II	41	N (NED)	PTFE graft	R0	N		Y	
		27	F	8.9 x 4.5 x 3.8	High	II	37	N (AWD)	PTFE graft	R0	Y/18		Y	
		63	F	8 x 6.8 x 4.3	Low	II	11	N (NED)	PTFE graft	R0	N		N	
		57	F	5 x 2.5 x 2	Moderate	II	6	N (NED)	PTFE graft	R1	N		N	
Kyriazi 2010	2	54	F	7 x 6 x 9		I/II	36	N (NED)	PTFE patch	R0	N		Y	
		56	F	6 x 4 x 8		II	12	Y/+	Primary repair		Y	N	Y	
Laskin 2010	33	39	F	12		I/II/III	1	Y/+		R2	Y			
		49	M	12	3	II	10	Y						
		62	F	7	1		7	Y			Y			
		73	F	10.5	3	II	3	Y/+		R1	Y			
		85	F	3.5		III	8	Y/+			Y			
		22	F	7	2	I/II	64	Y/+		R0	Y	Y	Y	
		32	F	5	2	I/II	144	Y/+			N			
		33	F	3.5	2	II	216	N (AWD)		R0	Y			
		36	M	6.7	1	II	96	Y/+			Y			
		45	F	10	2	I/II	81	Y/+			N			
		55	F	15	1	II/III	189	N (AWD)			Y	Y	Y	
		61	F	14	2	I	135	Y					Y	
		62	F		2	II	87	Y	Graft (unspecified)		Y			
		63	M	6	2	II	90	Y/+	Graft (unspecified)	R1	Y		Y	
		72	M	6	1	II	88	Y/+	Graft (unspecified)	R0	N			
		72	M	4	2	I	79	Y/-	Graft (unspecified)	R1				
		36	F	9	2	I/II	29	Y/+		R1	Y	Y	Y	
		44	F	8.5	1	I	29	Y/+	Graft (unspecified)	R0	Y		Y	
		44	F	14	2	I/II	14	N (AWD)			Y	Y		
		50	F	7.5	2	II	53	Y	Graft (unspecified)	R2				
		58	F	14	2	I	46	Y/+	Graft (unspecified)	R2	Y	Y		
		59	F	14	1	I/II	30	Y/+		R1	Y		Y	
		60	F	6	2	II	48	Y	Graft (unspecified)	R1	Y	Y		
		60	F	9	2	I/II	36	Y						
		61	M	10	2	II	27	N (AWD)		R1	Y			
		62	M	12	3	I	36	Y/+	Graft (unspecified)		Y		Y	
		80	F	6.5	2	I/II	31	Y						

Table 8. (Continued)

Paper	# Patients	Patient age (years)	Patient gender	Tumor size (cm)	Tumor grade (numerical or descriptive)	Region of IVC	Follow up (months)	Outcome	Vessel management	Margins	Recurrence/Time to recurrence (months)	Reresected	Any chemotherapy or radiation (Neo = neoadjuvant)	Notable Features
Laskin 2010		29	F	5	3	II/III							Y	
		45	M	6	2	I/II				R0				
		50	F	10	3	II			Graft (unspecified)					
		55	F	8	2	I								
		56	F	4.5	2	II							Y	
		60	F	12.5	1	I/II				R1			Y Neo	
Lee HM 2003	1	49	F	9 x 12	Moderate	I/II/III		N (AWD)	PTFE graft		Y/8			
Liu 2010	1	49	F	14.5 x 6.6 x 4.7		I/II	9	N (NED)	Ligation (occluded)		N			
Liu 2013	1	41	F				6	N (NED)	Dacron graft		N			Both kidneys attached to lower stump of IVC
Lotze 2012	1	54	F			I/II/III	0	Y periop						Removal from right atrium as well
Lovisetto 2013	1	78	M	5.5 x 5.7 x 7		I		N (NED)	Ligation		N		Y	
Luigi 2011	1	64	M	0.75 x 0.6 x 0.5	3	I	5	N (NED)	Primary repair	R0	N		Y	
Lygidakis 2007	1	55	F	4 x 20		I/II/III	7	N (NED)	Ligation		N			First case of tumor involving all segments treated with ligation alone
Madariaga 2000	3	45	F				65	N (AWD)	Dacron graft		Y/65			
		51	F				98	N (NED)	Dacron graft		N			
		54	F				156	N (AWD)	Dacron graft		Y/156			
Mann 2012	16	48	M		Moderate	II	30	Y/+	Primary repair		Y/9	2 of 4 reresected had prolonged survival, disease free 8 and 9 years later		
		29	F		High	III	39	Y/+	Primary repair		Y/5			
		55	F		High	I	60	Y/+	Primary repair		Y/10			
		62	M		Moderate	II	49	N (AWD)	Ligation		Y/10			
		63	M		Moderate	I	85	N (NED)	PTFE graft		N			
		48	M		High	I	55	N (AWD)	PTFE graft		Y/47			
		41	F		Moderate	II	48	N (NED)	PTFE graft		N			
		69	F		High	I	180	N (AWD)	Primary repair		Y/60			
		36	F		High	II	12	N (AWD)	Ligation		Y/2			
		45	F		Moderate	II	125	N (NED)	Ligation		N			
		31	F		High	II	125	N (AWD)	Vein patch (saphenous)		Y/12			
		79	F		Moderate	I	25	Y/+	PTFE graft		Y/16			
		45	F			I	52	N (NED)	PTFE graft		N		Y Neo	
		32	F		High	III	18	Y/+	PTFE graft		Y/8			Cardiopulmonary bypass for tumor extending to RA
		63	F		Moderate	I	29	N (NED)	PTFE graft		N			
		42	M		Moderate	I	2	N (NED)	Ligation		N			
Mayer 2007	1	57	F		3		11	N (NED)	Gore-Tex graft	R0	N		Y Neo	
Mingoli 1991	3	55	F	4 x 5 x 5	Low		78	N (NED)	Ligation		N			
		36	F	10	High		6	Y/+	Vein patch (jugular)	R2			Y	
		63	F	6.5	High		20	N (NED)			N			
Mondragon-Sanchez 1998	1	30	F		Moderate	II	12	N (NED)	Bovine pericardium graft	R0	N			
Monig 1995	3	47	F	8 x 4 x 6		I/II	10	N (NED)	PTFE graft	R0	N			
		66	F		High	I/II	14	N (NED)	Ligation		N			
		67	F			II	10	N (NED)	Primary repair		N			

Paper	# Patients	Patient age (years)	Patient gender	Tumor size (cm)	Tumor grade (numerical or descriptive)	Region of IVC	Follow up (months)	Outcome	Vessel management	Margins	Recurrence/Time to recurrence (months)	Reresected	Any chemotherapy or radiation (Neo = neoadjuvant)	Notable Features
Moorjani 2005	1	64	F	20 x 40		I/II/III					Y			Second reported case of intraluminal spread from uterine LMS
Mu 2011	1	74	F	8.1 x 5.5 x 3.6		I			Graft (unspecified)					
Munene 2011	4	47	F	7	Low	II		N	Vein patch (SFV)	R0			Y Neo	
		59	F	4	High	II		N	Vein patch (SFV)	R0			Y Neo	
		49	M	12.2	High	II		N	Graft (unspecified)	R0			Y Neo	
		46	F	9	High	II		N	Vein pqtch (SFV)	R0			Y Neo	
Nayyar 2010	2	48	M			II	6	N (NED)	Gore-Tex graft	R0	N			Left renal vein reconstruction using saphenous vein graft to infratumoral IVC
		45	F			I	9	N (NED)	Gore-Tex graft	R0	N		Y	Left renal vein reconstruction using saphenous vein graft to iliac vein
Ohman 2013	1	51	F	5.4 x 6.8 x 7.8	High	I			PTFE graft	R0				
Padilla-Fernandez 2012	1	38	F	22	2	I/II	12	N (NED)	PTFE graft		N		Y	Double IVC. Resected one, replaced with PTFE graft, and anasotomosed them together end-to-side left to right
Perera 2004	1	56	F		Low		90	Y/-	PTFE graft		N	Y	Y	Brachytherapy also used. Case of duodenocaval fistula. Likely late complication from postoperative radiation and brachytherapy.
Praseedom 2007	1	62	F			II/III	24	N (NED)	Banked aortic homograft	R0	N			
Ramponi 2012	1	31	M	1.2	Low	II	12	N (NED)	Primary repair	R0	N			
Rascanu 2011	1	62	F		I	I	53	N (AWD)	Vein patch	R0	Y/35	Y		
Reddy 2010	1	68	F	8 x 4		II/III	60	N (NED)	Primary repair	R0	N		Y	
Reges 2008	1	56	F	8.5 x 6.7		II	14	N (NED)	Ligation	R0	N			Deep hypothermic circulatory arrest for resection of extension into right atrium
Ridwelski 2001	4	57	F	5	Moderate	II	36	N (AWD)	Gore-Tex patch	R0	Y/18	Y		
		62	F	5	Moderate	II	12	N (NED)	Gore-Tex patch	R0				
		61	F	6.5	High	II	18	N (NED)	Gore-Tex patch	R1	N		Y	
		59	F			II	32	Y/+	Plastic patch		Y/32			
Rodriguez-Caulo 2012	1	81	F			II	12	N (NED)	Ligation	R0	N			
Ruh 2006	3	67	M	12 x 6.5 x 4	High	II	4	Y/+	Dacron graft	R0	Y/3			
		67	F	9 x 6 x 6	1	II/III	9	N (NED)	Dacron graft	R0	N			
					2		33	N (NED)	Dacron graft	R0	N			
Sarkar 1998	7	56	F			I	10	N	PTFE graft					
		58	M			II	7	N	PTFE graft					
		72	F			I/II/III	18	Y	PTFE graft					

Table 8. (Continued)

Paper	# Patients	Patient age (years)	Patient gender	Tumor size (cm)	Tumor grade (numerical or descriptive)	Region of IVC	Follow up (months)	Outcome	Vessel management	Margins	Recurrence/Time to recurrence (months)	Reresected	Any chemotherapy or radiation (Neo = neoadjuvant)	Notable Features
Sarkar 1998		41	F			I	9	Y	PTFE graft					
		43	F			I	48	N	PTFE graft					
		66	F			I	32	N	PTFE graft					
		45	F			I	19	N	PTFE graft					
Satheesan 2008	1	25	F	9 x 6 x 6	2 to 3				Ligation		Y/3			
Shen 2005	1	48	F	17 x 14 x 8	Moderate	II	9	N (NED)	PTFE graft		N			
Shindo 2002	2	64	M		Low	II	84	N (AWD)	Primary repair	R1	Y/36	Y		
		32	M				6	N (AWD)	Primary repair	R2	Y/0		Y	
Shvarts 2004	1	62	F	13	High	II				R2				
Singh 2010	1	50	F	6 x 7.4			9	N (NED)	Primary repair		N		Y	
Smith 1984	1	55	F			II	10	N (NED)	PTFE patch		N			
Soejima 2013	1	62	M	7 x 6.5 x 6		I	8	N (NED)	Tube cavoplasty using left IJV and left EIV	R0	N			
Sokolich 2008	1	60	F	17.6 x 8 x 13	3	II			Dacron graft	R0	Y/3		Y	
Spinelli 2008 Eur J	1	27	M	10 x 8 x 6	2	I/II/III	24	N (NED)	PTFE patch	R0	N			
Spinelli 2008 J Cardiovasc	12	Mean 58 (38-72)	M x 6		High x 12		0 x 2	Y periop x 2	Primary repair x 2		37% at 4 years			
			F x 6				Mean 35 months		PTFE patch x 4					
							1, 3, 5 year survival 83, 62, 51%		Ligation x 2					
							1, 3, 5 year disease-free survival 100, 77, 47%		PTFE x 4					
Staley 1967	1	65	F	16 x 15 x 11	Low	II	12	N (AWD)	Primary repair		Y			
Stauffer 2009	1	39	M	15 x 6 x 5	High	II	12	N (AWD)	PTFE graft	R0	Y	Y	Y Neo	First case of IVC reconstruction in combination with pancreatectomy. Also prior C4 corpectomy for disease.
Stuart 1973	1	58	F	3		II	51	Y/+	Ligation		Y/16	Y		
Suffat 2007	2	49	F	10 x 6 x 6	Moderate	II			PTFE graft	R0	Y/15			
		42	F	10 x 8 x 5	Moderate	II	7	Y/+	PTFE graft	R0	Y/4			
Suzmann 2000	1	52	M	14 x 12 x 11	High	II			Peritoneofascial Patch	R0				
Tan 2009	1	64	F	7 x 6.3		I	21	N (AWD)	Ligated (duplicated IVC)	R1	Y/12	Y		Duplicated IVC
Tameo 2010	2	60	F			I	16	N (NED)	PTFE graft	R0	N			
		58	F			I/II/III	4	N (NED)		R0	N			
Tilkorn 2010	1	41	F	8.8 x 6 x 5	1		64	N (NED)	Primary repair	R0	N			
Tranchart 2008	1	55	M		High	II	30	N (NED)	PTFE graft	R0	N			Implantation of right renal vein into portal vein
Ueda 2013	1	65	M	1.8			37	Y/+	Primary repair		Y/12			
Wang 2007	1	64	F	13 x 6.5 x 6.6										Functional adrenal tumor
Wang 2012	2	53	F	12 x 12 x 10		II	27	N (NED)	Ligation	R0	N		Y	Renal veins connected by graft to proximal portion of IVC
		66	M			II	9	N (NED)	Ligation	R0	N		Y	Left renal vein connected by graft to proximal portion of IVC

Paper	# Patients	Patient age (years)	Patient gender	Tumor size (cm)	Tumor grade (numerical or descriptive)	Region of IVC	Follow up (months)	Outcome	Vessel management	Margins	Recurrence/Time to recurrence (months)	Reresected	Any chemotherapy or radiation (Neo = neoadjuvant)	Notable Features
Wong 2005	1	57	M		High		6	Y/+			Y/6			Surgery done on emergency basis due to PE from tumor. Also rare LMS of adrenal involving IVC. Required cardiopulmonary bypass.
Yadav 2012	4	65	F			II			PTFE graft		?			
		60	M			I		N (NED)	Vein patch		N			
		62	F			II	0	Y periop	PTFE graft		?			
		45	M			II	6	Y/+	PTFE graft		Y/6			
Yamaguchi 1998	1	69	F	8.8 x 7.5		II	33	N (AWD)	Primary repair		Y			Preserved right renal vein by performing end-to-end anastomosis with gonadal vein to IVC (first report of this technique of salvaging the right kidney with vein instead of artificial graft.
Yoshidome 2005	2	65	F				21	Y/+	Ligation		Y/21			
		44	F				88	Y/+	Ligation		Y/88			
Yanaga 1991	1	50	F			II	20	N (NED)	Gore-Tex graft		N			
Yuzer 2004	1	39	M	6	2				Dacron graft	R0			Y	
Zaenkert 2013	2	34	F	4 x 2.9 x 1.8	3	II	6	N (NED)	Gore-Tex graft --> thoracic aorta homograft on POD 7	R0	N		Y Neo	
		59	F	12	1	II	6	N (NED)	Gore-Tex graft	R0	N			
Zhang 2010	1	36	F	13 x 9 (then median of 8 cm)	High	II	84	N (AWD)	Unspecified but later resection used PTFE graft		Y/11 and multiple times at median of every 15 months	Y x 7	Y	

Table 9. Leiomyosarcoma of the Aorta

Paper	# Patients	Patient age (years)	Patient gender	Tumor size (cm)	Tumor grade (numerical or descriptive)	Follow up (months)	Outcome	Vessel management	Margins	Recurrence/ Time to recurrence (months)	Reresected	Any chemotherapy or radiation (Neo = neoadjuvant)
Demers 1992	1	42	F		III	23	Y	Graft (unspecifed)	R1	Y/17		Y

Table 9. (Continued)

Paper	# Patients	Patient age (years)	Patient gender	Tumor size (cm)	Tumor grade (numerical or descriptive)	Follow up (months)	Outcome	Vessel management	Margins	Recurrence/ Time to recurrence (months)	Reresected	Any chemotherapy or radiation (Neo = neoadjuvant)
Dew 2005 (also in Mann 2012)	1	66	F		Low	127	Y/-	Graft (unspecifed)		N		
Freyrie 2008	1	53	F			10	Y/+	Graft (unspecifed)		Y		Y
Malone 1996	1	51	F	4 x 2.5 x 2.3	High	18	N (AWD)	Ligated		Y/6		Y
Millili 1981	1	64	M	4 x 5 x 3		4	Y/+	Dacron bifurcted graft	R0	Y/2		
Munene 2011	1	47	F	7	Low		N	Dacron graft	R0			Y
Ohman 2013	1	51	F	5.4 x 6.8 x 7.8	High			Dacron graft	R0			
Presti 2012	1	41	M	12 x 20	Low	19	Y/+	Intravascular stent graft before aortic resection with graft later covered by bovine pericardium		Y/6		
Spinelli 2008	1				High			Dacron bifurcted graft				
Stambo 2008	1	71	M					Endovascular graft for ruptured aorta from tumor but tumor not resected				
Szekely 2000		50	F			5	Y/+	Unspecified		Y		
Testini 1996	1	69	M	4.3 x 3.3		50.4	Y/+	Dacron bifurcted graft		Y		

Table 10. Leiomyosarcoma of the Renal Vessels

Paper	# Patients	Patient age (years)	Patient gender	Tumor size (cm)	Tumor grade (numerical or descriptive)	Vessel	Follow up (months)	Outcome	Margins	Recurrence/ Time to recurrence (months)	Reresected	Any chemotherapy or radiation (Neo = neoadjuvant)
Aguilar 2005	1	76	F	8 x 5 x 5	Moderate	Left renal vein	24	N (AWD)		Y/5		Y
Appell 1977	1	60	F	5		Left renal vein	16	Y/+		Y		Y
Arkadopoulos 2012	1	58	F	3 x 8		Right renal vein						
Bhathena 1972/ Montgomery 1976	1	50	F	7.5 x 7 x 6		Left renal vein	48	N (AWD)	R0	Y/36		
Brandes 1996	3	70	M	6.4 x 5 x 4.2		Right renal vein	51	N (NED)	R0	N		
		71	M	10 x 7.5 x 6.3		Left renal vein	22	Y/+		Y/3	Y	
		27	F	15 x 4 x 7.5		Left renal vein	49	Y/+		Y/3		Y
Douma 2012		43	F	10.7 x 8.5 x 12	High	Left renal vein	24	N (NED)		N		
Farah 1989	1	40	M	7 x 6 x 7.5	Moderate	Right renal vein						
Gierson 1976	1	54	F				78	N (NED)		N		
Gill 2000	1	76	F	10 x 8 x 5	High	Left renal vein	30	N (NED)		N		
Grignon 1991	1	61	F	5		Right renal vein		Y/+		Y	Y	Y

Table 10. (Continued)

Paper	# Patients	Patient age (years)	Patient gender	Tumor size (cm)	Tumor grade (numerical or descriptive)	Vessel	Follow up (months)	Outcome	Margins	Recurrence/ Time to recurrence (months)	Reresected	Any chemotherapy or radiation (Neo = neoadjuvant)
Herman 1981	1	48	F	5		Left renal vein	40	N (AWD)		Y/23	Y	
Ikegami 2009	1	40	F	8 x 5.4 x 4.2		Left renal vein						
Imao 2011	1	43	F	5.5			24	N (NED)		N		
Lemos 2003	1	47	M			Left renal vein						
Lopez Varela 1967	1	40	F	8		Right renal vein						
Lipton 1995	1	64	F	23 x 15 x 11	High	Left renal vein						
Maeda 2006	1	67	F	5.3 x 4 x 4.5		Right renal vein	24	N (NED)		N		
Martin 1989	1	48	F	5		Left renal vein	48	N (NED)		N		
Pelton 1990	1	27	F	15 x 14 x 7.5		Left renal vein	12	N (NED)		Y		Y
Polsky 1997	1	56	F	6 x 5 x 4		Left renal vein						
Radhakrishnan 1978	1	88	F			Left renal vein	90	Y/-		Y/60	Y	
Shindo 2002	1	32	M			Left renal vein	6	N (AWD)	R2			Y
Singh 2010	1	50	F	6 x 7.4		Right renal vein	9	N (NED)		N		Y
Vos 1988	1	65	F	6 x 6 x 4.5		Right renal vein	48	Y/+				

Table 11. Leiomyosarcoma of the Superior Mesenteric Vein

Paper	# Patients	Patient age (years)	Patient gender	Tumor size (cm)	Tumor grade (numerical or descriptive)	Follow up (months)	Outcome	Vessel management	Recurrence/Time to recurrence (months)	Reresected	Any chemotherapy or radiation (Neo = neoadjuvant)
Celdran 2003	1	66	M	4		6	N	Saphenous vein interpositional graft	N		
Goldin 2002	1	40	F	6.5	3	12	N (NED)	Saphenous vein interpositional graft	Y/6	Y	Y
Kuma 2008	1	62	F	13 x 10 x 7	3	33	N (AWD and almost dead)	Primary anastomosis	Y		Y
Leporrier 2006	1	50	F	3		18	N (NED)	Gore-Tex graft	N		

Table 12. Leiomyosarcoma of the Inferior Mesenteric Vein

Paper	# Patients	Patient age (years)	Patient gender	Tumor grade (numerical or descriptive)	Follow up (months)	Outcome	Vessel management	Recurrence/Time to recurrence (months)	Any chemotherapy or radiation (Neo = neoadjuvant)
Cimino 2013	1	64	M	Low	13	N (AWD)	Oversewn	Y/6	
Choquart 1976	1	83	F					Y/12	
Clemente 2009	1	66	F		24	N	Oversewn	N	Y

Table 13. Leiomyosarcoma of the Portal Vein

Paper	# Patients	Patient age (years)	Patient gender	Tumor size (cm)	Tumor grade (numerical or descriptive)	Follow up (months)	Outcome	Vessel management	Margins	Recurrence/Time to recurrence (months)	Any chemotherapy or radiation (Neo = neoadjuvant)
Madariaga 1995	1	28	F	7	Low	72	N (AWD)	Venous reconstruction (unspecified)	R1	Y/48	Y
Sundaresan 1990	1	67	F					No definitive resection			
Wilson 1987	Same as Madariaga										

Table 14. Leiomyosarcoma of the Splenic Vein

Paper	# Patients	Patient age (years)	Patient gender	Tumor size (cm)	Tumor grade (numerical or descriptive)	Follow up (months)	Outcome	Vessel management	Margins	Recurrence/ Time to recurrence (months)	Any chemotherapy or radiation (Neo = neoadjuvant)
Aguilar 2013	1	66	F	12 x 9 x 6	High	12	N (NED)	Resection	R0	N	Y
Gage 2012	1	58	F	3.5 x 3 x 3		15	N (NED)	Saphenous vein patch	R0	N	
Niver 2011 (same as Gage 2012)											
NEJM 1950	1	33	M	20			N (Patient has "done well")				

Table 15. Ex Vivo Resection of Leiomyosarcoma

Paper	# Patients	Patient age	Patient gender	Tumor size (cm)	Tumor grade	Vessel	Survival (months)	Death/Disease (+) or Other (-)	Surgery performed (En bloc resection plus:	Vessel management	Venovenous bypass	Margins	Recurrence/Time to recurrence (months)	Reresected	Chemo-therapy	Complication	Postoperative hospitalization (days)
Brekke 2003	1	64	M	6 x 6 x 7		IVC	24	N (NED)	Backtable IVC resection, reconstruction of hepatic veins, transplantation of liver	PTFE graft	Y (femoral and IMV to brachiocephalic)		N				11
Chiche 2003	1	46	M		High	Aorta	18	Y	Celiac and SMA also bypassed, left kidney autotransplanted to iliac fossa	Graft (unspecified)		R1	Y			Paraplegia, acute renal failure, chylothorax, sepsis	
Fabre 1995	1	75	F	20 x 15	High	IVC	15	N (NED)	Ex situ but in vivo surgery in which total vascular occlusion, venovenous bypass, and hypothermic solution perfused used	Gore-Tex graft	Y		N				21
Gruttadauria 2005	1	58	M			IVC				IVC previously resected	Y	R0	Y (but not of this case, had recurrence of previous cases twice)	Y	N		10
Kim JT 2012	1	30	F	20	High	IVC	25	N (AWD)	Hepatic vein venoplasty performed on back bench due to tumor invasion of left hepatic vein	PTFE graft		R0	Y/3		N		17
Kraybill 1997	1	49	F	4.5	Moderate	IVC, aorta	26	N (AWD)	Aortic and IVC reconstruction, left kidney autotransplanted onto iliacs	Dacron graft (both vessels, 20mm)		R0	Y/23		Y	Prolonged ileus and chronic diarrhea due to enteric denervation during dissection around SMA), required jejunostomy tube feeds to keep up with losses	
Kato 2012	1	63	F	7.6 x 6.4		Aorta, celiac, SMA	38	N (NED)	En bloc resection of entire intestinal tract from stomach to distal transverse colon, aorta, IVC, liver, spleen, pancreas. Reimplantation of vessels on graft.	Aorta: PTFE graft. IVC: ringed PTFE graft. Kidneys reimplanted on grafts. Common hepatic artery and SMA reconstructed with bifurcated thin-walled Gore-Tex graft.	N	R0	N		Y Neo		21
Weiner et al. (first reported here)	5	45	M	18 x 12.9 x 6.5	3	IVC	0.5	Y (periop)	Left hepatectomy, Whipple	Gore-Tex graft	N	R0	N			Hemorrhage, death	11
		45	F	10.1 x 7.5 x 4	High	IVC		Y/+	Ex vivo liver, retroperitoneal dissection	Temprary Gore-Tex, then native IVC returned	Yes (with temporary Gore-Tex)	R1	Y/6	Y	Y Neo	Transient delirium, pleural effusions, requiring ventilator support and diuresis, large blood volume loss requiring hemodynamic support and blood products, and an intraabdominal abscess requiring antibiotics and drainage	31
		53	F	30.5 x 20.2 x 11	High	IVC	5	N (NED)	Ex vivo hepatectomy and Whipple procedure, right nephrectomy, appendectomy	Gore-Tex graft		R0	N			Abscess, pneumonia, non-occlusive IVC thrombus	43
		46	F	21.5 x 14 x 8.5	High	IVC	21	N (AWD)	Ex-vivo partial central hepatectomy, Whipple, portocaval shunt, gastrojej, feeding tube, IVC and renal vein reconstruction	Gore-Tex graft		R0	Y/10	Y	Y Neo	Pleural effusion, bile leak	21
		65	M	7.5 x 7.5 x 4.5	High	SMV, SMA	61	N (NED)	Ex vivo resection of mesenteric tumor, autotransplantation of the intestine, insertion of venous graft	Dacron graft		R0			Y Neo	Self-limited pancreatic ascites, non-ST elevation myocardial infarction, seizures of unknown etiology, atrial fibrillation, and high-output stoma requiring gastrostomy feeding tube	64

Ligation versus Replacement

The most important decision is whether the vessel can simply be ligated or whether it must be replaced. The major advantages of ligation are 1) decreased operative time, 2) increased ease of operation, 3) elimination of graft infection risk, 4) and elimination of graft thrombosis risk.

Eliminating the risk of graft thrombosis therefore eliminates the potential need for long-term anticoagulation as well as the need for arterio-venous fistula to lower thrombotic risk (see more detailed discussion of both anticoa-gulation and arterio-venous fistula below) (Daylami 2010, Munene 2011, Lovisetto 2013).

Ligation is not always a feasible option, however. Graft replacement becomes necessary if patients have severe venous congestion symptoms, especially renal failure, or hemodynamic instability due to decreased venous return (Yoshidome 2005). Graft replacement can serve its purpose even if the graft later thromboses because it allows initial drainage of the lower body postoperatively and avoids morbidity during this critical period (Kraybill 1997). This is especially important if the vascular reconstruction requires the kidney to be autotransplanted to the iliac vessels. In this case, IV replacement, even if previously thrombosed, would allow drainage of the kidney until collaterals develop, as has been described (Kraybill 1997).

The decision to ligate is largely based on the tumor location and the presence of good collaterals. Ligation is easiest and has best results if it involves region I of the IVC (Dew 2005). The more superior IVC is harder to ligate due to renal flow and higher flow in general due to venous return from the visceral inflow (Hopson 1968, Luigi 2011), but good results are obtained with graft replacement (Illuminati 2006). Edema (Spinelli 2008) and renal failure (Yoshidome 2005) are the most common problems. On the other hand, the literature is replete with cases of successful IVC ligation without serious sequelae or even without any sequelae at all.

Even more important than the region of IVC involved is the presence of collaterals. There is ample evidence that the presence of good collaterals minimizes or eliminates the morbidity of IVC ligation (Spinelli 2008, Lovisetto 2013, Mingoli 1991, Mingoli 2010, Daylami 2010). This is why IVC thrombosis is not automatically an indication for graft replacement to restore flow. To the contrary, it often indicates that ligation is possible since good collaterals have probably developed (Hollenbeck 2003). In fact, IVC ligation outcomes are worse in patients who had patent IVC prior to ligation (Hollenbeck 2003). The presence of good collaterals can be confirmed pre-operatively using 3D imaging. Cina et al. show how CT angiographic imaging can be used to produce an excellent map of collaterals (Cina 2013).

The superior IVC can even be ligated in some cases if good enough collaterals exist. In one particularly sharp exchange, Mingoli et al. on behalf of the International Registry responded to one study that claimed to be the first reported operation with replacement of the IVC, reanastomosis of the left renal vein, and venovenous bypass all together by calling these steps unneccesary and pointing out that most patients in the registry did not experience major hemodynamic problems or renal or visceral congestion from clamping or ligating segments II or III of the IVC (Mingoli 1994, Yanaga 1993).

However, it is clear that one cannot always assume that collaterals are good, even when all preoperative indications point in that direction.

A retroperitoneal tumor can disrupt collaterals making replacement of IVC essential (Soejima 2013, Illuminati 2006).

Similarly, Yoshidome et al. argue that extensive retroperitoneal dissection with IVC resection may disrupt those collaterals that have formed, predispo-sing to venous complications (Yoshidome 2005).

In support of their point, 2 of their 8 patients with IVC ligation developed late venous complications, namely lower extremity edema, although they did not see any acute venous complications while none of their patients with IVC replacement had venous sequelae. In addition to the disruption of collaterals that occurs with retroperitoneal dissection, intentional ligation of lumbar veins and other collaterals during IVC dissection also potentially disrupts collaterals that would otherwise allow IVC occlusion (Yanaga 2013).

Therefore, ligation should not be used cavalierly. Ligation without good enough collaterals can have serious consequences. While edema is the most common complication (Illuminati 2006), more serious complications may also develop. In one case, Lygidakis et al. ligated the IVC from the iliac veins to the hepatic veins in a patient who seemingly had good hepatic vein, left renal vein, and paravertebral collaterals seen on preoperative MRI angiogram.

However, the patient required dialysis and pressors in the initial postop period due to low blood return and volume overload in the lower body and continued to require pressors for 2 months until the left kidney could develop adequate collaterals (Lygidakis 2007). These complications probably would not have occurred with graft replacement. While the authors conclude that it is safe to resect a very long IVC segment if there are good collaterals seen on imaging and to just dialyze if needed afterwards, this is probably too simplistic. It is better to monitor for venous congestion in some way intra-operatively if possible when ligating the IVC. The kidney can be observed for signs of congestion-related renal failure intraoperatively, and the problem fixed if necessary, as was done in one report (Arkadopoulos 2012).

Additionally, one can test clamp the IVC to measure back-pressure prior to ligating. Ligating the IVC with pressures greater than 30-40 mmHg is not recommended (Kieffer 2006, Kwon 2003, Sokolich 2008).

Finally, it is worth noting the one paper that discusses ligation of the aorta. Malone et al. present a case in which an aortic segment with tumor was resected without aortic reconstruction. This was done since 1) the aorta was distally reconstituted and 2) the authors were worried about anastomotic healing in the setting of radiation (Malone 1996). In this case, there were no bad consequences for the patient.

Choices of Graft Material

If graft replacement is necessary, the question then becomes which graft material to use.

Is there ideal graft material? The easy answer is that using autologous vein is the best option for the obvious reason that it is the most physiologic and avoids the disadvantages of prosthetics, which include thrombosis, infection, and fistula formation (Munene 2011, Soejima 2013, Fiore 2008, Fiore 2012, DiBennedeto 2012).

After that, there are several graft material options that have been shown to work well but which contain their own unique advantages and disadvantages. As of yet, there is no consensus as to which of these graft materials is best, if any. The advantages and disadvantages of each option will now be presented.

Autologous Vein

The advantages of autologous vein have just been enumerated above. This is the optimal graft or patch material. If the defect is small enough, autologous vein can be used as patches (Munene 2011). Otherwise, several portions of a vein can be opened and sutured to each other to form a larger tube cavoplasty graft, which is the most physiologically similar in nature and size to the native IVC (Soejima 2013). The most significant critique of tube cavoplasty is that its use has thus far been limited to a single case report, making its value difficult to judge.

Peritoneofascial Patch (Fascio-Peritoneal Patch)

Also under the category of autologous tissue is the option of peritoneofascial (also known as fascio-peritoneal) patch, in which a flap of posterior rectus sheath is mobilized and sutured to the edges of the IVC defect. Thus far, this technique has been described in only 2 case reports with a combined 3 patients (Chin 1999, Suzman 2000). It has been used to patch a defect up to 70% of the IVC diameter (Chin 1999). Reported advantages include its physiologic nature as "self" tissue, its safe track record thus far, its ability to patch defects even bigger than those using large vein patches since one can take as large a piece of rectus sheath as needed, ease of use, wide availability, lack of cost, avoidance of ligation with its associated complica-tions, avoidance of luminal narrowing, avoidance of reconstruction challenges, and avoidance of graft material with its associated complications (i.e., thrombosis and infection) (Chin 1999, Suzman 2000). Essentially, these are the same advantages of autologous vein grafts except the additional benefit of covering larger defects. Despite these advantages, experience is too limited thus far to draw a firm conclusion about its use.

Allogenic Homograft

Slightly less physiologic but still avoiding the use of prosthetics is banked allogenic homograft, whether cryopreserved iliac vein (n = 8) (Fiore 2008, Fiore 2012), cryopreserved and depopulated IVC (n = 1) (DiBenedetto 2012), cryopreserved aortic homograft (n = 1) (Praseedom 2007), or fresh cadaveric IVC homograft (n = 1) (Guerrero 2007). Advantages of banked homografts mostly involve avoiding prosthetic material and thus thrombotic and infectious risks (Fiore 2008). The depopulated grafts in particular have the additional advantages of having less intimal ingrowth, subendothelial fibrosis, and early calcification (DiBenedetto 2012). However, these hypotheses cannot yet be supported by the data. In the four papers to date that report on homograft use, together containing a total of 10 patients receiving homograft, there are no infections among any of the graft types, homograft or prosthetic, and while none of the 2 prosthetic grafts thrombosed, 4 (50%) of the homografts did.

That experience, combined with the scarcity of homograft supply, the increased cost, and the paucity of use thus far, prevents consensus about the value of homografts. Even the authors of all three papers believe further study is necessary before homografts can be recommended.

Bovine Pericardium

Even less physiologic but still avoiding synthetic graft use is bovine pericardium, utilized in two case reports consisting of a total of two patients. Proposed advantages include their inert state, their current acceptance for use in cardiac repair, their less thrombogenic nature compared to prosthetic grafts (therefore longer patency, allowing for development of more collaterals), and decreased needle hole bleeding and greater malleability compared to synthetic material. Disadvantages, however, include wall calcification and loss of strength as well as the obvious criticism that there is a dearth of data (Mondragon 1998, Binamigo 2003). Clearly a larger study is necessary to evaluate the use of bovine pericardium.

Polytetrafluoroethylene (PTFE)

PTFE is the most commonly used synthetic graft for IVC replacement after resection for LMS. PTFE has the advantage of being readily available for those who choose to stock it, and the most often described advantage is how well it resists compression from respiration and from neighboring structures (Suffat 2007), particularly if one uses ringed PTFE and anastomoses to a ring (Dalaunay 1991).

However, as a synthetic graft material, PTFE has the familiar disadvan-tages of higher infectious and thrombotic complications (Kieffer 2006, Stauufer 2009, Shindo 2002).

In addition, it is thought that rigid grafts are more poorly incorporated and have increased risk of perforation or fistulae (Illuminati 2006), particularly if they are ringed. In one case, rings were cited as a suspected cause of bowel injury by rubbing back and forth (Zaenkert 2013), and this risk was also proposed theoretically in another study (Angiletta 2011).

It is also worth noting that the infection issue is not limited to using artificial grafts with LMS of the IVC. One report of SMV LMS specifically mentioned avoiding the infectious risk of artificial grafts with bowel resection that often accompanies SMV resection (Celdran 2003), and the only reported case of abscess after resection of IMV LMS occurred in the only patient who received an artificial graft (Leporrier 2006).

On the other hand, there is evidence that these risks might be over-estimated. For example, despite the theoretically higher risk of infection, several large case series show very low incidence of graft infection with PTFE for LMS IVC replacement (Kieffer 2006, Hines 1999, Dew 2005, Illuminati 2006), and steps can be taken to decrease infectious risk such as using perioperative antibiotics, antibiotic irrigation of abdomen, and covering the graft with omentum (Illuminati 2006 and Stauffer 2009).

However, Yoshidome et al. note that the risk of infection grows larger with any bowel, pancreatic, or hepatobiliary resection due to the risk of bacterial or pancreatic leak, and one of their two patients who received a prosthetic IVC graft under these conditions developed a graft infection (Yoshidome 2005). In our large series, there was a single report of synthetic IVC graft infection.

Similarly, the risk of thrombosis might be overestimated compared to actual outcomes (Fiore 2012), and there are adjunct therapies to decrease thrombotic risk, such as anticoagulation and creation of arterio-venous fistulae (AVF) (Kieffer, Stauufer 2009). These other therapies will be discussed in more depth below.

Finally, it is worth considering that when graft thrombosis (which tends to be a late complication) does occur, it is almost never clinically significant (Stauffer 2009).

Dacron

While PTFE is widely discussed, and several authors express their preference for its use, Dacron is used frequently but without much discussion. To the extent that it is discussed, it is in the context of being compared to PTFE.

PTFE Versus Dacron

Several authors state their preference for PTFE and call it the most accepted material for replacement of the IVC after resection for LMS (Spinelli Eur J Surg Onc 2008, Spinelli J Cardiovac Surg 2008, Sokolich 2008, Kieffer 2006, Hines 1999, Dew 2005, Illuminati 2006). However, none support PTFE over other graft materials with more than anecdotal evidence and certainly without a true superiority study.

Liu et al. note the lack of superiority studies supporting the preference for PTFE in IVC LMS resection, which they attribute to its rarity (Liu 2013).

However, they cite a metaanalysis of 99 patients receiving open abdomi-nal aortic aneurysm repair showing no advantage of PTFE over Dacron (Stollwerck 2011).

If anything, the LMS literature discusses the theoretical disadvantage of PTFE potentially causing bowel injury or fistulae as discussed above. Overall, there is therefore no evidence to favor one over the other.

Gore-Tex

Gore-Tex grafts are also used for IVC replacement but less frequently than PTFE and Dacron and with less discussion in the literature. The collected experience with Gore-Tex is anecdotal at best. Madariaga et al. speculate that Gore-Tex might be less thrombogenic than other materials. They had a thrombosis rate of 2/4 patients with Dacron and switched to Gore-Tex with no thrombotic events in 4 patients (Madariaga 2000). These authors also prefer Gore-Tex to vein homograft due to its elastic wall strength. They quote a graft infection rate of 8-28% in the literature, although they had none.

Size of Graft Material

When choosing the size for a synthetic graft, there is a debate. Some argue for choosing a larger size than the native IVC, which could help avoid development of a thick pseudointima that narrows or occludes the vessel lumen with time (Glovicski 1984, Liu 2013, Tameo 2010). Others advocate choosing a smaller size graft, which has higher flow velocity and thus lower risk for thrombosis (Liu 2013, Bonamigo 2003, Kieffer, Suffat 2007). Besides avoiding stagnation, faster flow decreases interaction of the blood with the graft material, decreasing thrombotic risk ((Ruh 2006). Thus, these proponents recommend choosing a graft slightly smaller than the native IVC (Spinelli Eur J Surg Oncol 2008, Sarkar 1998). Others simply try to match the graft to the native IVC size (Manzanet 2005, Padilla-Fernandez 2012).

Vessel Summary

Having presented the data regarding different methods of managing the IVC, we now reiterate that our data, comprising the largest review of cases to data, do not support any one method.

We also emphasize that a true randomized controlled study would most likely be necessary to make a valid conclusion.

As they currently exist, the data are simply too sparse and heterogeneous to compare, and the choice of graft materials (or even whether to graft versus ligate) is rarely justified by any author.

Arterio-Venous Fistula Creation

Since one other major concern about grafts is their risk of thrombosis, another tactic used to lower the risk is to increase flow through he graft by creating an arterio-venous fistula in a vessel feeding the graft. Almost all authors use the iliac or femoral vessels for this fistula. Some recommend this modality especially when replacing IVC region II or III since this area depends on high flow from the renal vessels, which are often resected during the surgery (Hardwigsen 2005, Lovisetto 2013). The major potential complication of these fistulas is high-output cardiac failure, which can be addressed by banding or otherwise occluding the fistula (Illuminati 2006, Kieffer 2006). This risk appears to be small, however. In one large case series, fistula creation led to deceased graft thrombosis rate without any instances of high-output cardiac failure (Kieffer 2006). The risk can be further decreased by creating a fistula between the aorta and a relatively small vein, such as the lumbar or ovarian veins, to improve IVC flow with less risk of high-output cardiac failure (Spinelli Eur J Surg Onc 2008). Of note, the creation of fistulas does not always prevent graft thrombosis, and there are scattered reports of thrombosis in the presence of a patent fistula as early as 3 months (Dzsinich 1992) and as late as 3 years (Bonamigo 2003) after surgery.

Venovenous Bypass

Venovenous bypass is occasionally used during IVC resection, especially when dealing with regions II and III. The idea is not only to maintain hemodynamic stability while clamping the IVC for a prolonged period, but also to decreases hepatic ischemia through vascular exclusion (sometimes in concert with hypothermic hepatic perfusion (Fabre 1995) by making the anastomoses easier, less bloody, and therefore quicker (Kieffer 2006). Further hemodynamic support can be provided in extreme cases by clamping the infrarenal aorta as well, although this idea is not widely advocated (Kieffer 2006). Venovenous bypass seems to have been used more in earlier cases, just as it was used more in the early era of liver transplantation surgery, and has since been seen to be unnecessary in most cases. This trend can be seen in Mingoli's response to Yanaga et al. on behalf of the International Registry regarding their claim to be the first reported operation with replacement of the IVC with anastomosis of the left renal vein and venovenous bypass. Mingoli's letter to the editor in response points out the many successful cases in the registry performed without venovenous bypass and recommends bypass only in cases with major hemodynamic problems or renal or visceral congestion from clamping segments II or III of the IVC (Yanaga 1993, Mingoli 1994). Indeed, almost every one of the few cases reporting the use of venovenous bypass for IVC resection in our analysis were at least 1-2 decades old.

Brief Consideration of Anticoagulation

Anticoagulation is another tactic described in the literature for lowering thrombotic risk after graft replacement. However, while many authors debate whether to use anticoagulation after IVC resection for LMS, none take a firm position on this question, and there is no evidence in any case series providing a definitive answer and no consensus practice (Illuminati 2006, Dull 2013). Those who take a position base their practice and recommendation on their own customs and acknowledge the lack of evidence. Some pick arbitrary lengths of time for anticoagulation, such as 6 months (Liu 2013, Spinelli J Cardiovasc Surg 2008).

Others anticoagulate only in cases with special risk factors (Sarkar 1998, Suffat 2007). While the use of anticoagulation is debated for LMS of the IVC, its use is so infrequently recorded in case reports that we cannot make any conclusions based on our data (see above).

A larger randomized controlled study is required.

Renal Drainage Issues

If the IVC must be resected in the area of the renal veins, a special consideration concerns the management of these vessels (Tranchart 2008). In this discussion, the most basic tenet is that, while drainage through the right renal vein must be restored to avoid compromising the kidney due to congestion, the collateral drainage of the left kidney through the gonadal, adrenal, and lumbar veins is robust enough that the left renal vein can usually be ligated without affecting the kidney (Kyriazi 2010, Kraybill 1997, Mingoli 1991, Yamaguchi 1998, Yoshidome 2005, Mann 2012). This, along with the relative proximity of the right kidney to the IVC compared to the left kidney, is why typical resections in this region often take the IVC en bloc with the right kidney without reanastomosis of the left renal vein (Kraybill 1997).

If the right renal vein cannot be reconstructed, nephrectomy must be performed (Liu 2013). However, there are multiple ways of restoring right renal vein drainage. One obvious possibility is to anastomose to the IVC itself or to the IVC graft either directly or by using an interpositional graft (Liu 2013, Mingoli 1991, Yamaguchi 1998). This is one benefit of reconstructing region II of the IVC if the right kidney needs to be preserved (Mingoli 1991). If the IVC is ligated, the renal vein can be drained into the upper stump, if convenient, or even into a well-collateralized lower IVC stump using an interpositional graft (Liu 2013). Besides the IVC, the right renal vein can be drained into other nearby veins. Successful drainage into the gonadal vein (Yamaguchi 1998) and portal vein (Tranchart 2008) has been described. This provides the extra benefit of allowing continued drainage even if the IVC graft thromboses. A more extreme possibility is autotransplantation of the kidney to another location (Kraybil 1997).

While the left renal vein does not usually require reanastomosis, there are case reports of severe renal congestion despite the left-sided collaterals. In one case, the left renal vein was ligated, but the kidney became congested with poor renal function, requiring anastomosis to splenic vein with subsequently improved function (Satheesan 2008). In another case, the left renal vein was ligated, leading to venous congestion manifested by decreased UOP and macroscopic hematuria. Kidney function improved after end-to-side anasto-mosis of the left renal vein to the IMV (Arkadopoulos 2012).

This shows that the left renal vein cannot always be ligated in cases when the IVC is also ligated. In particular, ligation of the left renal vein should be performed cautiously if the right kidney has been resected, leaving only the left kidney for renal function, or if the LMS has not obstructed venous flow, therefore not favoring the development of enlarged collaterals (Nayyar 2010).

If the left renal vein must be preserved, it can be reanastomosed directly to the IVC graft (Kwon 2003), the iliac vein (Nayyar 2010), or to the lower stump of a ligated IVC, which avoids a large, difficult, invasive reconstruction in the upper IVC zone and lowers the risk of pulmonary embolism if the cephaled IVC is ligated (Liu 2013). This can be done with or without an interpositional graft, either synthetic or saphenous (Nayyay 2010).

In judging whether the left renal vein can be ligated safely, Satheesan et al. write that stump pressure of > 30-40 mm water should preclude ligation (Satheesan 2008). However, most do not measure stump pressures, and some authors simply reanastomose the left renal vein in all cases to be safe (Wang 2012).

Margins

As discussed above, it is well established that full resection is the standard of care and only chance for cure for LMS (Mingoli 1991, Keiffer 2006, Hollenbeck 2003, Hines 1999). Only those with tumor resection have any chance for long term survival (Staley 1967), and in their study of 14 patients with resection of IVC LMS, Hines et al. reported a 68% 5-year survival in those with negative margins versus 0% for those with positive margins ($p < 0.03$) (Hines 1999). In a different series of 40 patients with IVC resection for LMS, negative margins correlated with better survival, and the 2 longest survivors had negative margins (Laskin 2010). Another series found negative margins to be the only factor the correlated with prolonged disease-free survival (Hollenbeck 2003). This is not to say that outcomes with positive versus negative margins cannot have similar outcomes in a small sample set (Kim JT 2012), but this is not the rule. In our data review, we found that positive margins correlated highly significantly with disease-specific mortality as well as recurrence. There is no consensus on the appropriate width of margins. One study recommended 2-3 cm margins, but no justification is provided for this number (Aguilar 2013). In fact, it seems to be almost as important as achieving negative margins to not take overly large margins due to the high associated morbidity. Mingoli et al., on behalf of the International Registry, write that there is no lymphatic drainage of the IVC wall, so a more technically demanding and morbid wider resection is not necessary since the tumor is usually limited to the site.

They find no survival advantage in the registry to wider margins and higher morbidity. In the 2010 registry update, for example, there were more complications with wider resection (including all three perioperative deaths) but no difference in long-term survival or recurrence rates (Mingoli 2010). They therefore recommend leaving a cuff of less than 1 cm of tumor-free IVC (Mingoli 1993, Mingoli 1997, Mingoli 2010, Daylami 2010).

Finally, it is worth noting that margins are only as reliable as the choice of histological samples that are analyzed. Many of these tumors cover a large surface area, and it is difficult to sample the whole perimeter. It is likely that some samples reported as R0 margins may not have been truly negative if the positive regions were not examined. We bear this in mind as we analyze the results in the literature.

Recurrence, Reresection, and Palliative Resection

Having established the ideal treatment for LMS of the major abdominal vessels, it is perhaps less clear how to treat disease recurrence and what role there is for palliative resection.

Even with negative margins, LMS recurrence rates are high (Rascanu 2011). In the initial report of the International Registry, Mingoli et al. described a 52.4% recurrence rate after resection.

In their series of 19 patients resected with R0 margins, Ito et al. reported a 13/19 (68.4%) recurrence rate (Ito 2007). In pooled data, recurrence rates ranged roughly from 25-50% (Munene 2011, Praseedom 2007).

Our data showed a recurrence rate of 55.7%, and we also found that recurrence correlated highly with increased disease-specific mortality and decreased survival time.

Most often, those with recurrence died without resection. In one series, 9 of 22 patients recurred, and all died (median 36 months) (Kieffer 2006). On the other hand, there are many reports of successful extensions of survival after reresection for recurrence. The basis for this is likely the fact that sarcomas as a whole tend to be amenable to reresection (Shvarts 2004). The first example of successful IVC LMS reresection was described by Cope et al. in 1954, when a patient had 2 recurrences resected and survived an additional 19 months (Cope 1954). Other examples abound.

For example, of the 13 recurrences in Ito's series, 4 of these were reresected. Three died of their disease after living an additional 61, 56, and 50 months, while another was still living 24 months later (Ito 2007).

In another series, 2 patients recurred and were reresected with good results. The first patient, who first recurred at 3 years, survived an additional 8 years with repeated interventions for multiple recurrences; the second recurred at 3 years and survived an additional 4 years after reresection (Sindo 2002). Zhang et al. report 7 separate resections for the primary tumor and recurrences, with the patient still alive at 7 years (Zhang 2010). Cho et al. report 1 patient reresected and still alive 53 months later (Cho 2008). Mann et al. report 2 patients with recurrence as isolated liver mets, both alive without disease 8 and 9 years after metastasectomy (Mann 2012). Radhakrishnan et al. report the case of a 93-year-old woman with resection of a renal vein LMS who lived an additional 2.5 years disease free after resection of liver metastases 5 years after her initial surgery (Radhakrishnan 1978). Hilliard et al. report 1 patient with recurrences resected at 36 months resected and an additional recurrence at 5 years treated with radiofrequency ablasion, who survived to 5.5 years after initial surgery (Hilliard 2005). Cho et al. report on 2 patients resected for recurrence, with one surviving an additional 53 months and still alive and the other living an additional 22 months before dying (Cho 2008). Therefore, it is clear that resection of recurrence is a feasible and often beneficial intervention and should be recommended where appropriate.

In fact, our pooled data, the largest series to date, show a trend towards decreased disease-specific mortality after reresection of recurrence and a significant increase in survival time. The indications for reresection should be the same as for the initial resection (Shindo 2002).

This lesson also applies to incompletely resected LMS tumors. Generally for retroperitoneal sarcomas as a whole, there are better survival and functional outcomes with surgery at high-volume centers, especially for large or high-grade tumors (Zaenkart 2013). One study showed that inadequate resection at non-specialized centers could later be successfully corrected by repeat resection at a high-volume center (Gutierrez 2007). There are several specific examples for LMS as well. Zaenkart et al. describe 2 patients who underwent R0 resections with good disease free survival up to 6 months (short follow up) after first being inadequately resected elsewhere (Zaenkert 2013). Demers et al. describe 2 patients first inadequately resected elsewhere and then resected successfully at a specialized center with survivals of 23 months and 6 years after the first surgery before dying of recurrence (Demers 1992).

Ridwelski et al. describe 1 patient whose IVC LMS was described as unresectable at initial laparotomy at a non-specialized center who was then resected at a high volume center and was still alive without evidence of disease 18 months later (Ridwelski 2001).

The success of completion resections at specialized centers is not limited to the IVC. Chiche et al. report on 1 patient with an aortic LMS tumor inadequately resected elsewhere who lived an additional 18 months after definitive *ex vivo* resection (Chiche 2003).

Additionally, Demers et al. describe another patient with inadequately resected aortic LMS who lived an additional 23 months after definitive resection at a specialized center (Demers 1992).

As a general rule, potential contraindications for resection of IVC LMS include metastases, extensive local invasion, and inability to tolerate surgery (Lovisetto 2013). However, even the presence of widespread metastases is not always a contraindication for resection of a primary LMS tumor in a major abdominal vessel (Cho 2008). Metastases are found in 35 to 50% of LMS patients at diagnosis (Guarino 2000). Several case reports describe resection of synchronous metastases with IVC LMS (Kulayat 1997, Hardwigsen 2005, Shvarts 2004).

Even if a tumor is judged not to be resectable, there may still be some value in palliative resection. IVC LMS is slow growing, so debulking may add to lifetime and decrease severe symptoms (Mingoli 1991, Mann 2012). For example, Shindo et al. report on a palliative resection of an IVC LMS in a 32-year-old man that extended his life by greater than 6 months and relieved his severe pain (Shindo 2002). A case of debulking of an LMS in the portal vein similarly failed to remove all tumor but prolonged survival by greater than 6 years (Madariaga 1995).

Brief Consideration of Chemotherapy and Radiation As Adjuvant or Neoadjuvant Therapy

Adjuvant therapies, such as chemotherapy and radiation, will be the focus of other chapters. This section serves as a very brief consideration of the role of these therapies in resection of LMS tumors of the great abdominal vessels.

Currently, there are no standard regimens for any adjuvant or neoadjuvant therapies. Moreover, we lack the data to make informed decisions about these therapies. This is because it is extremely difficult to analyze chemoradiation data in the literature since the use of these therapies varies highly. In each report, the indications for choosing these therapies is different as is the choice of medications, doses, amount of radiation, etc. (Ito 2007). Often, it is not clear why some authors have chosen to use adjuvant therapies while others have not. This makes comparison of outcomes almost impossible.

Moreover, when neoadjuvant therapy is used, pre and post-treatment tumor sizes are rarely described, so there are no metrics of how effective it was (Stauffer 2009). Nonetheless, we will present some of the relevant debates from the literature.

Some authors believe that neoadjuvant therapy helps achieve negative margins (Daylami 2010, Mann 2012, Munene 2011, Lovisetto 2013). One of the most often cited examples is the series assembled by Daylami et al. in which none of the 10 patients who received neoadjuvant therapy developed local recurrence (Daylami 2010). Besides decreasing recurrence, neoadjuvant therapy can also shrink the tumor, although this is almost never described for LMS of the major abdominal vessels. One example is a 40% decrease in size of an aortic LMS tumor in one case (Demers 1992). Proposed advantages of neoadjuvant therapy include that the pre-resection tumor is more sensitive to chemoradiation than residual tumor since it is more vascularized, a smaller radiation field is required, there are fewer complications compared to adjuvant radiation, and that theoretically more R0 resections are possible (Munene 2011, Mann 2012, Lovisetto 2013).

One way neoadjuvant theoretically promotes R0 margins is by acting as a "spacer." Due to the anatomy of the retroperitoneal region of the IVC, positive margins are very common, found in up to 2/3 of patients (Hollenbeck 2003). Neoadjuvant radiation theoretically acts as "sterilizer" of surrounding tissues, thus increasing the chances of negative margins (Mann 2012).

In addition, giving radiation while the tumor is present has the extra benefit of allowing the tumor to shield the surrounding healthy tissue from the beam in a way that would not occur in adjuvant therapy (Mann 2012).

However, in our large data review, we found no survival advantage or decrease in recurrence from neoadjuvant therapy, nor did neoadjuvant therapy correlate with negative surgical margins.

While there might be a debatable advantage to neoadjuvant therapy, adjuvant therapy is rarely regarded as useful for LMS. One study found that adjuvant therapy decreased recurrence rates by 35% (Hines 1999), but most studies found no beneficial effect (Laskin 2010, Mingoli 2010, Kulayat 1997), although good response to neoadjuvant therapy might predict a good response to adjuvant therapy (Kulayat 1997).

In our large data set, we found no survival advantage or decrease in recurrence associated with the use of any chemotherapy or radiation.

It is debatable that chemotherapy and radiation convey a significant therapeutic advantage, but it is clear that these therapies can have significant disadvantages.

Even in the often-quoted study by Daylami et al. showing decreased recurrence with neoadjuvant radiation, there was an unusually high level of acute renal failure and chylous leak (an otherwise very rare complication) after resection.

Both were potential side-effects, with the chylous leaks thought to result from lymphatic disruption due to dissection in the scarred radiation bed (Daylami 2010).

Radiation has also been linked to duodenocaval fistula as late complica-tion of radiation, especially when graft material and brachytherapy are used in the irradiated area (Perera 2004).

Because of this risk, some authors as a precaution will preferentially ligate the IVC if possible rather than use a graft or will interpose omentum to mini-mize infection and fistulae (Illuminati 2006, Spinelli J Cardiovasc Surg 2008, Stauffer 2009, Tameo 2010).

Finally, it is worth noting that resection can be curative even in cases where neoadjuvant therapy has failed to shrink the tumor (Zhang 2010) and that, similarly, reresections of recurrences can be curative without adjuvant therapy (Cho 2008).

Overall, it is clear that there is no definitive evidence regarding the benefit versus complications of chemotherapy and radiation as an adjunct to surgical therapy. A large randomized study remains necessary (Munene 2011), but the rarity of LMS involving major abdominal vessels has made this impossible to date.

The only major attempt thus far (American College of Surgeons Oncology Group Z9031) failed since it could not recruit enough patients (Mann 2012).

Therefore, regardless of whether chemotherapy and/or radiation is used, the only curative therapy is resection with negative margins (Mayer 2007).

Acknowledgments

The authors wish to thank Dr. Francis Lee for his review of this manuscript and Dr. Yojiro Kato for contributing images for the figures.

Reviewed by Francis Y. Lee, M.D., Ph.D. Professor with Tenure Robert Carroll and Jane Chace Carroll Laboratories Professor of Orthopaedic Surgery. 51 West 51st Street, Suite 370, New York, NY 10019, Phone: (212) 305-4565, Fax: (212) 305-8271, E-mail: fl127@cumc.columbia.edu.

References

Abisi, S., Morris-Stiff, G. J., Scott-Coombes, D., Williams, I. M., Douglas-Jones, A. G., Puntis, M. C. Leiomyosarcoma of the inferior vena cava: clinical experience with four cases. *World J. Surg. Oncol.* 2006 Jan. 4;4:1.

Aguilar, C., Socola, F., Donet, J. A., Gallastegui, N., Hernandez, G. A. Leio-myosarcoma of the splenic vein. *Clin. Med. Insights Oncol.* 2013 Oct. 15; 7:263-8.

Aguilar, I. C., Benavente, V. A., Pow-Sang, M. R., Morante, C. M., Meza, L., Destefano, V., Ruiz, E., Garcia, J. Leiomyosarcoma of the renal vein: case report and review of the literature. *Urol. Oncol.* 2005 Jan.-Feb.;23(1):22-6.

Alexander, A., Rehders, A., Raffel, A., Poremba, C., Knoefel, W. T., Eisenberger, C. F. Leiomyosarcoma of the inferior vena cava: radical surgery and vascular reconstruction. *World J. Surg. Oncol.* 2009 Jun. 26; 7:56.

Al-Saif, O. H., Sengupta, B., Amr, S., Meshikhes, A. W. Leiomyosarcoma of the infra-renal inferior vena cava. *Am. J. Surg.* 2011 Feb.;201(2):e18-20.

Ameeri, S., Butany, J., Collins, M. J., Nair, V., Korosh, K., Kandel, R., Rubin, B. Leiomyosarcoma of the inferior vena cava. *Cardiovasc. Pathol.* 2006 May-Jun.;15(3):171-3.

Angiletta, D., Fullone, M., Greco, L., Marinazzo, D., Frontino, P., Regina, G. Leiomyosarcoma of the inferior vena cava: resection and vascular reconstruction using a dacron graft and an Adam DeWeese clip-three-year follow-up. *Ann. Vasc. Surg.* 2011 May;25(4):557.e5-9.

Appell, R. A., Thistlethwaite, J. R. Leiomyosarcoma of renal vein. *Urology.* 1977 Jun.;9(6):680-1.

Arii, S., Teramoto, K., Kawamura, T., Takamatsu, S., Sato, E., Nakamura, N., Iwai, T., Mori, A., Tanaka, J., Imamura, M. Significance of hepatic resec-tion combined with inferior vena cava resection and its reconstructtion with expanded polytetrafluoroethylene for treatment of liver tumors. *J. Am. Coll. Surg*. 2003 Feb.;196(2):243-9.

Arkadopoulos, N., Karmaniolou, I., Ekonomopoulos, N., Vassiliu, P., Smyrniotis, V. Combination of total abdominal inferior vena cava resection with a novel technique of left renal outflow restoration. *Surgery*. 2012 Jul.;152(1):142-3.

Babatasi, G., Massetti, M., Galateau, F., Rossi, A., Bhoyroo, S., Khayat, A. Leiomyosarcoma of the inferior vena cava: novel surgical reconstruction preserves renal function.

Ball, A. B., Fisher, C. Leiomyosarcoma of the renal vein: a report of two cases. *Eur. Urol*. 1990;18(2):150-2.

Bathan, A. J., Constantinidou, A., Pollack, S. M., Jones, R. L. Diagnosis, prognosis, and management of leiomyosarcoma: recognition of anatomic variants. *Curr. Opin. Oncol*. 2013 Jul.;25(4):384-9.

Bertini, R., Suardi, N., Marone, E. M., Roscigno, M., Petralia, G., Strada, E., Cestari, A., Arrigoni, G., Guazzoni, G., Montorsi, F., Chiesa, R., Rigatti, P. Pregnant woman presenting with a gross retroperitoneal mass: surgical treatment with caval replacement. *Eur. Urol*. 2008 Sep.;54(3):677-80.

Bhathena, D., Vazquez, M. Primary renal vein leiomyosarcoma. *Cancer*. 1972 Aug.;30(2):541-4.

Bieliūniene, E., Kavaliauskiene, G., Mitraite, D., Jonaitiene, E., Basevicius, A., Lukosevicius, S., Pranys, D., Krasauskas, V., Juodzbaliene, E. Leio-myosarcoma of the inferior vena cava. *Medicina* (Kaunas). 2010;46(3): 200-3.

Bonamigo, T. P., Becker, M., Faccini, F. P., Cantisani, G. P., Pereira, W. M., de Napoli, G., de Oliveira Ilha, D. Leiomyosarcoma of the inferior vena cava--a case report. *Vasc. Endovascular Surg*. 2003 May-Jun.;37(3):225-8.

Bonura, A., Saade, C., Sharma, P. Leiomyosarcoma of the inferior vena cava. *Australas Radiol*. 2006 Aug.;50(4):395-9.

Brandes, S. B., Chelsky, M. J., Petersen, R. O., Greenberg, R. E. Leiomyo-sarcoma of the renal vein. *J. Surg. Oncol*. 1996 Nov.;63(3):195-200.

Brekke, I. B., Mathisen, Ø., Line, P. D., Hauss, H. J. Hepatic autotransplan-tation with ex situ neoplasm extirpation and vena cava replacement. *Hepatogastroenterology*. 2003 Nov.-Dec.;50(54):2169-72.

Brewster, D. C., Athanasoulis, C. A., Darling, R. C. Leiomyosarcoma of the inferior vena cava. Diagnosis and surgical management. *Arch. Surg*. 1976 Oct.;111(10):1081-5.

Cacoub, P., Piette, J. C., Wechsler, B., Ziza, J. M., Blétry, O., Bahnini, A., Kieffer, E., Godeau, P. Leiomyosarcoma of the inferior vena cava. Experience with 7 patients and literature review. *Medicine* (Baltimore). 1991 Sep.;70(5):293-306.

Caso, J., Seigne, J., Back, M., Spiess, P. E., Pow-Sang, J., Sexton, W. J. Circumferential resection of the inferior vena cava for primary and recurrent malignant tumors. *J. Urol*. 2009 Sep.;182(3):887-93.

Celdrán, A., Frieyro, O., del Río, A., Franco, A., Bosch, O., Sarasa, J. L. Leio-myosarcoma of the portal venous system: a case report and review of literature. *Surgery*. 2004 Apr.;135(4):455-6.

Chan, A. C., Chan, S. C., Yiu, M. K., Ho, K. L., Wong, E. M., Lo, C. M. Technical considerations for radical resection of a primary leiomyo-sarcoma of the vena cava. *HPB* (Oxford). 2012 Aug.;14(8):565-8.

Chen, T. W., Tsai, C. H., Chou, S. J., Yu, C. Y., Shih, M. L., Yu, J. C., Hsieh, C. B. Intrapericardial isolation of the inferior vena cava through a trans-diaphragmatic pericardial window for tumor resection without sternotomy or thoracotomy. *Eur. J. Surg. Oncol.* 2007 Mar.;33(2):239-42.

Chiarugi, M., Pressi, E., Mancini, R., Fattori, S., Galatioto, C., Seccia, M. Leiomyosarcoma of the right ovarian vein. *Am. J. Surg.* 2009 Apr.;197 (4):e36-7.

Chiche, L., Mongrédien, B., Brocheriou, I., Kieffer, E. Primary tumors of the thoracoabdominal aorta: surgical treatment of 5 patients and review of the literature. *Ann. Vasc. Surg.* 2003 Jul.;17(4):354-64.

Chin, P. T., Gallagher, P. J., Stephen, M. S. Inferior vena caval resection with autogenous peritoneo-fascial patch graft caval repair: a new technique. *Aust. N. Z. J. Surg.* 1999 May;69(5):391-2.

Cho, S. W., Marsh, J. W., Geller, D. A., Holtzman, M., Zeh, H. 3rd, Bartlett, D. L., Gamblin, T. C. Surgical management of leiomyosarcoma of the inferior vena cava. *J. Gastrointest. Surg.* 2008 Dec.;12(12):2141-8.

Cimino, M., Mussi, C., Colombo, P., Lutman, F., Quagliuolo, V. Leiomyo-sarcoma arising from the inferior mesenteric vein draining in the spleno-mesenteric angle with a tumour thrombus at the splenomesenteric confluence: a case report and review of the literature. *Updates Surg.* 2013 Dec.;65(4):313-6.

Cinà, C. S., Riccioli, V., Passanisi, G., Musumeci, G., Loreto, C., Castorina, S. Computerized tomography and 3-D rendering help to select surgical strategy in leiomyosarcoma of the inferior vena cava. *Updates Surg.* 2013 Dec.;65(4):283-8.

Clemente, G., Sarno, G., Barbaro, B., Nuzzo, G. Leiomyosarcoma arising from the inferior mesenteric vein. *BMJ Case Rep.* 2009.

Choquart, P., Leclerc, J. P., Modigliani, R., Celerier, M., Dubost, C., Manoux, D. [Leiomyosarcoma of the inferior mesenteric vein (author's transl)]. *Ann. Chir.* 1976 Feb.;30(2):161-3.

Cope, J. S., Hunt, C. J. Leiomyosarcoma of inferior vena cava. *AMA Arch. Surg.* 1954 Jun.;68(6):752-6.

Daylami, R., Amiri, A., Goldsmith, B., Troppmann, C., Schneider, P. D., Khatri, V. P. Inferior vena cava leiomyosarcoma: is reconstruction nece-ssary after resection? *J. Am. Coll. Surg.* 2010 Feb.;210(2):185-90.

Delis, S., Triantopoulou, C., Bakoyiannis, A., Tassopoulos, N., Dervenis, C. Leiomyosarcoma of the infrarenal portion of the inferior vena cava in a cirrhotic patient with hepatitis C. *Abdom. Imaging.* 2008 Mar.-Apr.;33 (2): 222-4.

Demers, M. L., Curley, S. A., Romsdahl, M. M. Inferior vena cava leiomyo-sarcoma. *J. Surg. Oncol.* 1992 Oct.;51(2):89-92.

Dew, J., Hansen, K., Hammon, J., McCoy, T., Levine, E. A., Shen, P. Leio-myosarcoma of the inferior vena cava: surgical management and clinical results. *Am. Surg.* 2005 Jun.;71(6):497-501.

Di Benedetto, F., D'Amico, G., Montalti, R., Ballarin, R., Tarantino, G., Pecchi, A., Gerunda, G. E. Banked depopulated vena caval homograft: a new strategy to restore caval continuity. *Surg. Innov.* 2012 Mar.;19(1): NP5-9.

Douma, S., Kamparoudis, A., Petidis, K., Anyfanti, P., Doumas, M., Gkaliagkousi, E., Triantafyllou, A., Gavriilaki, E., Gerasimidis, T., Zamboulis, C. Leiomyosarcoma of renal vein, initially resembling pheo-chromocytoma. *Clin. Exp. Hypertens.* 2012;34(6):429-31.

Dube, V. E., Carlquist, J. H. Surgical treatment of leiomyosarcoma of the inferior vena cava: report of a case. *Am. Surg.* 1971 Feb.;37(2):87-90.

Drukker, L., Alberton, J., Reissman, P. Leiomyosarcoma of the inferior vena cava: radical surgery without vascular reconstruction. *Vasc. Endovascular Surg.* 2012 Nov.;46(8):688-90.

Dull, B. Z., Smith, B., Tefera, G., Weber, S. Surgical Management of Retroperitoneal Leiomyosarcoma Arising from the Inferior Vena Cava. *J. Gastrointest. Surg.* 2013 Oct. 22.

Dzsinich, C., Gloviczki, P., van Heerden, J. A., Nagorney, D. M., Pairolero, P. C., Johnson, C. M., Hallett, J. W. Jr, Bower, T. C., Cherry, K. J. Jr. Primary venous leiomyosarcoma: a rare but lethal disease. *J. Vasc. Surg.* 1992 Apr.;15(4):595-603.

Eder, F., Halloul, Z., Meyer, F., Huth, C., Lippert, H. Surgery of inferior vena cava associated malignant tumor lesions. *Vasa.* 2008 Feb.;37(1):68-80.

Fabre, J. M., Domergue, J., Fagot, H., Guillon, F., Souche, B., Joswik, M., Baumel, H. Leiomyosarcoma of the inferior vena cava presenting as Budd-Chiari syndrome. Vena cava replacement under veno-venous bypass and liver hypothermic perfusion. *Eur. J. Surg. Oncol.* 1995 Feb.;21(1):86-7.

Farah, M. C., Shirkhoda, A., Ellwood, R. A., Bernacki, E., Farah, J. Leiomyo-sarcoma of the renal vein: radiologic pathologic correlation. *Clin. Ima-ging.* 1989 Dec.;13(4):323-6.

Fiore, M., Locati, P., Mussi, C., Guarino, A., Piva, L., Santinami, M., Gronchi, A. Banked venous homograft replacement of the inferior vena cava for primary leiomyosarcoma. *Eur. J. Surg. Oncol.* 2008 Jun.;34(6):720-4.

Fiore, M., Colombo, C., Locati, P., Berselli, M., Radaelli, S., Morosi, C., Casali, P. G., Gronchi, A. Surgical technique, morbidity, and outcome of primary retroperitoneal sarcoma involving inferior vena cava. *Ann. Surg. Oncol.* 2012 Feb.;19(2):511-8.

Forni, E., Meriggi, F. [Neoplastic obstruction of the vena cava inferior in general surgery]. *G Chir.* 1999 Jun.-Jul.;20(6-7):296-306.

Freyrie, A., Ferri, M., Testi, G., Paragona, O., Faggioli, G. L., Stella, A. Primary malignant tumors of the aorta: clinical and prognostic aspects of two treated cases. *J. Cardiovasc. Surg.* (Torino). 2008 Jun.;49(3):399-400.

Gage, M. J., Newman, E., Maldonado, T. S., Hajdu, C. H. Leiomyosarcoma of the splenic vein. *J. Vasc. Surg.* 2012 May;55(5):1485-7.

Gage, M. J., Patel, A. V., Koenig, K. L., Newman, E. Non-vena cava venous leiomyosarcomas: a review of the literature. *Ann. Surg. Oncol.* 2012 Oct.; 19(11):3368-74.

Gierson, E. D., Rowe, J. H. Renal vein leiomyosarcoma. *Am. Surg.* 1976 Aug.; 42(8):593-4.

Gill, I. S., Hobart, M. G., Kaouk, J. H., Abramovich, C. M., Budd, G. T., Faiman, C. Leiomyosarcoma of the main renal artery treated by laparosco-pic radical nephrectomy. *Urology.* 2000 Oct. 1;56(4):669.

Gloviczki, P., Hollier, L. H., Dewanjee, M. K., Trastek, V. F., Hoffman, E. A., Kaye, M. P. Experimental replacement of the inferior vena cava: factors affecting patency. *Surgery.* 1984 Feb.;95(2):160-8.

Goldin, S. B., Webb, T. H., Lillemoe, K. D. Leiomyosarcoma arising from the superior mesenteric vein. *Surgery.* 2002 Jul.;132(1):108-9.

Goto, J., Otsuka, F., Kodera, R., Miyoshi, T., Kinomura, M., Otani, H., Mimura, Y., Ogura, T., Yanai, H., Nasu, Y., Makino, H. A rare tumor in the adrenal region: neuron-specific enolase (NSE)-producing leiomyo-sarcoma in an elderly hypertensive patient. *Endocr. J.* 2008 Mar.;55(1): 175-81.

Grignon, D. J., Ro, J. Y., Papadopoulos, N. E., Ayala, A. G. Leiomyosarcoma of renal vein. *Urology*. 1991 Sep.;38(3):255-8.

Gruttadauria, S., Marsh, J. W., Bartlett, D. L., Gridelli, B., Marcos, A. Ex situ resection techniques and liver autotransplantation: last resource for otherwise unresectable malignancy. *Dig. Dis. Sci.* 2005 Oct.;50(10):1829-35.

Guerrero, M. A., Cross, C. A., Lin, P. H., Keane, T. E., Lumsden, A. B. Inferior vena cava reconstruction using fresh inferior vena cava allograft following caval resection for leiomyosarcoma: midterm results. *J. Vasc. Surg*. 2007 Jul.;46(1):140-3.

Gutierrez, J. C., Perez, E. A., Moffat, F. L., Livingstone, A. S., Franceschi, D., Koniaris, L. G. Should soft tissue sarcomas be treated at high-volume centers? An analysis of 4205 patients. *Ann. Surg*. 2007 Jun.;245(6):952-8.

Hardwigsen, J., Balandraud, P., Ananian, P., Saïsse, J., Le Treut, Y. P. Leio-myosarcoma of the retrohepatic portion of the inferior vena cava: clinical presentation and surgical management in five patients. *J. Am. Coll. Surg*. 2005 Jan.;200(1):57-63.

Hashimoto, M., Kobayashi, T., Tashiro, H., Amano, H., Oshita, A., Tanimoto, Y., Kuroda, S., Tazawa, H., Aikata, H., Chayama, K., Fujii, M., Arihiro, K., Ohdan, H. A huge metastatic liver tumor from leiomyosarcoma of the inferior vena cava: report of a case. *Surg. Today*. 2012 May;42(5):505-8.

Hassan, M., Ciancio, G., Shirodkar, S. P., Del Mazo, M. B., Barron, M., Salerno, T. A., Livingstone, A. S. Surgical technique of removal of inferior vena cava leiomyosarcoma extending into the right atrium without deep hypothermic circulatory arrest. *J. Card. Surg*. 2010 May;25(3):277-81.

Herman, C., Morales, P. Leiomyosarcoma of renal vein. *Urology*. 1981 Oct.; 18(4):395-8.

Hernandez, F. J., Stanley, T. M., Ranganath, K. A., Rubinstein, A. I. Primary leiomyosarcoma of the aorta. *Am. J. Surg. Pathol*. 1979 Jun.;3(3):251-6.

Hilliard, N. J., Heslin, M. J., Castro, C. Y. Leiomyosarcoma of the inferior vena cava: three case reports and review of the literature. *Ann. Diagn. Pathol*. 2005 Oct.;9(5):259-66.

Hines, O. J., Nelson, S., Quinones-Baldrich, W. J., Eilber, F. R. Leiomyo-sarcoma of the inferior vena cava: prognosis and comparison with leiomyosarcoma of other anatomic sites. *Cancer*. 1999 Mar. 1;85(5):1077-83.

Hollenbeck, S. T., Grobmyer, S. R., Kent, K. C., Brennan, M. F. Surgical treatment and outcomes of patients with primary inferior vena cava leio-myosarcoma. *J. Am. Coll. Surg*. 2003 Oct.;197(4):575-9.

Hopson, W. B. Jr, Burlison, P. E., Sherman, R. T. Leiomyosarcoma of the inferior vena cava. A case report. *Ann. Surg*. 1968 Aug.;168(2):290-3.

Ikegami, Y., Umemoto, Y., Kohri, K. Leiomyosarcoma of the renal vein. *Int. J. Urol*. 2009 Sep.;16(9):768.

Illuminati, G., Calio', F. G., D'Urso, A., Giacobbi, D., Papaspyropoulos, V., Ceccanei, G. Prosthetic replacement of the infrahepatic inferior vena cava for leiomyosarcoma. *Arch. Surg*. 2006 Sep.;141(9):919-24.

Imao, T., Amano, T., Takemae, K. Leiomyosarcoma of the renal vein. *Int. J. Clin. Oncol.* 2011 Feb.;16(1):76-9.

Inoue, K., Watanabe, H., Ohashi, Y., Morioka, M., Fujita, Y. Leiomyosarcoma of the renal vein: a case report. *J. Urol.* 1994 Jul.;152(1):153-5.

Ito, H., Hornick, J. L., Bertagnolli, M. M., George, S., Morgan, J. A., Baldini, E. H., Wagner, A. J., Demetri, G. D., Raut, C. P. Leiomyosarcoma of the inferior vena cava: survival after aggressive management. *Ann. Surg. Oncol.* 2007 Dec.;14(12):3534-41.

Kato, S., Tanaka, T., Kitamura, H., Masumori, N., Ito, T., Kawaharada, N., Tsukamoto, T. Resection of the inferior vena cava for urological malignancies: single-center experience. *Int. J. Clin. Oncol.* 2013 Oct.;18 (5):905-9.

Kato, T., Kato, T., Sakamoto, S., Kobayashi, T., Ikeda, R., Nakamura, T., Akakura, K., Hikage, T., Inoue, T. Primary adrenal leiomyosarcoma with inferior vena cava thrombosis. *Int. J. Clin. Oncol.* 2004 Jun.;9(3):189-92.

Kato, T., Lobritto, S. J., Tzakis, A., Raveh, Y., Sandoval, P. R., Martinez, M., Granowetter, L., Armas, A., Brown, R. S. Jr, Emond, J. Multivisceral ex vivo surgery for tumors involving celiac and superior mesenteric arteries. *Am. J. Transplant.* 2012 May;12(5):1323-8.

Kaushik, S., Neifeld, J. P. Leiomyosarcoma of the renal vein: imaging and surgical reconstruction. *AJR Am. J. Roentgenol.* 2002 Jul.;179(1):276-7.

Kawahara, T., Nakagawa, T. A case of leiomyosarcoma arising from the inferior vena cava. *Jpn. J. Clin. Oncol.* 2012 Jan.;42(1):83.

Kevorkian, J., Cento, D. P. Leiomyosarcoma of large arteries and veins. *Surgery* 1973;73:390-400.

Kieffer, E., Alaoui, M., Piette, J. C., Cacoub, P., Chiche, L. Leiomyosarcoma of the inferior vena cava: experience in 22 cases. *Ann. Surg.* 2006 Aug.; 244(2):289-95.

Kim, J. T., Kwon, T., Cho, Y., Shin, S., Lee, S., Moon, D. Multidisciplinary treatment and long-term outcomes in six patients with leiomyosarcoma of the inferior vena cava. *J. Korean Surg. Soc.* 2012 Feb.;82(2):101-9.

Kleisli, T., Raissi, S. S., Nissen, N. N., Cheng, W., Cohen, L., Sacks, S. A., Trento, A. Cavo-atrial tumor resection under total circulatory arrest without a sternotomy. *Ann. Thorac. Surg.* 2006 May;81(5):1887-8.

Kraybill, W. G., Callery, M. P., Heiken, J. P., Flye, M. W. Radical resection of tumors of the inferior vena cava with vascular reconstruction and kidney autotransplantation. *Surgery.* 1997 Jan.;121(1):31-6.

Krüger, T., Mustafi, M., Nadalin, S., Aebert, H. *Ann. Thorac. Surg.* 2010 Aug.;90(2):642-4.

Kulaylat, M. N., Karakousis, C. P., Doerr, R. J., Karamanoukian, H. L., O'Brien, J., Peer, R. Leiomyosarcoma of the inferior vena cava: a clinico-pathologic review and report of three cases. *J. Surg. Oncol.* 1997 Jul.;65 (3):205-17.

Kuma, S., Utsunomiya, T., Yano, S., Kameyama, T., Okamoto, M., Matsuyama, A., Hashimoto, K., Yamamoto, M., Ezaki, T., Fujihara, M., Ishida, T. Leiomyosarcoma originating from the superior mesenteric vein: a case report and review of the literature. *Ann. Vasc. Surg.* 2008 May-Jun.; 22(3):453-5.

Kwon, T. W., Sung, K. B., Cho, Y. P., Kim, D. K., Yang, S. M., Ro, J. Y., Kim, G. E. Pararenal leiomyosarcoma of the inferior vena cava. *J. Korean Med. Sci.* 2003 Jun.;18(3):355-9.

Kyriazi, M. A., Stafyla, V. K., Chatzinikolaou, I., Koureas, A., Chatziioannou, A., Kondi-Paphiti, A., Arkadopoulos, N., Smyrniotis, V. Surgical challenges in the treatment of leiomyosarcoma of the inferior vena cava: analysis of two cases and brief review of the literature. *Ann. Vasc. Surg*. 2010 Aug.;24(6):826.

Laskin, W. B., Fanburg-Smith, J. C., Burke, A. P., Kraszewska, E., Fetsch, J. F., Miettinen, M. Leiomyosarcoma of the inferior vena cava: clinicopatho-logic study of 40 cases. *Am. J. Surg. Pathol*. 2010 Jun.;34(6):873-81.

Lee, H. M., Jeong, D. S., Park, P. W., Kim, W. S., Sung, K., Lee, Y. T. Surgical treatment for an invasive leiomyosarcoma of the inferior vena cava. *Korean J. Thorac. Cardiovasc. Surg*. 2013 Oct.;46(5):373-6.

Lee, S. W., Yang, J. H., Yoo, S. J., Kim, S. H., Jang, H. J., Park, H. S., Park, S. J., Kim, D. Y., Hong, E. K., Moon, Y. S., Park, J. W., Kim, C. M. [A case of primary leiomyosarcoma of the inferior vena cava treated by surgical resection and reconstruction with synthetic graft replacement]. *Korean J. Gastroenterol*. 2003 Sep.;42(3):249-54.

Lemos, G. C., El Hayek, O. R., Apezzato, M. Leiomyosarcoma of the renal vein. *Int. Braz. J. Urol*. 2003 Jan.-Feb.;29(1):43-4.

Leporrier, J., Alkofer, B., Lebreton, G., Lepennec, V., Chiche, L. Leiomyo-sarcoma of the superior mesenteric vein: a diagnostic and therapeutic challenge. *J. Hepatobiliary Pancreat. Surg*. 2006;13(6):584-6.

Lipton, M., Sprayregen, S., Kutcher, R., Frost, A. Venous invasion in renal vein leiomyosarcoma: case report and review of the literature. *Abdom. Imaging*. 1995 Jan.-Feb.;20(1):64-7.

Liu, C., Zheng, Y., Yang, X., Shao, J., Song, X., Liu, B., Guan, H. Surgical resection of the inferior vena cava for leiomyosarcoma. *Ann. Vasc. Surg*. 2010 Aug.;24(6):822.e11-5.

Liu, Y., Sun, Y., Jiang, Y., He, X. Y., Kong, Q. X., Wu, J. X., Zhang, Y. S., Jin, X. A novel strategy of vascular reconstruction after radical resection of an inferior vena cava leiomyosarcoma. *Ann. Vasc. Surg*. 2013 Aug.;27 (6):803.e1-5.

López Varela, E. A., Pereira Garro, C. Leiomyosarcoma of the renal vein. Case report. *Int. Surg*. 1967 Apr.;47(4):340-3.

Lotze, U., Reponova, J., Muth, G., Oltmanns, G., Reich, H. C., Etzrodt, G., Kaiser, W. A., Mutschke, O., Ortmann, M., Stippel, D., Wahlers, T. Leio-myosarcoma of the inferior vena cava extending into the right atrium. A rare differential diagnosis of a right atrial tumor with fatal outcome. *Herz*. 2012 Aug.;37(5):573-8.

Lovisetto, F., Corradini, C., De Cesare, F., Geraci, O., Manzi, M., Emidi, R., Arceci, F. Leiomyosarcoma of the inferior vena cava incidentally detected. *Ann. Vasc. Surg*. 2013 Aug.;27(6):803.e15-9.

Luigi, M., Michele, G., Michele, S., Francesco, T., Raffaele, P., Gianmarco, R., Marianna, P., Bartolomeo, B., Natale, D. M. Leiomyosarcoma of inferior cava vein: en bloc resection and primary repair of vessel. *Am. Surg*. 2011 Jun.;77(6):e121-3.

Lygidakis, N. J., Bhagat, A. D., Sharma, S. K., Kefalourous, H., Porfiris, T., Grigorakos, L., Vrachnos, P., Mihalopoulos, A., Bleta, A., Bodozoglou, N., Voulgari, K., Vlachos, L. Leiomyosarcoma of the inferior vena cava--an unusual case. *Hepatogastroenterology*. 2007 Apr.-May;54(75):710-5.

Madariaga, J. R., Nalesnik, M. A., Iwatsuki, S., Starzl, T. E., Fung, J. J. Spindle cell tumor of the portal vein. *J. Surg. Oncol*. 1995 Jun.;59(2):139-41.

Madariaga, J. R., Fung, J., Gutierrez, J., Bueno, J., Iwatsuki, S. Liver resection combined with excision of vena cava. *J. Am. Coll. Surg*. 2000 Sep.;191 (3):244-50.

Maeda, T., Tateishi, U., Fujimoto, H., Kanai, Y., Sugimura, K., Arai, Y. Leio-myosarcoma of the renal vein: arterial encasement on contrast-enhanced dynamic computed tomography. *Int. J. Urol.* 2006 May;13(5):611-2.

Malone, M. D., Kerr, K., Kavanah, M., Menzoian, J. O. Primary leiomyo-sarcoma of the abdominal aorta. *J. Vasc. Surg.* 1996 Sep.;24(3):487-93.

Mann, G. N., Mann, L. V., Levine, E. A., Shen, P. Primary leiomyosarcoma of the inferior vena cava: a 2-institution analysis of outcomes. *Surgery.* 2012 Feb.;151(2):261-7.

Manzanet, G., Morón, R., Suelves, C., Calderón, R., Corell, R., Castell, L., Trías, A., Todolí, G., Navarro, J., Peiró, E., Clarós, A. Prosthetic replace-ment of the inferior vena cava. Current controversies. *Cir. Esp.* 2005 Mar.; 77(3):170-2.

Martin, J., Garcia, M., Duran, A., Forcada, P., Marco, V. Renal vein leiomyo-sarcoma: a case report and literature review. *Urol. Radiol.* 1989; 11(1):25-9.

Mayer, F., Aebert, H., Rudert, M., Königsrainer, A., Horger, M., Kanz, L., Bamberg, M., Ziemer, G., Hartmann, J. T. Primary malignant sarcomas of the heart and great vessels in adult patients--a single-center experience. *Oncologist.* 2007 Sep.;12(9):1134-42.

McCullough, D. L., Gittes, R. F. Ligation of the renal vein in the solitary kidney: effects on renal function. *J. Urol.* 1975;113:295-8.

Melchior, E. Sarkom der V cava inferior. *Deutsch Z Chir.* 1928;213:135-40.

Merlo, M., Varetto, G. F., Bitossi, O., Conforti, M., Rispoli, P. Leiomyo-sarcoma of the inferior vena cava: a clinicopathologic review and report of four cases. *Minerva Chir.* 2008 Jun.;63(3):209-21.

Millili, J. J., LaFlare, R. G., Nemir, P. Jr. Leiomyosarcoma of the abdominal aorta: a case report. *Surgery.* 1981 May;89(5):631-4.

Mingoli, A., Feldhaus, R. J., Cavallaro, A., Stipa, S. Leiomyosarcoma of the inferior vena cava: analysis and search of world literature on 141 patients and report of three new cases. *J. Vasc. Surg.* 1991 Nov.;14(5):688-99.

Mingoli, A., Cavallaro, A., Stipa, S., Feldhaus, R. J. Inferior vena cava leio-myosarcoma. *J. Vasc. Surg.* 1993 Feb.;17(2):451.

Mingoli, A., Cavallaro, A., di Marzo, L., Morelli, M. M., Feldhaus, R. J. Inferior vena cava replacement for primary tumor: is the use of venove-nous bypass necessary? *Surgery.* 1994 Mar.;115(3):409.

Mingoli, A., Sapienza, P., Cavallaro, A., Di Marzo, L., Burchi, C., Giannarelli, D., Feldhaus, R. J. The effect of extend of caval resection in the treatment of inferior vena cava leiomyosarcoma. *Anticancer Res.* 1997 Sep.-Oct.;17 (5B):3877-81.

Mingoli, A., Cavallaro, A., Sapienza, P., Di Marzo, L., Feldhaus, R. J., Cavallari, N. International registry of inferior vena cava leiomyosarcoma: analysis of a world series on 218 patients. *Anticancer Res.* 1996 Sep.-Oct.; 16(5B):3201-5.

Mingoli, A., Sapienza, P., Brachini, G., Tarantino, B., Cirillo, B. Surgical treatment of inferior vena cava leiomyosarcoma. *J. Am. Coll. Surg.* 2010 Jul.;211(1):145-6.

Mondragón-Sánchez, R., Orellana, H., Bernal-Maldonado, R., Ruíz-Molina, J. M. Resection of tumors of the pararenal inferior vena cava with in situ perfusion of the right kidney and graft replacement with bovine pericar-dium. *J. Am. Coll. Surg.* 1998 Jun.;186(6):717-9.

Moorjani, N., Kuo, J., Ashley, S., Hughes, G. Intravenous uterine leiomyo-sarcomatosis with intracardial extension. *J. Card. Surg.* 2005 Jul.-Aug.; 20(4):382-5.

Mönig, S. P., Gawenda, M., Erasmi, H., Zieren, J., Pichlmaier, H. Diagnosis, treatment and prognosis of the leiomyosarcoma of the inferior vena cava. Three cases and summary of published reports. *Eur. J. Surg.* 1995 Apr.; 161(4):231-5.

Montgomery, E. M., Litvak, A. S., McRoberts, J. W. Leiomyosarcoma of renal vein. *Urology.* 1976 Sep.;8(3):215-7.

Mu, D., Wang, D., Zhou, K., Zhu, B. Radiographic features of intraluminal leiomyosarcoma of the inferior vena cava: an atypical case report. *Abdom. Imaging.* 2011 Oct.;36(5):586-9.

Munene, G., Mack, L. A., Moore, R. D., Temple, W. J. Neoadjuvant radio-therapy and reconstruction using autologous vein graft for the treatment of inferior vena cava leiomyosarcoma. *J. Surg. Oncol.* 2011 Feb.;103(2):175-8.

Navarra, G., Occhionorelli, S., Mascoli, F., Santini, M., Benea, G., Marzola, A. Primary leiomyosarcoma of the aorta: report of a case and review of the literature. *J. Cardiovasc. Surg.* (Torino). 1994 Aug.;35(4):333-6.

Nayyar, R., Panda, S., Saini, A., Seth, A., Chaudhary, S. K. Leiomyosarcoma of inferior vena cava involving bilateral renal veins: Surgical challenges and reconstruction with upfront saphenous vein interposition graft for left renal vein outflow. *Indian J. Urol.* 2010 Jul.;26(3):438-40.

Niver, B. E., Megibow, A. J., Faust, M. J., Rosenkrantz, A. B. Multidetector CT appearance of leiomyosarcoma of the splenic vein. *Clin. Radiol.* 2011 Jul.;66(7):688-90.

Ohman, J. W., Chandra, V., Poultsides, G., Harris, E. J. Iliocaval and aortoiliac reconstruction following en bloc retroperitoneal leiomyosarco-ma resection. *J. Vasc. Surg.* 2013 Mar.;57(3):850.

Padilla-Fernandez, B., Lorenzo-Gomez, M. F., Herrero-Polo, M., Silva-Abuin, J. M., Martin-Izquierdo, M., Antunez-Plaza, P. Leiomyosarcoma of the inferior vena cava in a patient with double inferior vena cava. *Ann. Vasc. Surg.* 2012 Aug.;26(6):859.

Perl, L. Ein Fall von Sarkom der V cava inferior. *Virchows Arch. Pathol. Anat.* 1871;53:378-83.

Pelton, J. J., Palazzo, J. P., Peterson, R. O., Eisenberg, B. L. Renal vein leio-myosarcoma. *J. Surg. Oncol.* 1990 Oct.;45(2):131-3.

Perera, G. B., Wilson, S. E., Barie, P. S., Butler, J. A. Duodenocaval fistula: a late complication of retroperitoneal irradiation and vena cava replacement. *Ann. Vasc. Surg.* 2004 Jan.;18(1):52-8.

Phoa, S. S., van Rooij, W. J., Kox, C., Dijkstra, P. F. Leiomyosarcoma of the suprarenal and renal veins, report on two cases. *Rofo.* 1988 Jan.;148(1): 84-5.

Polsky, S., Goodloe, S. Jr, Peterson, S., Karakousis, C. P. Leiomyosarcoma of the renal vein. *Eur. J. Surg. Oncol.* 1997 Oct.;23(5):456.

Praseedom, R. K., Dhar, P., Jamieson, N. V., Wallwork, J., Bergman, I., Lomas, D. J. Leiomyosarcoma of the retrohepatic vena cava treated by excision and reconstruction with an aortic homograft: a case report and review of literature. *Surg. Innov.* 2007 Dec.;14(4):287-91.

Presti, C., Casella, I. B. Technique of aortic replacement through endovascular stenting before aortic wall resection for primary leiomyosarcoma of the abdominal aorta. *Ann. Vasc. Surg.* 2012 Oct.;26(7):1052-5.

Radhakrishanan, J., Alrenga, D. P., Ghosh, B. C. Isolated hepatic metastasis from renal vein leiomyosarcoma. *Arch. Pathol. Lab. Med.* 1978 Nov.;102 (11):606.

Ramponi, F., Kench, J. G., Simring, D. V., Crawford, M., Abadir, E., Harris, J. P. Early diagnosis and resection of an asymptomatic leiomyosarcoma of the inferior vena cava prior to caval obstruction. *J. Vasc. Surg*. 2012 Feb.; 55(2):525-8.

Rascanu, C., Duran, M., Grabitz, K., Weis-Müller, B., Sandmann, W. Success-ful surgical management of a recurrent leiomyosarcoma of the inferior vena cava. *Vasa*. 2011 Jan.;40(1):69-72.

Reddy, V. P., Vanveldhuizen, P. J., Muehlebach, G. F., Dusing, R. W., Birkbeck, J. P., Williamson, S. K., Krishnan, L., Meyers, D. G. Leiomyo-sarcoma of the inferior vena cava: a case report and review of the litera-ture. *Cases J*. 2010 Feb. 23;3:71.

Reges, R., Denardi, F., Matheus, W., Ferreira, U., Netto, N. R. Jr, Billis, A. Primary leiomyosarcoma of the inferior vena cava: How should it be treated and the vein anatomy re-established? *Int. J. Urol*. 2008 Mar.;15 (3):259-60.

Ridwelski, K., Rudolph, S., Meyer, F., Buhtz, P., Burger, T., Lippert, H. Primary sarcoma of the inferior vena cava: review of diagnosis, treatment, and outcomes in a case series. *Int. Surg*. 2001 Jul.-Sep.;86(3):184-90.

Rodríguez-Caulo, E. A., Velázquez, C., Ramírez, B., Barquero, J. M. Primary inferior vena cava leiomyosarcoma: reconstruction is not mandatory. *Asian Cardiovasc. Thorac. Ann*. 2012 Dec.;20(6):715-7.

Ruh, J., Lang, H., Paul, A., Dirsch, O., Broelsch, C. E. Surgical aspects in the therapy of primary sarcoma of the vena cava. *J. Am. Coll. Surg*. 2006 Mar.;202(3):559-62.

Sarkar, R., Eilber, F. R., Gelabert, H. A., Quinones-Baldrich, W. J. Prosthetic replacement of the inferior vena cava for malignancy. *J. Vasc. Surg*. 1998 Jul.;28(1):75-81.

Satheesan, B., Subramaniam, S. R., Kathiresan, N., Sunil, B. J. Postoperative renal failure following inferior vena caval tumor resection with right nephrectomy: A case report and review of literature. *Indian J. Urol*. 2008 Jan.;24(1):104-6.

Sharma, B. C., Saraswat, V. A., Dhiman, R. K., Ghoshal, U. C., Puri, A. S., Sikora, S. S. Unusual tumors causing extrahepatic portal venous obstruct-tion. *HPB Surg*. 1996;9(3):165-7.

Shen, Z. J., Zhou, X. L., Yu, Y. L., Li, M. One case of leiomyosarcoma of the inferior vena cava treated with radical resection and vascular reconstruct-tion. *Vasc. Med*. 2005 Aug.;10(3):225-7.

Shindo, S., Matsumoto, H., Ogata, K., Katahira, S., Kojima, A., Iyori, K., Ishimoto, T., Kobayashi, M., Tada, Y., Suzuki, T., Itakura, J., Iizuka, H., Matsumoto, Y. Surgical treatment of retroperitoneal leiomyosarcoma invading the inferior vena cava: report of three cases. *Surg. Today*. 2002; 32(10):929-33.

Shvarts, O., Han, K. R., Lam, J. S., Belldegrun, A. S. Primary leiomyosarcoma of the inferior vena cava presenting as a renal mass. *Rev. Urol*. 2004 Winter;6(1):39-42.

Singh, I., Joshi, M., Mishra, K. Capsular renal leiomyosarcoma with encase-ment of the inferior vena cava - Diagnosed by immunostaining and review of literature. *Urol. Ann*. 2010 Jan.;2(1):36-8.

Smith, B. M., Mulherin, J. L., Sawyers, J. L., Turner, B. I., Prager, R. L., Dean, R. H. Suprarenal vena caval occlusion. Principles of operative management. *Ann. Surg*. 1984 Jun.;199(6):656-68.

Soejima, Y., Matsumoto, T., Shirabe, K., Maehara, Y. Tube cavoplasty using autologous vein grafts for resected inferior vena cava reconstruction. *Surg. Today*. 2013 Apr.;43(4):452-5.

Sokolich, J., Mejia, A., Cheng, S., Dunn, E. Retroperitoneal leiomyosarcoma of the inferior vena cava mimicking a liver tumor. *Am. Surg*. 2008 May; 74(5):433-6.

Spinelli, A., Schumacher, G., Benckert, C., Sauer, I. M., Schmeding, M., Glanemann, M., Neumann, U. P., Jonas, S., Neuhaus, P. Surgical treat-ment of a leiomyosarcoma of the inferior vena cava involving the hepatic and renal veins confluences: technical aspects. *Eur. J. Surg. Oncol.* 2008 Jul.;34(7):831-5.

Spinelli, F., Stilo, F., La Spada, M., De Caridi, G., Benedetto, F. Surgical treatment of tumors involving the inferior vena cava. Personal experience. *J. Cardiovasc. Surg* (Torino). 2008 Jun.;49(3):323-8.

Staley, C. J., Valaitis, J., Trippel, O. H., Franzblau, S. A. Leiomyosarcoma of the inferior vena cava. *Am. J. Surg*. 1967 Feb.;113(2):211-6.

Stambo, G., Valentin, M., Kerr, T. M., Blanco, R. Endovascular treatment of an acutely ruptured abdominal aorta from tumor invasion by an unresec-table retroperitoneal leiomyosarcoma. *Ann. Vasc. Surg*. 2008 Jul.-Aug.; 22 (4):568-70.

Stauffer, J. A., Fakhre, G. P., Dougherty, M. K., Nakhleh, R. E., Maples, W. J., Nguyen, J. H. Pancreatic and multiorgan resection with inferior vena cava reconstruction for retroperitoneal leiomyosarcoma. *World J. Surg. Oncol*. 2009 Jan. 6;7:3.

Stollwerck, P. L., Kozlowski, B., Sandmann, W., Grabitz, K., Pfeiffer, T. Long-term dilatation of polyester and expanded polytetrafluoroethylene tube grafts after open repair of infrarenal abdominal aortic aneurysms. *J. Vasc. Surg*. 2011 Jun.;53(6):1506-13.

Stuart, F. P., Baker, W. H. Palliative surgery for leiomyosarcoma of the inferior vena cava. *Ann. Surg*. 1973 Feb.;177(2):237-9.

Suffat, L. P., Mazza, L., Farina, E. C., Cassine, D., Merlo, M., Limerutt, G., Fronda, G. Leiomyosarcoma of the inferior vena cava. Report of two cases and review of the literature. *Ann. Ital. Chir*. 2007 Jul.-Aug.;78(4):303-6.

Sundaresan, M., Kelly, S. B., Benjamin, I. S., Akosa, A. B. Primary hepatic vascular leiomyosarcoma of probable portal vein origin. *J. Clin. Pathol*. 1990 Dec.;43(12):1036.

Suzman, M. S., Smith, A. J., Brennan, M. F. Fascio-peritoneal patch repair of the IVC: a workhorse in search of work? *J. Am. Coll. Surg*. 2000 Aug.;191 (2):218-20.

Székely, E., Kulka, J., Miklós, I., Kaliszky, P. Leiomyosarcomas of great vessels. *Pathol. Oncol. Res*. 2000;6(3):233-6.

Tan, G. W., Chia, K. H. An unusual case of leiomyosarcoma of the inferior vena cava in a patient with a duplicated inferior vena cava. *Ann. Vasc. Surg*. 2009 Mar.;23(2):256.e13-8.

Tameo, M. N., Calligaro, K. D., Antin, L., Dougherty, M. J. Primary leio-myosarcoma of the inferior vena cava: reports of infrarenal and supra-hepatic caval involvement. *J. Vasc. Surg*. 2010 Jan.;51(1):221-4.

Testini, M., Todisco, C., Simone, M., Paradiso, V., D'Agostino, D., Ferlan, G., Testini, A., Caruso, G. Treatment of haemorrhage following rupture of aortic leiomyosarcoma. Survival for 4.2 years. *J. Cardiovasc. Surg*. (Torino). 1996 Dec.;37(6):593-6.

Thapar, V. B., Satoskar, R. R., Kanjan, G. M., Chaudhary, A. S. Leiomyo-sarcoma of the inferior vena cava: a case report and review of literature. *Int. Surg*. 2005 Nov.-Dec.;90(5):262-5.

Tilkorn, D. J., Hauser, J., Ring, A., Goertz, O., Stricker, I., Steinau, H. U., Kuhnen, C. Leiomyosarcoma of intravascular origin--a rare tumor entity: clinical pathological study of twelve cases. *World J. Surg. Oncol*. 2010 Nov. 22;8:103.

Tranchart, H., Carloni, A., Balzarotti, R., de Laveaucoupet, J., Chapelier, A., Smadja, C. Leiomyosarcoma of the inferior vena cava involving the renal veins: a simple method of right renal vein reimplantation. *J. Vasc. Surg.* 2008 Jan.;47(1):209-12.

Ueda, J., Yoshida, H., Mamada, Y., Taniai, N., Yoshioka, M., Kawano, Y., Mizuguchi, Y., Shimizu, T., Takata, H., Uchida, E. Surgical resection of a leiomyosarcoma of the inferior vena cava mimicking hepatic tumor. *Case Rep. Med.* 2013;2013:235698.

Varela-Duran, J., Oliva, H., Rosai, J. Vascular leiomyosarcoma: the malignant counterpart of vascular leiomyoma. *Cancer.* 1979 Nov.;44(5):1684-91.

Vos, P., Barwegen, M. G., Bakker, H. H., Dabhoiwala, N. F., Schipper, M. E. Leiomyosarcoma of the renal vein: a case report. *J. Urol.* 1988 May;139 (5):1042-4.

Wang, Q., Jiang, J., Wang, C., Lian, G., Jin, M. S., Cao, X. Leiomyosarcoma of the inferior vena cava level II involvement: curative resection and reconstruction of renal veins. *World J. Surg. Oncol.* 2012 Jun. 28;10:120.

Wang, T. S., Ocal, I. T., Salem, R. R., Elefteriades, J., Sosa, J. A. Leiomyo-sarcoma of the adrenal vein: a novel approach to surgical resection. *World J. Surg. Oncol.* 2007 Oct. 3;5:109.

WEEKLY clinicopathological exercises; leiomyosarcoma, retroperitoneal, with invasion of tail of pancreas, hilus of spleen and splenic vein. *N. Engl. J. Med.* 1950 Nov. 23;243(21):833-6.

Wilson, S. R., Hine, A. L. Leiomyosarcoma of the portal vein. *AJR Am. J. Roentgenol.* 1987 Jul.;149(1):183-4.

Wong, C., Von Oppell, U. O., Scott-Coombes, D. Cold feet from adrenal leio-myosarcoma. *J. R. Soc. Med.* 2005 Sep.;98(9):418-20.

Xu, T. B., Liu, W. Y., Chen, G., Wang, H. Z., Bie, P. *Primary leiomyosarco-ma of the inferior vena cava: a case report.*

Yadav, R., Kataria, K., Mathur, S. R., Seenu, V. Leiomyosarcoma of inferior vena cava: a case series of four cases. *Indian J. Pathol. Microbiol.* 2012 Jan.-Mar.;55(1):83-5.

Yamaguchi, R., Yamaguchi, A., Isogai, M., Hori, A., Kin, Y. Leiomyosarcoma of the inferior vena cava. Resection and reconstruction of the renal vein using the gonadal vein. *Surg. Today.* 1998;28(3):359-61.

Yanaga, K., Okadome, K., Ito, H., Matsumata, T., Makino, T., Okamura, H., Sugimachi, K. Graft replacement of pararenal inferior vena cava for leio-myosarcoma with the use of venous bypass. *Surgery.* 1993 Jan.;113 (1): 109-12.

Yoshidome, H., Takeuchi, D., Ito, H., Kimura, F., Shimizu, H., Ambiru, S., Togawa, A., Ohtsuka, M., Kato, A., Miyazaki, M. Should the inferior vena cava be reconstructed after resection for malignant tumors? *Am. J. Surg.* 2005 Apr.;189(4):419-24.

Yuzer, Y., Zeytunlu, M., Makay, O., Sozbilen, M., Yuce, G. Leiomyosarcoma of the inferior vena cava: report of a case. *Surg. Today.* 2004;34(4):370-3.

Zaenkert, E. K., Bruns, C. J., Winter, H., Rentsch, M., Jauch, K. W., Hardin, G., Angele, M. K. Resection of sarcoma involving the intrahepatic vena cava: report of 2 cases from a specialized center. *Ann. Vasc. Surg.* 2013 May;27(4):498.e9-13.

Zhang, H., Kong, Y., Zhang, H., He, X., Zhang, H. Y., Liu, C., Xiao, M., Xu, X. Leiomyosarcoma of the inferior vena cava: case report and treatment of recurrence with repeat surgery. *Ann. Vasc. Surg.* 2010 Apr.;24(3):417.e5-9.

In: Leiomyosarcoma
Editor: Rosemary H. Leach
ISBN: 978-1-63117-940-2

Chapter 2

Leimyosarcomas of the Genitourinary Tract

Eun-mi Yu,[1] Adam Kittai[2] and Jeanny B. Aragon-Ching[1,*]
[1]Department of Medicine, Division of Hematology/Oncology,
George Washington University Medical Center, Washington, DC, US
[2]Department of Internal Medicine, George Washington University Medical Center,
Washington, DC, US

Abstract

Leiomyosarcomas (LMS) are a common subtype of sarcoma that is frequently characterized by aneuploidy. However, leiomyosarcomas of the genitourinary (GU) tract make up less than 5% of all leiomyosarcomas. Areas of involvement includes bladder, prostate, seminal vesicle, and renal which will be discussed herein. Given rarity of these tumors, no consensus on treatment guidelines are available. However, a common unifying theme suggests that these are highly aggressive tumors that have a high propensity for metastasis even with adequate surgical extirpation. This review will discuss the common presentation, risk factors, treatment and prognosis associated with these GU tumors.

I. Introduction on Leiomyosarcomas

Leiomyosarcomas (LMS) are one of the most common subtypes of sarcomas derived from smooth muscle cells, accounting for around 11% of all soft tissue sarcomas (STS). [1] About half of all LMS occurs in the uterus, but other common sites include the

* Corresponding Author: Jeanny B. Aragon-Ching, M.D., F.A.C.P., Assistant Professor of Medicine, Department of Medicine, Division of Hematology and Oncology, George Washington University Medical Center, 2150 Pennsylvania Avenue, NW, Washington, DC 20037, USA. Tel: 202-741-2478; Fax: 202-741-2487. Email: jaragonching@mfa.gwu.edu.

gastrointestinal (GI) tract, retroperitoneum, skin, blood vessels, and bone. LMS of the genitourinary (GU) tract are extremely rare and comprise less than 5% of all LMS, about 2.1% of all soft tissue sarcomas and 1-2% of all malignant GU tumors. [2-4] In one recently published retrospective analysis of LMS cases, 5 out of 46 cases (11%) of extrauterine LMS were of the genitourinary tract, [5] and perhaps not as totally distinct from uterine LMS as was once believed. Typical histologic features of LMS include high cellularity, with cells having abundant pink to red cytoplasm on hematoxylin and eosin (H&E) staining and are arranged in fascicles. Nuclei are centrally located and often described as cigar-shaped. [6] One of the key features is the presence of longitudinal myofibrils that run along the length of the cell. Diagnosis of LMS is based on the assessment of cellular atypia, presence of necrosis, and mitotic activity which help differentiate LMS from other benign entities. [7] The most common histologic subtype of LMS is spindle-cell type, but other variants have been described including myxoid, inflammatory, and granular cell. The different anatomic variants of LMS are histologically similar, but have varying clinical behavior and prognosis. Hence, division into site-specific subgroups such as retroperitoneal or abdominal, somatic soft tissue, vascular and cutaneous are often employed. [6]

Most LMS appear to arise sporadically and have complex karyotypes. There are no known LMS-specific cytogenetic or molecular abnormalities, but many LMS have chromosomal aberrations in the form of gains, losses, and amplifications. Losses from chromosome regions in 3p21-23, 8p21-pter, 13q12-13, and 13q32-qter are often seen. [8] Gains from chromosomes 1, 15, 17, 19, 20, 22, and X and losses from 1q, 2, 4q, 9p, 10, 11q, 13q, and 16 have been detected via comparative genomic hybridization (CGH) techniques. [9-11] Some chromosomal aberrations tend to correlate with poor outcome, large tumor size, and increased propensity to metastasize. For instance, CGH data suggest that loss of 10q sequences and gain of 5p are associated with more aggressive clinical course. [12, 13] These cytogenetic abnormalities appear to affect multiple pathways, including the retinoblastoma (Rb) pathway, [13] as well as phosphatase and tensin homolog (PTEN) [12] which play a role in the development of LMS and also serve as potential therapeutic targets. An increasing number of genes and proteins are being identified with ongoing gene and protein expression studies that appear to be associated with poor prognosis and high metastatic risk in LMS.

LMS typically occur in middle-aged adults and the elderly. Clinical presentation depends largely on the anatomic location and size of the tumor. LMS involving the GU tract can present with pelvic pain, urinary obstruction, hematuria, and constipation. Diagnostic imaging can assist in making a diagnosis, but ultimately, definitive diagnosis is achieved by biopsy and pathologic examination of the tumor. Magnetic resonance imaging (MRI) and computed tomography (CT) scans are often used for staging and defining the exact location and extent of the disease.

There are no consensus guidelines for treatment of LMS, but it is well established that complete surgical resection is the only treatment with curative potential. Data are particularly lacking in genitourinary LMS, but adjuvant radiation and chemotherapy are often used on the basis of the evidence that is available in the management of uterine LMS and soft tissue sarcomas, in general. Radiotherapy is often used in the adjuvant setting for improved local control of recurrence when surgical margins are inadequate despite the apparent lack of a progression free survival (PFS) and overall survival (OS) benefit in uterine LMS. [14, 15] Radiation therapy is also used for palliation of symptoms in the metastatic setting. The role of systemic chemotherapy remains unclear at this time, as most studies to date show a possible delay in recurrence, but no improved overall survival benefit. [16, 17] However, more recent promising data suggests that the use of adjuvant chemotherapy may provide a progression-free survival benefit in selected uterine LMS patients, which hopefully will translate to an overall survival benefit. [18] First-line chemotherapy with ifosfamide with or without doxorubicin is used widely in the advanced/metastatic setting. A randomized phase III trial showed no significant difference in overall survival (OS) between doxorubicin alone versus doxorubicin plus ifosfamide although the combination did provide a PFS benefit as well as a higher response rate (RR). [19] A better-tolerated combination of gemcitabine and docetaxel is increasingly used in uterine LMS based on results of a phase II study showing an overall response rate (ORR) of 53% in 34 patients with unresectable uterine LMS, 16 of whom had progression on doxorubicin-based chemotherapy. [20] Conversely, the use of single agent gemcitabine versus the combination of gemcitabine plus docetaxel was further evaluated in 41 non-uterine LMS in what was known as the TAXOGEM study. [21] Combination chemotherapy in this setting did not appear to provide a survival advantage over monotherapy with gemcitabine alone. Median PFS and OS were 6.3 months and 15 months for the gemcitabine group and 3.4 months and 13 months, respectively, for the gemcitabine plus docetaxel group. There are ongoing clinical trials for advanced LMS studying the efficacy of trabectedin based on its apparent activity in LMS in several phase II trials. Eribulin, pazopanib, and ridoforolimus are among the newer, targeted agents currently under study for the treatment of LMS. Increasing knowledge of the underlying genetic and molecular mechanisms and pathophysiology of extra-uterine LMS will hopefully help guide clinicians in the optimal management of these aggressive malignancies and improve outcomes in those with rare genitourinary LMS.

a. Genitourinary Tract Sarcomas

Adult genitourinary (GU) tract sarcomas are rare tumors (see Table 1 for key findings). This poses a particularly complex problem since the limited availability of prospective clinical trials translates to lack of standard guidelines in the management of these patients. Physicians as well as patients alike often resort to information that is based on very little evidence that may be subject to publication bias as one does with cases of unusual or rare tumors. [22] Unlike sarcomas that occur in other areas where liposarcomas may be the more common histology, GU sarcomas most commonly comprise of LMS, of which 47% are renal, 50% bladder, 57% prostate and 19% paratesticular. [23-27] LMS was the most common histologic subtype that occurs in the GU tract in a single institutional series from a contemporary cohort of 131 patients. [28] In this patient series, presence of metastasis in 21% of patients at the time of referral strongly correlated with disease specific survival (1.4 vs 10.7 years, $p < 0.0001$). Factors that were associated with decline in disease-specific survival include incomplete initial resection, positive margins, bigger tumors, and metastasis. To some extent, the management of GU tract sarcomas follows the general principles of surgical management of sarcomas in these areas including that of the kidney, bladder, and prostate.

Table 1. Key Features of genitourinary (GU) tract leiomyosarcomas (LMS)

LMS Location	Typical Age at Presentation (y/o)	Symptoms	Radiographic Findings	Prognosis	Treatment
Bladder	50-60	Hematuria, urinary obstruction, abdominal pain	Well-circumscribed bladder mass	OS 62-84% at 5 years	Radical cystectomy +/- en bloc removal of prostate and seminal vesicles (men) and of uterus, cervix, vaginal cuff (women) +/- lymph node dissection
Prostate	50-80	Urinary obstruction, pelvic pain, urinary frequency	Enlarged prostate with heterogeneous, round or lobulated mass.	OS 26% at 5 years	Radical cystoprostatectomy +urinary diversion or pelvic exenteration +/- neoadjuvant/adjuvant chemotherapy and/or radiation
Kidney	40-70	Flank Pain, Abdominal Mass, Hematuria	Encapsulated solid mass with heterogeneous enhancement on CT	OS 29-36% at 5 years	Radical Nephrectomy +/- Adjuvant Chemoradiation
Seminal Vesicle	37-68	Pelvic pressure, Dysuria, Bladder outlet obstruction	Large Mass on CT/ MRI	Unclear	Radical Resection
Paratesticular	40-70	Large, Discrete, Painless mass, Separate from Scrotum	Heterogeneous Mass on ultrasound	OS 50-80% at 5 Years	Radical Orchiectomy +/- Adjuvant Radiotherapy

Surgical resection, whenever possible, remains the standard of care and utility of chemotherapy or radiation in the adjuvant setting remains controversial although some would consider these patients as suitable candidates for adjuvant treatment protocols and further consideration for these multimodal therapies should occur on an individualized basis. Treatment for metastatic cases follows that of leiomyosarcomas in general.

II. Leiomyosarcoma of the Bladder

The most common malignant mesenchymal tumor of the bladder is LMS, but comprises <1% of all bladder malignancies. LMS of the bladder was first reported in 1929. [29] Known risk factors include history of pelvic radiation therapy and cyclophosphamide use for treatment of other cancers. [30] In one of the largest case series reported thus far of 20 LMS patients, the mean age was 58 years (range of 29 to 84 years old) and the male to female ratio was 2:1. [31] Criteria for distinguishing leiomyoma from LMS in the bladder have not been clearly established. Historically, any degree of mitotic activity, increased cellularity, or pleomorphism in a bladder smooth muscle tumor has resulted in the diagnosis of LMS because the morphologic features predictive of malignant behavior are not as well-characterized as it is for uterine leiomyosarcomas which are far more commonly occurring smooth muscle neoplasms. Histologic features were examined in all cases and clinical follow-up information was obtained in 15 of these cases. LMS cases were subclassified into low-grade (8/20) and high-grade (12/20) based on mitotic counts, 1 to 4/10 HPF (high power field) and 4-17/10 HPF, respectively. In addition to the typical spindle-cell pattern of LMS, 5 of 20 cases showed epithelioid features. Other more common features that were noted were tumor cell necrosis in 11 cases and mucosal ulceration in 7 cases. Of the cases where the tumor-muscularis propria interface could be assessed, an infiltrative border was seen in 4 of 6 high-grade and 2 of 6 low-grade LMS. None of the 20 cases of LMS had areas resembling benign leiomyoma.

Given the rarity of presentation of bladder leiomyosarcomas, therapeutic guidelines remain poorly defined and complete surgical extirpation has remained the cornerstone of treatment for these patients. [32]

Treatment of LMS of the bladder with curative intent should consist of aggressive surgical extirpation with a radical cystectomy whenever feasible. Radical resection of the tumor with en-bloc removal of the bladder, prostate, and seminal vesicles in men, and the uterus, cervix, and vaginal cuff in women, similar to that of bladder transitional cell carcinoma treatment, have resulted in lower rates of local recurrence. One retrospective case series analyzed the outcomes of 7 bladder LMS patients who underwent surgical resection with negative margins. [2] Pathologic stage was assigned using the Memorial Sloan-Kettering Cancer Center (MSKCC) soft-tissue sarcoma staging system. Six patients were assigned with MSKCC stage 3 and one patient, with stage 2 disease. Tumor grade was also assessed and all but one patient were diagnosed with high-grade LMS. Six of these patients underwent a radical cystectomy and one patient was treated with partial cystectomy; all patients were also treated with radical pelvic lymph node dissection. Negative surgical margins was achieved in all seven patients, but three patients were found with lymph nodes positive for bladder LMS. Two of the three patients with lymph node positivity underwent adjuvant chemotherapy; the third patient declined adjuvant therapy and died 9 months later with lung and liver metastases. Two patients had local pelvic recurrence after surgery and adjuvant chemotherapy and 36 Gy of radiation therapy. The chemotherapy that was used was doxorubicin plus ifosfamide in one patient whereas cisplatin and gemcitabine was used to treat the other patient. While both patients achieved a complete response at 25 and 28 months, respectively, both passed away 3 months after developing lung and liver metastasis despite treatment with salvage chemotherapy. Two patients developed distant metastasis 4 and 6 months, respectively, after surgery and adjuvant chemotherapy. The four patients who did not have lymph node positivity on pathologic examination after definitive surgery were not treated with adjuvant therapy and were alive with no evidence of disease at 74, 61, 33, and 8 months.

Another larger series reported the outcomes of 19 bladder sarcoma cases from January 1985 to July 2004, 14 of whom had leiomyosarcomas. [33] The primary treatment was surgery in 16 patients and the median disease specific survival (DSS) was 11.6 years and median recurrence free survival (RFS) was 3.4 years. Eight of these patients underwent radical cystectomy, 3 patients were treated with transurethral resection of bladder tumor, 3 patients had a partial cystectomy, and 2 patients underwent pelvic exenteration. 12 patients treated with surgery achieved negative surgical margins and the median DSS for this group was 11.6 years, with a median RFS of 7.6 years. Margin status was available for 2 of 3 patients treated with a partial cystectomy, who both had negative margins and did not develop local recurrence. However, both patients eventually developed metastases to the lung and one had died of disease by the time of publication. Primary systemic chemotherapy was used for two patients who had metastatic disease at presentation. One patient received doxorubicin and dacarbazine and the other was treated with vincristine, doxorubicin, and cisplatin. The median DSS and RFS for these patients were 6 months. 4 patients received neoadjuvant therapy with either chemotherapy (n=3) or external-beam radiotherapy (n=1), whereas 3 patients were treated with chemotherapy in the adjuvant setting. Neoadjuvant and adjuvant therapy were both associated with the doubling of DSS, but this was not found to be statistically significant due to the small number of patients treated. A total of 10 patients were treated with salvage therapy for development of distant metastases, 9 with systemic chemotherapy, 1 with radiation therapy, and 1 with surgery. 9 of the patients treated with salvage therapy died of disease and the median survival for this group was 20 months.

In summary, the mainstay of therapy in leiomyosarcoma of the bladder is surgical resection with radical cystectomy and lymph node dissection with the goal of achieving negative margins. There is inadequate evidence to support the use of neoadjuvant or adjuvant therapy, and it is also unclear if these approaches provide any survival benefit in certain high-risk settings such as high-grade tumor, higher stage of disease, lymph node involvement, positive surgical margins, or in the presence of lymphovascular invasion. Salvage therapy with current available modalities do not provide a durable response in those who develop local recurrence or distant metastases after primary therapy.

III. Leiomyosarcoma of the Prostate

Leiomyosarcoma is the most common primary sarcoma that occurs in the prostate, but as with other sarcomas that occur in the GU tract, it accounts for less than 0.1% of all cancers that originate in the prostate. [34] It is an extremely rare entity with only around two-hundred cases reported in the literature to date. LMS of the prostate typically occurs in the fifth to eighth decade of life. Presenting symptoms mimic those of other more common prostatic lesions such as benign prostatic hyperplasia and adenocarcinoma, including urinary obstruction, pelvic pain, and urinary frequency. Diagnosis is usually made by transrectal needle biopsy or transurethral resection of the prostate. Serum prostate specific antigen (PSA) levels are usually within normal limits unless there is concomitant conventional adenocarcinoma of the prostate in the specimen. Tumor size varies greatly, with the majority of reported lesions measuring 5 to 10 cm. Histologically, LMS have similar characteristics to those of other organs, but most reported cases of prostatic LMS have been high-grade tumors that frequently have high mitotic activity, necrosis, and cause obliteration of the normal architecture of benign prostatic glandular tissue. Tumors are positive for actin, desmin, and calponin on IHC studies. Epithelioid LMS is one of the more commonly-reported subtypes that can also arise from the prostate and can show focal positivity for keratin on IHC. The American Joint Committee on Cancer (AJCC) stage of LMS of the prostate is determined by imaging with computed tomography (CT) or magnetic resonance imaging (MRI) scans. Chest CT should be included in the staging work-up given that the most common site of metastases involves the lungs. Given the aggressive biology of prostatic LMS, most patients present with advanced-stage disease. Overall prognosis is poor and 50-75% of affected patients die within 2-5 years. [35, 36] In one retrospective analysis of 54 cases of LMS of the prostate, [37] 23.5% of patients had metastatic disease upon initial diagnosis. The most common sites of metastases were the lung, liver, and bone. Median survival was 17 months and the 5-year survival rate was 26% for the 34 patients for whom outcome data was available. Compared to other genitourinary LMS such as those arising in the kidney and bladder, prostate LMS is seemingly associated with much shorter survival. [2, 38] Negative surgical margins and the absence of metastases appear to be predictors of longer survival. [24, 37]

There are currently no standard treatment guidelines for prostatic LMS. Multimodality therapy is commonly used and includes surgery, neoadjuvant and adjuvant chemotherapy, and radiation. Metastatic disease is most often treated with systemic chemotherapy. Definitive surgical approaches have included radical retropubic prostatectomy, radical cystoprostatectomy, suprapubic prostatectomy, and pelvic exenteration, but it is unclear if more aggressive surgery provides a survival benefit. Moreover, there is also lack of data to support the use of adjuvant chemotherapy and/or radiation. The most commonly-used chemotherapy regimens for LMS, in general, have included doxorubicin or epirubicin in combination with cyclophosphamide, ifosfamide, or dacarbazine and/or a vinca alkaloid. [24, 39-41] A retrospective analysis of 25 prostate sarcoma patients, 10 of whom had LMS of the prostate, revealed that surgery with or without adjuvant therapy is feasible for this disease. [42] In this series, 4 of these patients underwent definitive surgery and 3 of them underwent adjuvant therapy: 2 had systemic chemotherapy and one had radiation alone. Interestingly, the one patient who did not receive adjuvant therapy survived the longest at 29 months. The 3 patients that received adjuvant therapy had an overall survival between 23 and 27 months. Another retrospective analysis of 21 prostate sarcoma patients treated from 1972-2000 at the M.D. Anderson Cancer Center included 12 LMS patients, 6 of whom underwent initial surgery for high-grade, AJCC Stage II-III disease. [24] Four of these patients died of disease with their survival time ranging from 15-41 months. One patient was alive with no evidence of disease at 96 months, and another, alive with no evidence of disease at 12 months. One patient with AJCC stage III, high-grade LMS with tumor size of 14 cm was initially treated with preoperative therapy with doxorubicin, dacarbazine, and 50 Gy of external beam radiotherapy which resulted in a 46% decrease in the size of the tumor. This patient subsequently underwent total pelvic exenteration and ileal loop urinary diversion with negative surgical margins and was alive with no evidence of disease at 88 months. There were a total of 5 LMS patients that were treated only with systemic chemotherapy, 4 of whom had stage IV disease, 1 had stage II disease. All stage IV patients died after a survival time ranging from 3-18 months and the stage II patient treated with chemotherapy only died at 30 months. As a whole, patients with prostate sarcoma appeared to benefit from combined modality therapy consisting of pre-operative therapy in this series. 4 out of 5 patients with stage III prostate sarcoma treated with pre-operative therapy were alive and free of disease at a mean of 70 months. There also appeared to be an added survival benefit for those with large tumor size greater than 10 cm. 4 out of 7 patients with stage III prostate sarcoma and tumor size greater than 10 cm had an increased mean survival of 85 months after combined modality therapy in comparison to the other 3 patients treated with either chemotherapy or surgery alone who had a mean survival of 39 months. In this series of 21 prostate sarcoma patients, there were no differences in survival between histologic subtypes. There was no survival advantage appreciated for patients with low grade or tumor size equal to or less than 5 cm, similar to the general experience with other soft tissue extremity sarcoma treatment. The only factor that appeared to be a significant indicator of decreased disease specific survival was the presence of metastatic disease.

In summary, LMS of the prostate is difficult to cure with current approaches given the aggressive nature of the disease, but it is clear that definitive surgery and achievement of negative surgical margins offers the only probability for prolonged overall survival. Based on the retrospective data that is available, select patients may benefit from a combined modality approach, particularly with neoadjuvant chemotherapy and/or radiation. There is no clear role for adjuvant therapy, even though it is commonly used. Metastatic LMS of the prostate is universally fatal with a median survival of 5 months despite the use of systemic chemotherapy.

IV. Leiomyosarcoma of the Kidney

LMS of the kidney is an uncommon entity with a very aggressive feature and portends a poor prognosis. It accounts for about 1% of all renal malignancies, and accounts for 50-60% of sarcomas that occur in the kidney, making it the most common histologic sarcoma subtype. [43] They tend to affect patients between the ages of 40-70 years, both men and women equally. Typically presenting as abdominal mass, flank pain, and hematuria, it is a rare diagnosis that should be kept in mind when this triad of symptoms occur. [44, 45] Renal LMS commonly arises from the renal capsule, renal pelvis, or the vessels of the kidney, tending to envelop the kidney or take over the renal parenchyma itself. Histopathologically, it consists mainly of spindle cells in a fascicular, plexiform/ haphazard growth pattern with interspersed connective tissue. Nuclear pleomorphism, mitoses, and necrosis differentiate LMS from benign leiomyomas and the immunohistochemical stains are typically positive for actin, desmin, and calponin.

On CT scans, they present as large (average 13.4 cm), well circumscribed, encapsulated solid or multinodular masses with heterogeneous enhancement. [46] Similar to what's seen on CT, MRI imaging of LMS appears as a soft-tissue mass with heterogeneous signal intensity. LMS tends to have low signal intensity areas on T1 and T2 weighted images with delayed enhancement; corresponding to areas of fibrous connective tissue. Furthermore, even as it presents radiographically as large tumors, diagnosis is often not achieved until the post-operative setting, [47] as it may not be easily distinguishable from that of conventional clear cell renal cell carcinomas. [48]

The pattern of spread is dictated by the origin of the tumor. For instance, LMS from the renal capsule has a tendency to envelop the kidney, whereas if parenchymal in origin, it may replace the renal parenchyma. Furthermore, renal pelvic LMS can extend into the collecting system, and renal vein LMS can extend in the IVC. [44] Ninety percent of renal LMS will go on to metastasize to the lungs, liver and bone. Prognostically, grade, age and stage have been shown to be key determinants of overall survival. In one case series that included 10 patients with LMS of the kidney, a correlation between tumor grade and mortality was seen with all 3 of the patients with high grade 3 LMS who died of their disease, as opposed to 2 out of the 7 with lower grade disease surviving at the time of reporting. [49] The study concluded that it is important to grade renal LMS, as it clearly played a role in prognosis in their case series. Using the Surveillance, Epidemiology and End Results (SEER) database, a series of 112 cases of renal LMS was studied and they found that the patients exhibited an overall survival of 25 months, with a 25% 5-year overall survival. [38] In this large series, stage and age were once again shown to be the strongest predictor for overall survival, followed by histological grade, histological subtype, tumor size, and gender. However, one criticism for this particular series was inclusion of a mixed population of patients, although their results were very similar to previously published studies. In another comprehensive case series from 3 institutions that included 27 cases of primary LMS of the kidney, [50] only tumors with classic signs of LMS on H+E stain were included. The rarity of this tumor was exemplified by case assignment of only 27 individuals over a 23-year search period. Consistent with what has been already described, the average age at diagnosis was 58.5 years, but women were slightly more affected than men (59% women), and all tumors had typical histopathology. Average length of follow-up was 2.8 years, with 75% of the patients described eventually dying of tumor burden. Distant metastases were seen in majority of patients, about 90%, having metastasized most commonly to the lungs, followed by the liver, bone, skeletal muscle, pericardium, chest wall, skin and colon in the most common order of frequency.

LMS of the kidney is a very aggressive tumor, with a 5 year survival of rate of 29-36%, and a median survival cited as 18 months. [44, 50] Radical resection of the kidney is the standard of treatment, [51] as irradiation and chemotherapy alone have proven ineffective and unlikely to alter clinical course. [52] The role of adjuvant chemotherapy and/or radiation in these patients have remained indeterminate to date, although may have a role in patients who otherwise have not successfully undergone complete resections. [53] The combination of gemcitabine and docetaxel has shown promise in patients with leiomyosarcomas, particularly uterine LMS in the metastatic setting, but median survival continues to remain unchanged. [54]

V. Leiomyosarcoma of the Testes/ Paratesticular Site

LMS arising in the paratesticular tissue is a particularly rare tumor. Conversely, only about 10% of all paratesticular sarcomas are histologically leiomyosarcomas. [55] Of the tumors that occur in the scrotal region, majority are testicular in origin and only 3% arises from the parastesticular structures. [56] The paratesticular structures include the spermatic cord, epididymis, testicular tunic, or the scrotum, with the spermatic cord being the most common part affected in about 80-90% of the time. To date, there are approximately only 100 cases reported. [57] As the name LMS suggests, the tumor typically arises from the muscle cells of each paratesticular structure; the vas deferens and cremasteric muscle in the spermatic cord, the smooth muscle basement membrane of the epididymis, and the dartos layer of the scrotum. LMS typically presents as a large, discrete, painless scrotal mass, separate from the testicle, in adults aged 40-70 years. [58] Given the rarity of the tumor, epidemiological studies to elucidate risk factors become problematic although it has been suggested that high-dose hormones can predispose patients to the development of this tumor as illustrated in one case report. [59] On gross resection, LMS are solid, grey, and rubbery. Histology is variable; they can be well differentiated, pleomorphic or undifferentiated. [58] As imaging with ultrasound only reveals a heterogeneous mass, diagnosis occurs histopathologically. Classically, histology shows the classic whorl pattern with a fascicular architecture, foci of cytologic atypia, mitoses, with areas of necrosis in high-grade tumors. Immunohistochemical stains are typically positive for alpha actin, smooth muscle myosin, desmin and vimentin. [60]

The historical treatment for LMS of the spermatic cord remains to be surgery with radical orchiectomy, [61, 62] especially since local recurrence can occur as high as 90% following simple excision alone and as high as 75% even in the setting of radical resection. [63] Although difficult to assess, five-year survival and overall survival have been cited as anywhere from 50-80%. [57] Prognosis can be determined using the Fédération Nationale des Centres de Lutte Contre le Cancer (FNCLCC) or the National Cancer Institute (NCI) grading system as with other sarcomas. [64] Radiotherapy as adjunctive therapy has been shown to be beneficial in spermatic cord sarcoma as exhibited in a study where patients who underwent surgery alone was compared to those who had surgery plus adjuvant radiation. [65] Patients who received adjunctive radiation had no signs of regional failure as opposed to 56% of those who received surgery alone. Although this study involved other histopathologic subtypes of sarcomas (apart from the 7 cases of LMS, 7 had liposarcomas, 2 had malignant fibrous histiocytomas, and 1 patient had mesothelioma), it alludes to evidence that radiotherapy may be useful in LMS, which is now often used in the treatment of LMS. There is controversy around prophylactic lymph node dissection in the setting of LMS, as classically LMS tumors spread hematogenously and not through the lymphatics. Thus far, the data has not shown a remarkable survival benefit in support of retroperitoneal lymph node dissection. [66] In addition, there is practically no data to support adjunctive chemotherapy in this setting. [61] Hence, radical resection alone continues to be the standard of care for treatment.

VI. Leiomyosarcoma of the Seminal Vesicle

LMS of the seminal vesicle is another extremely rare tumor. A review of the English literature yields very few reported cases. [4, 67-72] Age at diagnosis ranged from 37 to 68 years and generally presents as pelvic pressure, dysuria, and bladder outlet obstruction. [69] The tumors were typically large, at an average of about 8 cm in size. Given the large size at presentation, the mass would be palpated while doing a digital rectal examination, which would ultimately lead to a fine needle biopsy revealing the diagnosis. Following CT and MRI staging, all of the cases underwent complete radical resection of the tumor and the surrounding organs, including but not limited to the prostate, bladder, rectum, and lymph nodes. Five of the cases showed no metastases or involvement of the surrounding tissue after initial resection, although the tumors did abut the surrounding organs significantly. Micro-invasion to the surrounding tissues of the prostate or bladder was seen in 3 cases. [67, 70, 72] When described, pathological appearance was high-grade, whorled with foci of necrosis, and included atypical spindle cells. [67-69] Two cases found the tumor to stain positive for actin, whereas they had opposing findings when stained for cytokeratin, and AE-3. [68, 69]

Radical resection made up the treatment for all cases. Only 1 patient utilized adjuvant chemo-radiation therapy, and the patient was tumor free at 20 months. [67] In another case adjuvant radiation therapy was used, and the patient developed metastases at 29 months. [69] The cases had a median follow-up of 22 months, with a range from 6 to 51 months. In the three cases with the longest patient follow up at 24, 29, and 51 months, all patients eventually developed metastases. Metastases eventually were described at about 24 months in one patient who developed metastases to the kidney at which time he received chemo-radiation. Another developed metastases to the lungs at 29 months and was treated with doxorubicin, and another developed metastases to the scalp, liver and lung also at 29 months. He received doxorubicin and ifosfamide, without tumor response. He then received gemcitabine and docetaxel, and his tumor burden was stabilized 51 months later. [69]

Given the rarity of LMS of the seminal vesicle it is hard to generalize and prognosticate this particular tumor. As in other cases of LMS, radical resection of the tumor is the treatment of choice. The role of adjuvant chemo-radiation remains unclear to date.

Conclusion

The presentation, diagnosis, treatment, and prognoses for GU LMS are altogether rare, challenging, and guarded with complete surgical extirpation as the major cornerstone of treatment, as with other soft tissue sarcomas. Understanding the typical presentation and appropriate utilization of a multimodality approach achieves the best possible outcomes for this patient population where standard treatment does not uniformly exist. Increasing exploration of unique molecular pathways will hopefully pave the way for better opportunities for therapeutic intervention.

References

[1] Ducimetiere F, Lurkin A, Ranchere-Vince D, et al: Incidence of sarcoma histotypes and molecular subtypes in a prospective epidemiological study with central pathology review and molecular testing. *PLoS One* 6:e20294, 2011.

[2] Labanaris AP, Zugor V, Meyer B, et al: Urinary bladder leiomyosarcoma in adults. *Int. Urol. Nephrol.* 40:311-6, 2008.

[3] Stojadinovic A, Leung DH, Allen P, et al: Primary adult soft tissue sarcoma: time-dependent influence of prognostic variables. *J. Clin. Oncol.* 20:4344-52, 2002.

[4] Russo P, Brady MS, Conlon K, et al: Adult urological sarcoma. *J. Urol.* 147:1032-6; discussion 1036-7, 1992.

[5] Farid M, Ong WS, Tan MH, et al: The influence of primary site on outcomes in leiomyosarcoma: a review of clinicopathologic differences between uterine and extrauterine disease. *Am. J. Clin. Oncol.* 36:368-74, 2013.

[6] Weiss S, Goldblum J: Leiomyosarcomas, Enzinger and Weiss's soft tissue tumours. Philadelphia, Elsevier Saunders, 2008.

[7] Gadducci A: Prognostic factors in uterine sarcoma. *Best Pract. Res. Clin. Obstet. Gynaecol.* 25:783-95, 2011.

[8] Yang J, Du X, Chen K, et al: Genetic aberrations in soft tissue leiomyosarcoma. *Cancer Lett.* 275:1-8, 2009.

[9] Wang R, Lu YJ, Fisher C, et al: Characterization of chromosome aberrations associated with soft-tissue leiomyosarcomas by twenty-four-color karyotyping and comparative genomic hybridization analysis. *Genes Chromosomes Cancer* 31:54-64, 2001.

[10] Otano-Joos M, Mechtersheimer G, Ohl S, et al: Detection of chromosomal imbalances in leiomyosarcoma by comparative genomic hybridization and interphase cytogenetics. *Cytogenet. Cell Genet.* 90:86-92, 2000.

[11] Derre J, Lagace R, Nicolas A, et al: Leiomyosarcomas and most malignant fibrous histiocytomas share very similar comparative genomic hybridization imbalances: an analysis of a series of 27 leiomyosarcomas. *Lab. Invest.* 81:211-5, 2001.

[12] Hu J, Rao UN, Jasani S, et al: Loss of DNA copy number of 10q is associated with aggressive behavior of leiomyosarcomas: a comparative genomic hybridization study. *Cancer Genet. Cytogenet.* 161:20-7, 2005.

[13] Wang R, Titley JC, Lu YJ, et al: Loss of 13q14-q21 and gain of 5p14-pter in the progression of leiomyosarcoma. *Mod. Pathol.* 16:778-85, 2003.

[14] Mahdavi A, Monk BJ, Ragazzo J, et al: Pelvic radiation improves local control after hysterectomy for uterine leiomyosarcoma: a 20-year experience. *Int. J. Gynecol. Cancer* 19:1080-4, 2009.

[15] Reed NS, Mangioni C, Malmstrom H, et al: Phase III randomised study to evaluate the role of adjuvant pelvic radiotherapy in the treatment of uterine sarcomas stages I and II: an European Organisation for Research and Treatment of Cancer Gynaecological Cancer Group Study (protocol 55874). *Eur. J. Cancer* 44:808-18, 2008.

[16] Pervaiz N, Colterjohn N, Farrokhyar F, et al: A systematic meta-analysis of randomized controlled trials of adjuvant chemotherapy for localized resectable soft-tissue sarcoma. *Cancer* 113:573-81, 2008.

[17] Woll PJ, Reichardt P, Le Cesne A, et al: Adjuvant chemotherapy with doxorubicin, ifosfamide, and lenograstim for resected soft-tissue sarcoma (EORTC 62931): a multicentre randomised controlled trial. *Lancet Oncol.* 13:1045-54, 2012.

[18] Hensley ML, Wathen JK, Maki RG, et al: Adjuvant therapy for high-grade, uterus-limited leiomyosarcoma: results of a phase 2 trial (SARC 005). *Cancer* 119:1555-61, 2013.

[19] Van Der Graaf W, Judson I, Verweij J: Results of a randomised phase III trial (EORTC 62012) of single agent doxorubicin versus doxorubicin plus ifosfamide as first line chemotherapy for patients with advanced or metastatic soft tissue sarcoma: a survival study by the EORTC Soft Tissue and Bone Sarcoma Group, Program and Abstracts of the 37th European Society for Medical Oncology Congress. Vienna, Austria, 2012.

[20] Hensley ML, Maki R, Venkatraman E, et al: Gemcitabine and docetaxel in patients with unresectable leiomyosarcoma: results of a phase II trial. *J. Clin. Oncol.* 20:2824-31, 2002.

[21] Pautier P, Floquet A, Penel N, et al: Randomized multicenter and stratified phase II study of gemcitabine alone versus gemcitabine and docetaxel in patients with metastatic or relapsed leiomyosarcomas: a Federation Nationale des Centres de Lutte Contre le Cancer (FNCLCC) French Sarcoma Group Study (TAXOGEM study). *Oncologist* 17:1213-20, 2012.

[22] Raghavan D: A structured approach to uncommon cancers: what should a clinician do? *Ann. Oncol.* 24:2932-4, 2013.

[23] Srinivas V, Sogani PC, Hajdu SI, et al: Sarcomas of the kidney. *J. Urol.* 132:13-6, 1984.

[24] Sexton WJ, Lance RE, Reyes AO, et al: Adult prostate sarcoma: the M. D. Anderson Cancer Center Experience. *J. Urol.* 166:521-5, 2001.

[25] Vogelzang NJ, Fremgen AM, Guinan PD, et al: Primary renal sarcoma in adults. A natural history and management study by the American Cancer Society, Illinois Division. *Cancer* 71:804-10, 1993.

[26] Sen SE, Malek RS, Farrow GM, et al: Sarcoma and carcinosarcoma of the bladder in adults. *J. Urol.* 133:29-30, 1985.

[27] Coleman J, Brennan MF, Alektiar K, et al: Adult spermatic cord sarcomas: management and results. *Ann. Surg. Oncol.* 10:669-75, 2003.

[28] Dotan ZA, Tal R, Golijanin D, et al: Adult genitourinary sarcoma: the 25-year Memorial Sloan-Kettering experience. *J. Urol.* 176:2033-8; discussion 2038-9, 2006.

[29] Hager BH, Hunt VC: A report of a case of leiomyosarcoma of bladder. *J. Urol.* 21:129-133, 1929.

[30] Helpap B: Nonepithelial neoplasms of the urinary bladder. *Virchows Arch.* 439:497-503, 2001.

[31] Lee TK, Miyamoto H, Osunkoya AO, et al: Smooth muscle neoplasms of the urinary bladder: a clinicopathologic study of 51 cases. *Am. J. Surg. Pathol.* 34:502-9, 2010.

[32] Wilson TM, Fauver HE, Weigel JW: Leiomyosarcoma of urinary bladder. *Urology* 13:565-7, 1979.

[33] Spiess PE, Kassouf W, Steinberg JR, et al: Review of the M.D. Anderson experience in the treatment of bladder sarcoma. *Urol. Oncol.* 25:38-45, 2007.

[34] Miedler JD, Maclennan GT: Leiomyosarcoma of the prostate. J. Urol. 178:668, 2007.

[35] Cheville JC, Dundore PA, Nascimento AG, et al: Leiomyosarcoma of the prostate. Report of 23 cases. *Cancer* 76:1422-7, 1995.
[36] Lee G, Lee SY, Seo S, et al: Prognostic factors and clinical outcomes of urological soft tissue sarcomas. *Korean J. Urol.* 52:669-73, 2011.
[37] Vandoros GP, Manolidis T, Karamouzis MV, et al: Leiomyosarcoma of the prostate: case report and review of 54 previously published cases. *Sarcoma* 2008:458709, 2008.
[38] Kendal WS: The comparative survival of renal leiomyosarcoma. *Can. J. Urol.* 14:3435-42, 2007.
[39] Suppiah R, Wood L, Elson P, et al: Phase I/II study of docetaxel, ifosfamide, and doxorubicin in advanced, recurrent, or metastatic soft tissue sarcoma (STS). *Invest. New Drugs* 24:509-14, 2006.
[40] Serrone L, Zeuli M, Gamucci T, et al: A phase II study of dose-intense ifosfamide plus epirubicin with hematopoietic growth factors for the treatment of patients with advanced soft tissue sarcomas; a novel sequential schedule. *Cancer Chemother. Pharmacol.* 47:206-10, 2001.
[41] Le Cesne A, Judson I, Crowther D, et al: Randomized phase III study comparing conventional-dose doxorubicin plus ifosfamide versus high-dose doxorubicin plus ifosfamide plus recombinant human granulocyte-macrophage colony-stimulating factor in advanced soft tissue sarcomas: A trial of the European Organization for Research and Treatment of Cancer/Soft Tissue and Bone Sarcoma Group. *J. Clin. Oncol.* 18:2676-84, 2000.
[42] Wang X, Liu L, Tang H, et al: Twenty-five cases of adult prostate sarcoma treated at a high-volume institution from 1989 to 2009. *Urology* 82:160-5, 2013.
[43] Bonsib SM: Pathology and Genetics of Tumours of the Urinary System and Male Genital Organs. Lyon, France, IARC, 2004 pp. 61.
[44] Katabathina VS, Vikram R, Nagar AM, et al: Mesenchymal neoplasms of the kidney in adults: imaging spectrum with radiologic-pathologic correlation. *Radiographics* 30:1525-40, 2010.
[45] Raman SP, Hruban RH, Fishman EK: Beyond renal cell carcinoma: rare and unusual renal masses. *Abdom. Imaging* 37:873-84, 2012.
[46] Ochiai K, Onitsuka H, Honda H, et al: Leiomyosarcoma of the kidney: CT and MR appearance. *J. Comput. Assist. Tomogr.* 17:656-8, 1993.
[47] Sharma D, Pradhan S, Aryya NC, et al: Leiomyosarcoma of kidney: a case report with long term result after radiotherapy and chemotherapy. *Int. Urol. Nephrol.* 39:397-400, 2007.
[48] Kurugoglu S, Ogut G, Mihmanli I, et al: Abdominal leiomyosarcomas: radiologic appearances at various locations. *Eur. Radiol.* 12:2933-42, 2002
[49] Deyrup AT, Montgomery E, Fisher C: Leiomyosarcoma of the kidney: a clinicopathologic study. *Am. J. Surg. Pathol.* 28:178-82, 2004.
[50] Miller JS, Zhou M, Brimo F, et al: Primary leiomyosarcoma of the kidney: a clinicopathologic study of 27 cases. *Am. J. Surg. Pathol.* 34:238-42, 2010.
[51] Miettinen M, Fetsch JF: Evaluation of biological potential of smooth muscle tumours. *Histopathology* 48:97-105, 2006.
[52] Dominici A, Mondaini N, Nesi G, et al: Cystic leiomyosarcoma of the kidney: an unusual clinical presentation. *Urol. Int.* 65:229-31, 2000.

[53] Raut CP, Pisters PW: Retroperitoneal sarcomas: Combined-modality treatment approaches. *J. Surg. Oncol.* 94:81-7, 2006.
[54] Maki RG: Gemcitabine and docetaxel in metastatic sarcoma: past, present, and future. *Oncologist* 12:999-1006, 2007.
[55] Lopes RI, Leite KR, Lopes RN: Paratesticular leiomyosarcoma treated by enucleation. *Int. Braz. J. Urol.* 32:66-7, 2006.
[56] Mechri M, Ghozzi S, Khiari R, et al: A rare cause of a scrotal mass: primary leiomyosarcoma of epididymis. *BMJ Case Rep.* 2009, 2009.
[57] Weinshank LB, Kellner D, Nash I: Paratesticular leiomyosarcoma: case report and review. *Conn. Med.* 75:399-403, 2011.
[58] Khoubehi B, Mishra V, Ali M, et al: Adult paratesticular tumours. *BJU Int.* 90:707-15, 2002.
[59] Froehner M, Fischer R, Leike S, et al: Intratesticular leiomyosarcoma in a young man after high dose doping with Oral-Turinabol: a case report. *Cancer* 86:1571-5, 1999.
[60] Fisher C, Goldblum JR, Epstein JI, et al: Leiomyosarcoma of the paratesticular region: a clinicopathologic study. *Am. J. Surg. Pathol.* 25:1143-9, 2001.
[61] Watanabe J, Soma T, Kawa G, et al: Leiomyosarcoma of the spermatic cord. *Int. J. Urol.* 6:536-8, 1999.
[62] Gigantino V, La Mantia E, Franco R, et al: Testicular and testicular adnexa tumors in the elderly. *Anticancer Drugs* 24:228-36, 2013.
[63] Blitzer PH, Dosoretz DE, Proppe KH, et al: Treatment of malignant tumors of the spermatic cord: a study of 10 cases and a review of the literature. *J. Urol.* 126:611-4, 1981.
[64] Coindre JM: Grading of soft tissue sarcomas: review and update. *Arch. Pathol. Lab. Med.* 130:1448-53, 2006.
[65] Fagundes MA, Zietman AL, Althausen AF, et al: The management of spermatic cord sarcoma. *Cancer* 77:1873-6, 1996.
[66] Enoch S, Wharton SM, Murray DS: Management of leiomyosarcomas of the spermatic cord: the role of reconstructive surgery. *World J. Surg. Oncol.* 3:23, 2005.
[67] Agrawal V, Kumar S, Sharma D, et al: Primary leiomyosarcoma of the seminal vesicle. *Int. J. Urol.* 11:253-5, 2004.
[68] Amirkhan RH, Molberg KH, Wiley EL, et al: Primary leiomyosarcoma of the seminal vesicle. *Urology* 44:132-5, 1994.
[69] Cauvin C, Moureau-Zabotto L, Chetaille B, et al: Primary leiomyosarcoma of the seminal vesicle: case report and review of the literature. *BMC Cancer* 11:323, 2011.
[70] Muentener M, Hailemariam S, Dubs M, et al: Primary leiomyosarcoma of the seminal vesicle. *J. Urol.* 164:2027, 2000.
[71] Schned AR, Ledbetter JS, Selikowitz SM: Primary leiomyosarcoma of the seminal vesicle. *Cancer* 57:2202-6, 1986.
[72] Upreti L, Bhargava SK, Kumar A: Imaging of primary leiomyosarcoma of the seminal vesicle. *Australas Radiol.* 47:70-2, 2003.

In: Leiomyosarcoma
Editor: Rosemary H. Leach

ISBN: 978-1-63117-940-2

Chapter 3

Reconstructive Challenges in Leiomyosarcoma

John A. M. Paro, M.D., Eric J. Wright, M.D., Tiffany Chen, B.S. and Gordon K. Lee, M.D., FACS
Stanford University Hospital and Clinics, Palo Alto, CA, US

Abstract

Leiomyosarcoma represents a particular subset of malignant connective tissue neoplasms arising from smooth muscle. Soft tissue sarcomas themselves are relatively uncommon, and leiomyosarcomas represent less than 10% of this group of cancers. These tumors are traditionally quite resistant to radiation and chemotherapy, and surgical intervention remains the best option for affected patients. Smooth muscle is located throughout the entire body, including intra-abdominal organs, blood vessel walls and skin. Many of these cancers occur in the gastrointestinal tract and uterus, with extirpation and wound closure performed by the primary surgical team. They can also be found in the abdominal wall, retroperitoneum, thorax, and pelvic viscera which introduces certain reconstructive challenges. As plastic and reconstructive surgeons, we are often called upon to assist our oncologic surgical colleagues to help restore the integrity of the abdominal wall, chest wall, and pelvis following excision. Techniques utilized range in complexity from primary closure and local tissue rearrangement to free microvascular tissue transfer. In this chapter we will speak to the basics of leiomyosarcoma tumor biology and then highlight some of the principles of reconstructive surgery as well as challenges specific to defects created by soft tissue sarcoma resection.

Background

Sarcomas are rare, malignant tumors that arise from mesenchymal tissue and comprise less than 1% of all adult malignancies diagnosed annually in the United States [1]. About 20% of sarcomas originate from the bone while the remaining 80% are of soft tissue origins. Soft tissues are found throughout the entire body and include adipose, muscle, fibrous tissues, blood vessels, deep skin tissues, and nerves. As such, soft tissue sarcomas can develop all over the body, although they are most commonly found in the extremities, chest wall, and retroperitoneum [1]. The American Cancer Society estimates that 11,410 new cases of soft tissue sarcomas, with 6,290 male and 5,120 female cases, will be diagnosed in the United States in 2013. Of these, approximately 4,400 deaths will occur, 2,500 in males and 1,890 in females [2].

Soft tissue sarcomas are classified based on the tissue of origin of the tumors. Due to the embryonic mesenchymal origins, there are over 50 distinct histological subtypes of soft tissue sarcomas. Leiomyosarcomas in particular are derived from smooth muscle and represent 13.4% of soft tissue sarcoma cases, which make it the second most common subtype after fat-derived liposarcomas [3]. Approximately 50% of leiomyosarcomas are found in the uterus [4], with a large proportion of the remaining tumors found in the retroperitoneum and larger blood vessels such as the inferior vena cava. Cases of rare primary tumors in the thyroid gland, gallbladder, base of tongue, liver, bronchus, kidney, and pancreas have also been reported [5-12].

As with many cancers, the incidence of leiomyosarcomas increases with age, although childhood cases have been reported [13]. Most cases of retroperitoneal and inferior vena cava leiomyosarcomas are in women [14], while cutaneous and subcutaneous leiomyosarcomas are more common in men [15].

There are no known direct causes of leiomyosarcomas, although some factors may be associated with development of the disease. Post-irradiation sarcomas have been increasing in number recently, but they are still rare, and leiomyosarcomas do not appear to be one of the more frequent subtypes that develop [16]. A number of Epstein-Barr virus related smooth muscle tumors have been reported among severely immunosuppressed patients due to AIDS, post-transplant immunosuppression, or autoimmune disease [17]. Patients with concurrent EBV and HIV infections were of younger age and had multifocal tumors of smooth muscle characteristics that most often involved the central nervous system [18].

Survivors of hereditary retinoblastoma appear to have a higher risk of developing subsequent primary malignancies including soft tissue sarcomas due to germline mutations in *RB1*. A study in 2007 showed that the most frequent subtype represented was leiomyosarcomas in 23 out of a total of 69 observed soft tissue sarcomas [19]. Another report has shown that some leiomyosarcoma patients carry the *TP53* mutation, although this is not causative and appears to be exclusively among those greater than 20 years of age [20]. Similarly, patients with mutations in *NF1* exhibiting familial neurofibromatosis may develop leiomyosarcomas, yet this is uncommon and occur less often in leiomyosarcomas than other malignancies [21].

The predominance of women with retroperitoneal and inferior vena cava leiomyosarcomas suggests that estrogen may play a role in smooth muscle proliferation; however, this has not been confirmed. Furthermore, there is little evidence that support the development of leiomyosarcomas from their benign leiomyoma counterparts; rather, the tumors are believed to arise de novo without an apparent cause. [22]

Leiomyosarcomas are generally found as painless, enlarging masses with well-defined borders, although invasion into surrounding tissues may also be present. Larger tumors may lead to hemorrhaging and necrosis and more frequently develop in the abdominal regions than elsewhere in the body [1].

Staging of leiomyosarcomas was developed by the International Union Against Cancer [UICC] American Joint Committee on Cancer [AJCC], and takes into account histologic grade, tumor size, depth [superficial or deep], regional lymph node involvement, and distant metastases. Unfortunately, staging does not incorporate histology and location information, which are important for prognosis. The grade of tumors is based on differentiation, mitotic rate, and amount of tumor necrosis as outlined by the French Federation of Cancer Centers Sarcoma Group [FNCLCC] [1]. Grading provides information on the degree of malignancy, the likelihood of distant metastases, and disease-specific survival, with higher grades associated with more aggressive tumors [23, 24]. Leiomyosarcomas arising in the extremities have overall better prognoses than those from the retroperitoneum as they are generally smaller and do not metastasize [25]. On the other hand, in addition to tumor size and grade, involvement of the bone or neurovasculature is indicative of poorer outcomes [23].

The primary predictor of local recurrence is surgical resection margins, which depends on the type of the surrounding tissue and anatomic proximity to other structures [25]. Complete surgical excision of the tumor with wide negative margins leads to the best chance for a cure, although this is often difficult. Unlike other cancers, such as cutaneous malignancies, there is not a universally agreed upon standard for the margin necessary during surgical excision. It is highly dependent on it's location within the body and anatomic considerations may preclude wide margins. For cutaneous leiomyosarcoma, there is evidence that adequate oncologic control is possible with 1 cm margins [26]. Grade and size of tumor are also significant predictors of local recurrence, metastases, and survival [24]. Pulmonary metastases are by far the most common, and typically treated with wedge excision if the location in the lung allows for this [25].

There is currently little consensus in terms of the role of chemotherapy and radiation as pre- or post-operative adjuncts to sarcoma resection. Post-operative radiotherapy is typically considered if there are microscopically positive margins within the surgical specimen. Many centers are also trialing the use of intra-operative radiation therapy. [27]. The use of chemotherapy, especially in the post-operative period, remains controversial with experts from across the world disagreeing on the utility of any particular regimen [28]. Surgical resection remains the only potentially curative therapy for this time of tumor.

Wide local excision is possible in a number of anatomic locations. Uterine and many intra-abdominal/retroperitoneal tumors can be resected and closed primarily by the oncologic team without the need for reconstruction. Since the mesenchymal cell in question – smooth muscle in this case – is found throughout the body, surgical excision can occasionally present reconstructive challenges that require the help of a plastic surgeon. In the remainder of the chapter we will speak to the approach taken to reconstruction of leiomyosarcoma defects that result after wide local excision.

Reconstructive Principles

When faced with a wound or defect, a reconstructive surgeon must consider a number of details regarding the specific problem. Important factors include: wound size and depth, location, quality of surrounding tissues, exposure of structures such as organs, bone, nerve, or tendons, and presence of contamination or infection. The goal when faced with any wound is to achieve closure without undue tension. Based on the size of the defect, suturing alone may not be sufficient or even possible. Plastic surgeons utilize a number of other approaches when faced with this situation. These are often described as following a stepwise approach – akin to progressing along rungs of a "reconstructive ladder." [Figure 1]

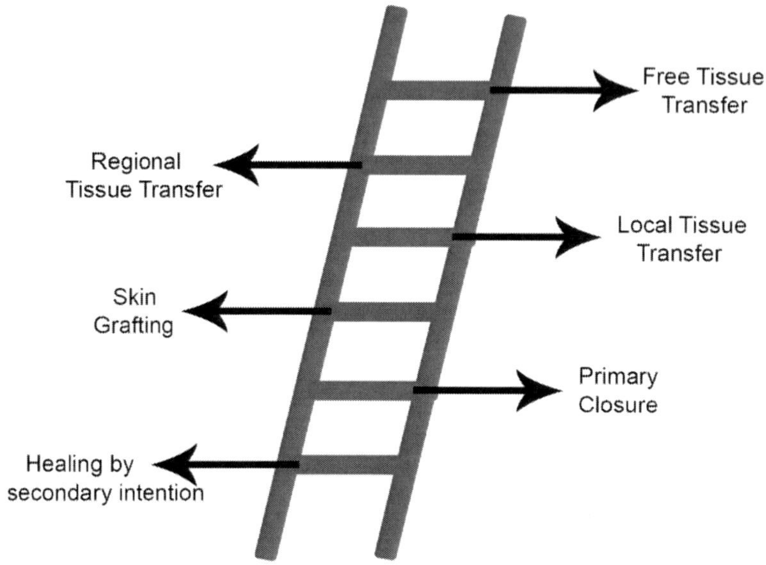

Figure 1. The "Reconstructive Ladder."

The rungs of this ladder are typically described as going from most simple to most complex and include healing by secondary intention, direct tissue closure, skin grafting, local tissue transfer, regional tissue transfer, and free tissue transfer. Traditionally, the simplest option would be chosen, moving up the ladder only as necessary. Plastic surgeons occasionally make modifications based on the clinical scenario, prompting some to refer to this as more of a "reconstructive elevator."

Plastic surgeons are often consulted by other surgical services for wound management when direct tissue closure will not be possible. One standard option that sometimes can be of use is skin grafting. This involves transfer of the epidermis with some or all of the dermis from one portion of the body to the wound. Full thickness skin grafts involve excising tissue with 100% of the dermis and closing the donor site primarily. This provides a hearty skin graft that will limit contracture at the recipient site and can regain hair growth – the size of possible grafts is limited given the needed for donor site closure. Split thickness skin grafts are taken with a dermatome skin shaver, allowing the surgeon to harvest epidermis with a portion of the dermis – enough to allow the skin graft to adequately cover and close the wound, but leaving behind enough dermal cells to cause epithelialization of the donor site. Donor sites are bountiful for split thickness skin grafts, and can be enlarged by meshing the graft to create a larger surface area. This will result, however, in a larger amount of wound contraction. Skin grafts are good options for smaller wounds on the extremity where there is a healthy soft tissue bed of muscle remaining and when only skin has been resected. A skin graft survives initially on the diffusion of nutrients from the surrounding recipient site – so this is not a good option if there are exposed structures such as bone, nerve, or tendon within the wound. The process of skin graft "take" involves imbibition (diffusion of nutrients), followed by inosculation (connection of small blood vessels) and finally revascularization. [Figure 2]

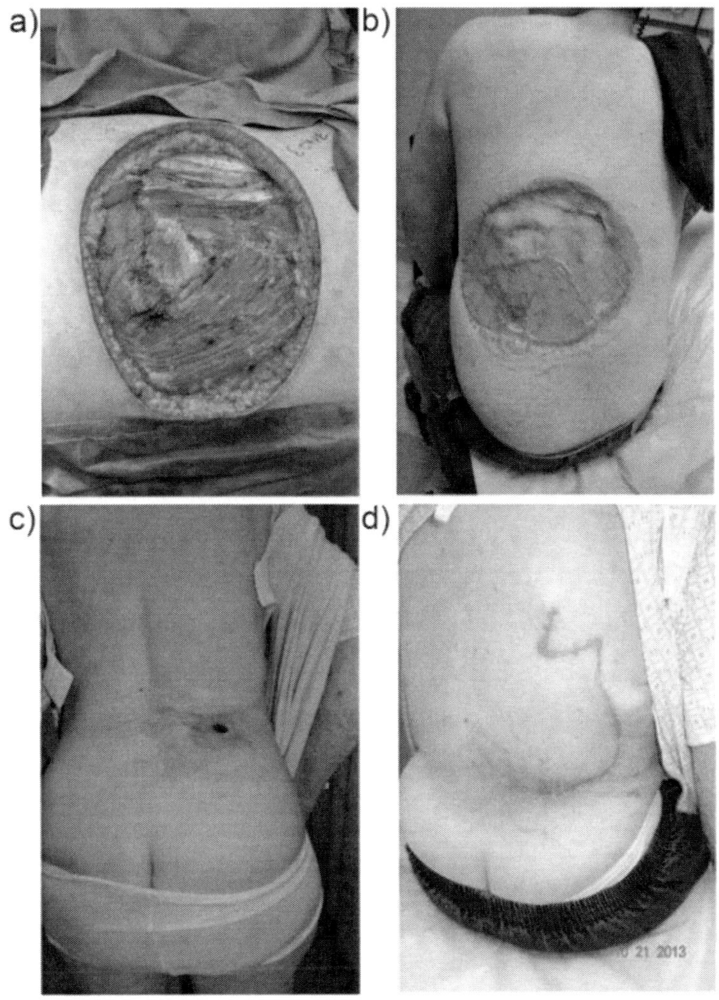

Figure 2. a-b) Large soft tissue defect of posterior trunk, treated with split thickness skin grafting; c-d) Lower trunk wound treated with local rotational flap.

While a graft is transferred without its own blood supply, reconstructive surgeons often utilize "flaps" for more robust tissue transfer and when defects extend beyond just a simple skin excision. A flap has its own blood supply and can be comprised of a number of tissue components including skin, fat, muscle, and even bone. These flaps can be based locally or regionally on a blood supply and re-oriented through advancement or rotation to fill an adjacent defect. Occasionally, if an ideal donor site exists at a distant location, a flap can be completely removed from its blood supply and hooked up through microsurgical anastomosis to blood vessels in the recipient site. This constitutes what plastic surgeons refer to as a "free flap."

There are a number of fundamental principles that a reconstructive surgeon keeps in mind when evaluating any wound. The reconstructive ladder provides a framework for an organized approach to most surgical problems. Given the variety of presentations possible in leiomyosarcoma, the surgeon may be required to consider his or her full complement of wound closure options. Leiomyosarcomas can occur in any portion of the body, including the head and neck as well as the extremities. This chapter cannot be an exhaustive discussion of reconstructive principles of all anatomic regions. For the remainder of the text we will focus on three particular challenges that we have encountered in our clinical practice: reconstruction of the abdominal wall, chest wall, and pelvis.

Abdominal Wall Reconstruction

Anatomy

The abdominal wall is a broad term for the boundaries of the abdominal cavity, and can be thought of as having anterior, posterior, and lateral components. We are most commonly asked to direct our reconstructive efforts to the anterior or lateral portions of the abdominal wall. The superior, inferior and lateral extents of the abdomen are comprised of the xiphoid process and costal margins, the inguinal ligaments and pubic tubercle, and the mid axillary line respectively. From superficial to deep, the surgeon will encounter skin, subcutaneous fat, a superficial fascial system including Camper's and Scarpa's fasciae, and the abdominal wall musculature. The prominent rectus abdominis muscles are juxtaposed at the midline (linea alba) and extend from the pubic symphysis to the xiphoid/costal cartilages. Lateral to the rectus abdominis, we find the linea semilunaris, which mark the border of the lateral musculature. These are comprised of the external and internal obliques as well as the transversus abdominis muscles [29]. The blood supply to the rectus abdominis muscle is predominantly from the superior and inferior epigastric arteries, with important lateral contributions from multiple intercostal arteries. Other smaller vessels from the circumflex iliac, lumbar and pudendal systems provide additional inflow to the inferior abdomen. Perforating vessels pierce the rectus muscle from the epigastric arterial system to bring blood flow to the overlying skin and subcutaneous fat of the abdominal wall [30]. Recognizing the vascular anatomy is critical to ensure that your reconstructive efforts will have adequate perfusion.

Walking Up the Reconstructive Ladder

The ultimate goal of abdominal wall reconstruction is to reestablish form and function. Resections of tumors such as leiomyosarcomas will often necessitate full thickness resections of the abdominal wall, including fascia and muscle. The tumor may or may not involve the skin – if the skin is spared, they can be elevated as flaps and replaced following the reconstruction. If there is cutaneous involvement, the skin becomes part of the oncologic specimen and the surgeon will have to consider soft tissue coverage as well as fascial reconstruction.

Much like any reconstructive problem, we will often think of this in terms of our "ladder" discussed above. Healing by secondary intention is not a practical option in this situation as this results in unnecessarily prolonged healing and potential disability for the patient. However, occasionally negative pressure wound therapy is utilized as a staging or intermediate measure if the reconstruction needs to be delayed for any reason, such as when margins need to be confirmed prior to definitive flap reconstruction. Primary closure of the fascia is possible in some instances but typically the defect is too large to allow this. To avoid an abdominal hernia, the musculofascial defect after tumor resection must be reconstructed to maintain abdominal wall integrity. A piece of mesh used as a "bridge" does not restore the patient's original core strength, but does prevent an abdominal hernia. There are descriptions of procedures such as skin grafting directly over bowel, but this should be avoided since this results in a large fascial defect and hernia. In terms of abdominal reconstruction, surgeons are often faced with local or regional tissue transfer or beyond.

Components Separation/Mesh Repair

One excellent option that we utilize for abdominal reconstruction – both for oncologic reconstructions as well as complex hernia repairs – is a technique called the separation of components. This technique was first introduced by Ramirez as a way to advance the bilateral abdominal wall musculature to facilitate the closure of large defects. With this procedure, the surgeon can span abdominal defects of 10 cm, 20 cm and 6 cm in the upper, mid, and lower abdomen, respectively [31].

Understanding the abdominal wall anatomy allows the surgeon to selectively advance parts of the abdominal wall musculature and maintain fascial continuity. In this technique, the external oblique is released at its insertion to the lateral border of the rectus sheath (the linea semilunaris). The neurovascular bundles from the intercostals run between the internal oblique and transversus abdominis, so this is a safe plane for dissection and also allows vascular and functional preservation in the reconstruction. The surgeon is then able to advance a flap consisting of the rectus, internal oblique, and transversus abdominis. We utilize a stepwise approach, and attempt to close the fascia primarily without a separation of components. This technique is particularly effective for tumors that are directly in the midline where there is sufficient tissue remaining to allow for this technique to be performed. Obviously, when the abdominal wall is resected and the components are missing, there may be no remaining components to separate. This is particularly true for cancer cases where the abdominal wall may be resected and the only viable option is a piece of mesh that is used to "bridge" the defect [32]. [Figure 3]

One topic of persistent debate in the literature revolves around the use of implantable materials for abdominal wall reconstruction. A variety of meshes are commercially available including synthetic and biologic materials. The authors prefer to use reinforcement during our repairs, but would argue that hernia repair failure rates (i.e., recurrent hernias) are more related to surgical technique rather than implantable material. Each case must be assessed on an individual basis. In general, if there is exposed bowel with the possibility of bacterial contamination (for example, an enterocentaneous fistula or an enterostomy, for example) a biologic mesh is preferentially utilized given the possibility for vascular ingrowth. If the case is considered "clean," then a piece of synthetic mesh is acceptable. Surgeons should consider the higher cost of biologic mesh compared to synthetics [33]. For a more thorough review of the literature, please refer to a recent Nova Sciences publication on the subject matter [34].

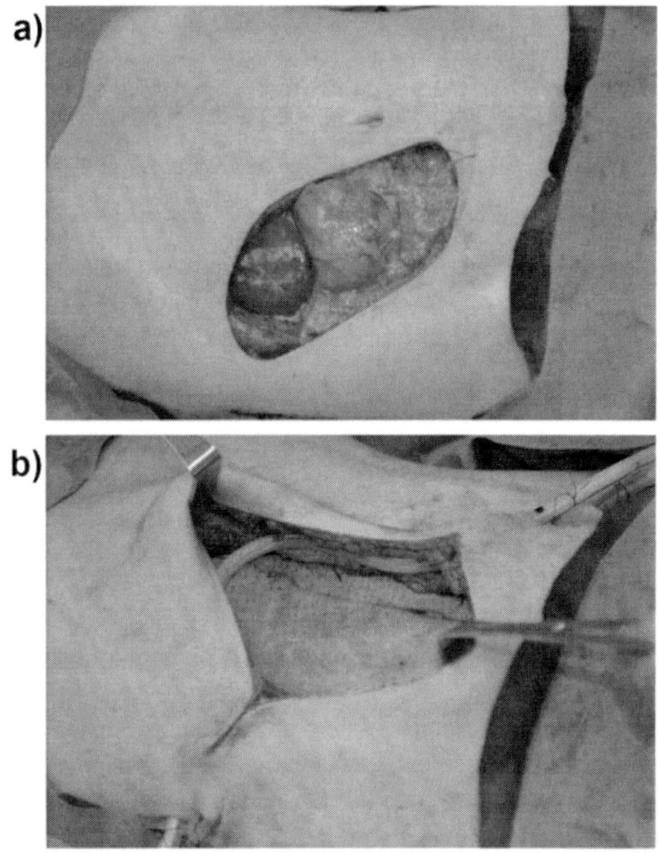

Figure 3. a) Photograph of an abdominal wall sarcoma resection with exposed viscera – there is adequate skin, but missing fascia; b) After placement of biological mesh for reconstruction.

Autologous Tissue Repair

If the separation of components is insufficient, other tools can help restore facial continuity. A reconstructive surgeon often strives to "replace like with like" – and in this case, healthy vascularized fascia can be transferred from other parts of the body. One common donor site is the tensor fascia lata (TFL) of the lateral thigh. The TFL originates from the anterior iliac crest, inserting onto the iliotibial band. The muscle itself is small, but is encircled by the deep fascia of the thigh (fascia lata) and is a strong, thick layer. This has been utilized in abdominal wall reconstruction in a variety of ways. Most simply, the TFL can be harvested as a graft and transferred to the abdomen. The fascia lata has minimal metabolic demand and can be bought over as a broad sheet to the recipient site. TFL grafts as large as 28 x 14 cm can be harvested [35].

The TFL muscle can also be rotated into the defect as a pedicled musculofascial flap with preservation of its bloody supply based on the transverse branch of the lateral circumflex femoral artery. This type of flap can be designed with or without a skin paddle depending on the clinical situation. [Figure 4]. An even larger defect can be spanned if the TFL is mobilized as a free flap using microsurgical technique. In this situation, the blood supply of the flap is often connected to intraperitoneal vessels.

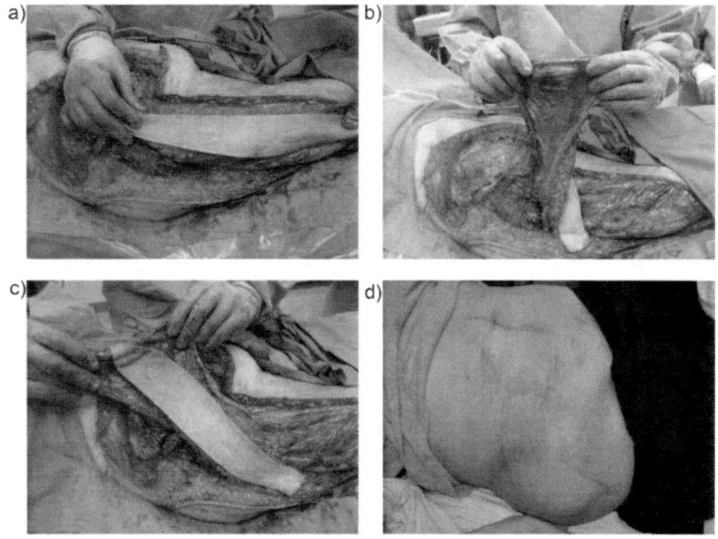

Figure 4. a-c) This patient had an abdominal wall defect requiring skin and vascularized fascia. A pedicled tensor fascia lata (TFL) flap was harvested and transposed into the defect. Intraoperative photographs shown; d) Post-operative result at six weeks.

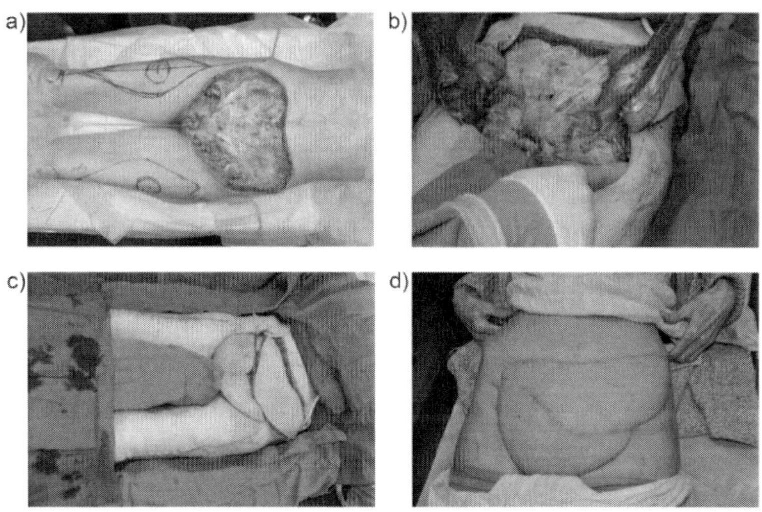

Figure 5. This patient has a large cutaneous resection – the fascia was intact, but soft tissue needed; b) This photograph demonstrates the inset of the flaps and the vascular pedicle; c) Here, the flaps are in place prior to being sutured; and d) Post-operative results at two months

If a large portion of abdominal skin has been removed as part of the resection then soft tissue coverage will need to address the skin deficit. Skin grafts directly over fascia can be quite unsightly and is not recommended. The authors have had success with using an

Anterolateral Thigh (ALT) free flap (harvesting skin, fat and fascia from the leg, with at most a small cuff of muscle) based on the descending branch of the lateral circumflex femoral artery. This can be transferred as a pedicled flap or even as a free flap via microsurgical technique to provide a bulkier soft tissue coverage of the abdominal wall. [Figure 5]

Chest Wall Reconstruction

Following resection of the tumor with adequate margins, restoration of the chest wall must be performed. The chest wall, or thorax, is composed of numerous layers. Externally, the skin covers the muscles of respiration. The skeletal thorax provides protection of vital organs as well as support for respiration. The inner thin pleural layer surrounds the internal organs. A multidisciplinary team working together in a collaborative allows for determination of the optimal oncologic treatment. Involving the oncologist, surgical oncologist and the reconstructive surgeon preoperatively allows for appropriate expectations regarding surgery and possible adjuvant treatments. Knowledge of the planned defect and possibility of subsequent radiation can help determine the needed reconstructive needs. As well, involvement of the reconstructive surgeon gives the oncology surgeon the comfort to appropriately obtain wide margins, despite the large residual defect. Reconstruction must allow for continued respiratory function and stability of the shoulder and upper extremity, protection of internal organs, closure of the external wound and lastly, restoration of normal body contours.

Chest Wall Stabilization

Though each defect following tumor resection is different, the fundamentals of reconstruction remain the same. Rigid fixation of defects involving multiple ribs or sternum has been shown to improve initial respiration, thus decreasing ventilator dependence [36]. The exact size of the defect that requires reconstruction is debated but many surgeons believe defects involving 4-5 ribs or with diameters greater than 5 cm would benefit from fixation. The location is also important. Lateral and posterolateral skeletal defects are more likely to affect respiratory function [37]. Posterior, back musculature and scapula can provide sufficient support to minimize changes in respiratory function. The need for fixation must be individualized for each patient [38].

Options for reconstruction include both autologous tissue and alloplastic materials. Autologous reconstructions include the use of bone or fascial grafts with the most common being tensor fascia lata. Numerous prosthetic materials have been developed that are used in chest wall surgery. Polypropylene mesh, Vicryl mesh, Marlex mesh, polyglycolic acid, polylactic acid, Dacron, methymethacrylate, Gore-Tex and others have been described in the literature as being used for providing stability of the chest. These materials can also be used in combination to improve overall outcome. Use of these prosthetic materials is essential in very large defects. The benefits include no donor site morbidity at the harvest site or increased operative time, no size limitations and overall maintenance of the integrity of the repair [39]. However, there are drawbacks to their use. As a foreign material, synthetic mesh material may have minimal vascular incorporation. As such, the risk of infection is higher with synthetic material. It can be incorporated within the surrounding tissue due to fibroblast infiltration, but this leads to significant adhesion formation [40]. Though conservative management of infected material is possible, surgical removal of the densely adherent material is most likely.

An alternative to synthetic materials is the use of biologic mesh, which is being used with increased frequency [41]. Biologic mesh serves as scaffolding to facilitate vascularization and incorporation within the surrounding tissue. As described in the previous section, there is extensive literature regarding their use in abdominal wall reconstruction. Animal models show similar chest wall stabilization when comparing biologic mesh to synthetic mesh [42]. Benefits to this type of mesh are that it has been shown to have less infection rates as well as have less growth restriction when used with children, thus decreasing chances of scoliosis or other growth disturbances [43]. There are higher costs associated with biologic mesh and an increased risk of postoperative seromas. However, infections can be managed with antibiotics with greater success with biologic mesh than with synthetic materials [44]. Similar to synthetic meshes, there are numerous types available for use including both cadaveric allografts and xenografts. Each of the biologic meshes has inherent property differences, depending on the origin and processing technique.

The choice of either biologic or synthetic mesh depends on surgeon preference and the defect needing reconstructed. Once the structural integrity has been restored, the remaining soft tissue defect can be addressed. [Figure 6].

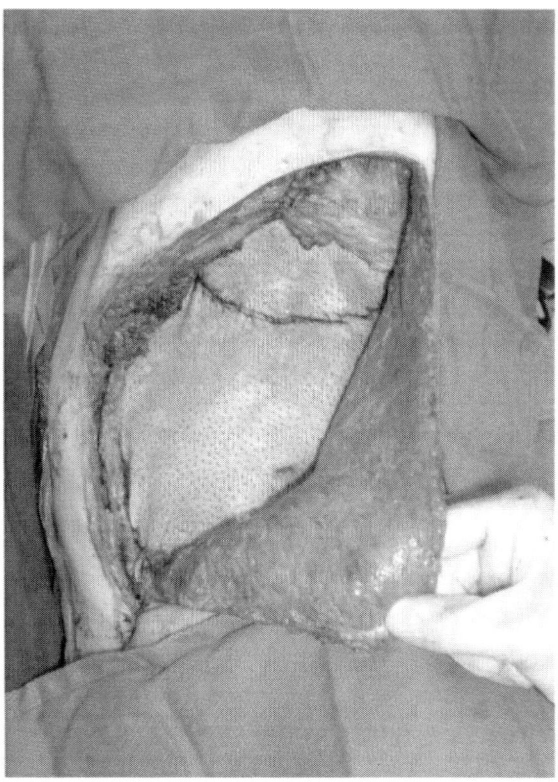

Figure 6. Intraoperative photograph of a left-sided chest wall defect repaired with a piece of biologic mesh.

Soft Tissue Coverage of Chest

Common to many oncologic resections, there is a need for soft tissue coverage. The chest wall has several local muscle and fasciocutaneous flaps that can be recruited for wound closure. Knowledge of the blood supply to these flaps is critical to ensure survival. Often oncologic resection can injure the blood supply to local tissue flaps, which can preclude their use, and thus dictates a working knowledge of all available options.

The pectoralis major muscle flap can be utilized for anterior chest wall defects. With the main vascular supply, the thoracoacromial artery and vein, entering superolateral to the muscle, this flap can be rotated and advanced to cover defects. Disinsertion of the muscle from the superomedial humerus can add in advancing this muscle. Medially the pectoralis major receives segmental blood supply from the internal mammary artery perforators. Due to this vascularity, the muscle can be turned over. The muscle can be skin grafted or harvested with a cutaneous segment. Harvest of this muscle is well tolerated though weakness can be noted in internal rotation and adduction of the humerus.

The latissimus dorsi muscle is the second common muscle flap used for chest wall reconstruction. The thoracodorsal artery supplies this large, flat muscle of the back. With release of the insertion at the intertubercular groove of the humerus, this muscle can be rotated across the axilla to reach defects as far anteriorly as the sternum. As with the pectoralis muscle, a skin paddle or skin grafting of the muscle can be performed. The latissimus dorsi harvest can cause shoulder weakness, but surrounding muscles can with time compensate for the majority of patients [45].

Supplied by both the lateral thoracic artery and the serratus branch of the thoracodorsal artery, the serratus anterior muscle is a thin, broad lateral chest wall muscle that can be rotated to cover both posterior and anterior defects. Including the underlying rib if needed can create an osteomyocutaneous flap. It is important to note that only the inferior three to four slips of serratus anterior muscle can be used for coverage, use of more superior muscle risks developing winging of the scapula.

The rectus abdominus muscle can be used to cover lower anterior chest wall defects. Rotated superiorly on the superior epigastric vessels, a large amount of subcutaneous tissue can be transferred with this muscle. Variations of this muscle flap are commonly used for breast reconstruction, taking advantage of the ability to transfer the lower abdominal adipose tissue to the superior chest wall. The rectus flap cutaneous portion can be harvest in a vertical or transverse fashion, depending on the defect. Muscle-sparing techniques can be performed, thus minimizing abdominal wall weakness associated with harvest of the rectus abdominus muscle. Adequate fascial closure is also important due to the risk of abdominal bulge and hernia formation following this muscle harvest. [Figure 7]

If local muscle or fasciocutaneous muscle flaps are not available, the highly vascularized omentum can be harvested. With two dominant arterial pedicles, the right and lateral gastroepiploic arteries, division of one pedicle allows for a long arc of rotation. The omentum can be tunneled through the diaphragm or draped over the costal margin. The obvious disadvantage of this flap is the need for entry into the abdominal cavity for harvest. Previous abdominal surgeries could have caused injury to the omentum or caused significant formation of adhesions, thus making the harvest more challenging. Skin grafting of the omentum is required.

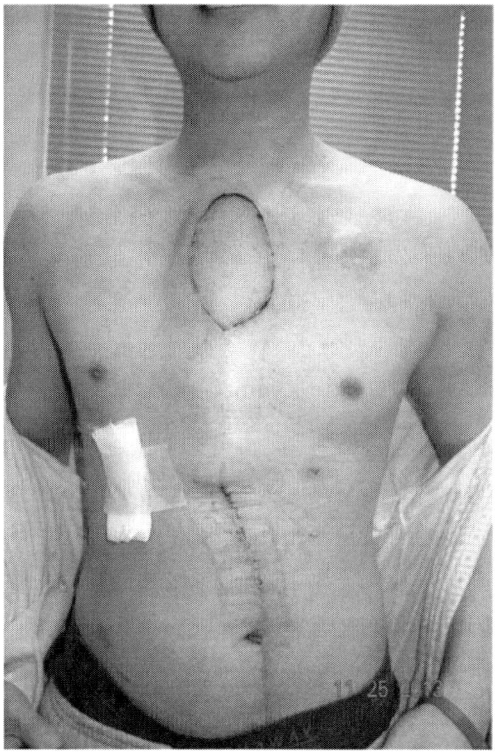

Figure 7. Post-operative result of a "pedicled" Vertical Rectus Abdominis Myocutaneous (VRAM) flap for check wall reconstruction. Note the donor site incision closed primarily, and the skin paddle overlying the central chest.

Though muscle flaps are commonly used, several local fasciocutaneous can be used, which negate the need for muscle. Several flaps are based upon the branches of the subscapular vessels. The dorsal thoracic fascia flap based upon the circumflex scapular artery provides a large thin flap that can be rotated based upon the arc of the vascular pedicle. Smaller flaps, such as the scapula, parascapular, and thoracodorsal artery perforator flaps are also located in this area and can easily be transposed to cover posterior and lateral chest wall defects [46]. The benefit of these flaps is that there is minimal donor site morbidity. With improved knowledge of artery perforator perfusion, these flaps can offer alternatives to the workhorse muscle flaps that have been described.

The vast majority of chest wall defects can be reconstructed utilizing one of the techniques described above. However, in a small number, the defect may be too extensive or the locoregional flap options are not available due to either the flap itself or vascular pedicle being resected. In these circumstances, microvascular free flap coverage is a valuable option [47]. Microvascular free flap surgery involves the use of an operating room microscope to repair blood vessels too small to otherwise manipulate, thus restoring blood flow to the transferred flap. When performing a microvascular free flap reconstruction, there are several options that are available. Contralateral muscles, such as the latissimus dorsi muscle, can be harvested and transferred to the defect. There are also options from the extremity, such as the anterolateral thigh flap, which can be transferred to the chest wall for reconstruction [48].

Due to the vast armamentarium of reconstructive options available, aggressive resection with wide margins of the tumor can be performed without concern of possible reconstruction problems. Knowledge of the surrounding anatomy and blood supply allow successful wound closure.

Pelvic Reconstruction

Anatomy and Principles

Leiomyosarcomas can often involve genitourinary and gastrointestinal organs, which are often included in a surgical resection. This can be taken with or without the surrounding skin of the perineum, and often the patient is left with considerable a considerable cavity or "dead space." The goal of reconstruction is to provide soft tissue bulk within this cavity to prevent the accumulation of fluid or intestinal contents and thereby reduce the risk of pelvic abscess, wound breakdown, and bowel obstruction.

The perineum can be though of as the diamond-shaped outflow tract of the pelvis. The boundaries include the ischial tuberosities laterally, the inferior margin of the pubic symphysis, and the coccyx/sacrotuberous ligaments [49]. This is further subdivided into an anterior urogenital triangle and a posterior anal triangle [29]. The primary goal of reconstruction is to heal the resultant wound in a one-stage operation while considering as much of a return to function as possible given the defect [49].

Regional Tissue Transfer

In the setting of sarcoma, often the first rungs of the reconstructive ladder are not available to the plastic surgeon assisting with wound closure. There are a number of excellent options for perineal reconstruction utilizing regional flaps, using either skin only or myocutaneous flaps.

For certain defects, the surgeon can utilize fasciocutaneous flaps to reconstruct the defect without requiring the donor site morbidity of a muscle harvest. A number of nearby areas have been described for reconstruction, including a gluteal flaps, posterior thigh flaps, and smaller perforator or "propeller" flaps based on small blood vessels. The ALT flap described above can also be utilized as a "pedicled" flap without disrupting its blood supply and transposed into the defect. [Figure 8].

Other options for regional flap coverage include myocutaneous flaps, including muscles such as the recuts abdominis and gracilis muscles. Long considered a workhorse flap for perineal reconstruction, the Vertical Rectus Abdominis Myocutaneous (VRAM) can be harvested and brought into the perineal defect for closure of the wound. This flap has a hearty blood supply based on the inferior epigastric artery and brings a large volume of soft tissue to help obliterate the dead space of the pelvic cavity. A skin paddle is typically brought with the flap to assist with cutaneous closure of the wound.

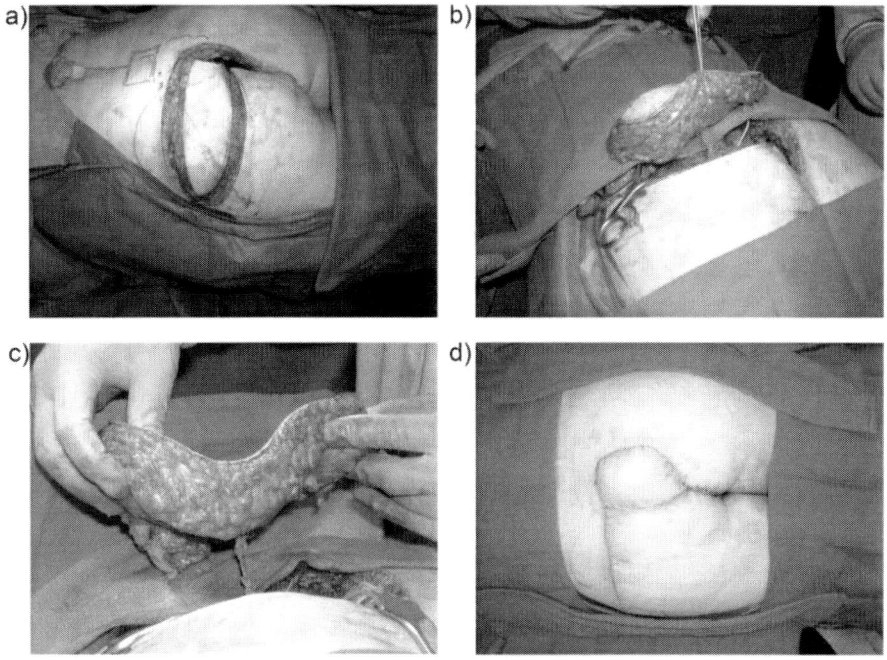

Figure 8. a-c) This patient had a pelvic defect requiring the obliteration of deadspace; as well as skin coverage. A left-sided gluteal fasciocutaneous flap was performed, based on the superior gluteal artery (seen in picture c); d) Immediate post-operative result.

The gracilis flap has the benefit of decreased donor site morbidity compared to a VRAM, but is limited by a shorter vascular pedicle and an unreliable skin paddle. The gracilis can be harvested an inset while the patient lays prone without reposition in the middle of an operation. In other instances, the recuts abdominis may be an unsuitable choice for a muscular flap if the muscle of blood supply was resected during the tumor operation, or if an ostomy was required and was placed through the muscle. Retrospective results have showed that this flap is associated with fewer complications than flaps utilized from the thigh [50].

The flaps described above are excellent options for achieving a healed wound and limiting post-operative complications. Although beyond the scope of this chapter, it is worth noting that plastic surgeons have also made progress in providing comprehensive reconstruction following perineal resections. Utilizing modifications of the flaps described above, we are able to create a neovagina or phallus – often even with sensation – to provide a true return to both form and function for the patient.

Conclusion

Leiomyosarcomas represents a particular subset of malignant connective tissue neoplasms arising from smooth muscle. Surgical intervention remains the best option for affected patients given the limited efficacy of chemotherapy and radiation. Since these particular tumors can be found throughout the body, requiring aggressive resections, they can pose particular challenges for the reconstructive surgeon. Physicians need to be aware of the important features of this rare tumor group and understand the key principles that are involved in planning reconstructive surgeries for these patients. For the abdominal wall, mesh is often required to bridge the musculofascial defect when primary fascial closure is not feasible with or without the use of the component separation technique. Flaps can provide vascularized soft tissue for skin coverage when the remaining abdominal skin cannot be closed primarily. In a similar fashion, involvement of the chest wall by leiomyosarcomas often require bony stability with the use of mesh, along with soft tissue coverage using a flap. Pelvic defects can be treated with variety of regional flaps, allowing for restoration of form and function. Coordination between surgical oncologists and reconstructive plastic surgeons will allow for optimal management.

References

[1] Fletcher C.D.M., Unni K.K., Mertens F. (Eds.): World Health Organization Classification of Tumours. Pathology and Genetics of Tumours of Soft Tissue and Bone. IARC Press: Lyon 2002.

[2] Siegel R, Naishadham D, Jemal A. Cancer statistics, 2013. CA*: A Cancer Journal for Clinicians* 2013; 63:11–30.

[3] Ries LAG, Kosary CL, Hankey BF, Miller BA, Clegg L, Edwards BK (eds). SEER Cancer Statistics Review, 1973-1996, National Cancer Institute. Bethesda, MD, 1999.

[4] Farid M, Ong WS, Tan MH, et al. The influence of primary site on outcomes in leiomyosarcoma: a review of clinicopathologic differences between uterine and extrauterine disease. *Am J Clin Oncol* 2013; 36:368-74.

[5] Bathan AJ, Constantinidou A, Pollack SM, et al. Diagnosis, prognosis, and management of leiomyosarcoma: recognition of anatomic variants. *Curr Opin Oncol* 2013; 25:384-89.

[6] Mouaqit O, Belkacem Z, Ifrine L, et al. A rare tumor of the thyroid gland: report on one case of leiomyosarcoma and review of literature. *Updates Surg* 2013.

[7] Park EY, Seo HI, Yun SP, et al. Primary leiomyosarcoma of gallbladder. *J Korean Surg Soc* 2012; 83:403–07.

[8] Croce A, Moretti A, Laus M, Crescenzi D. Leiomyosarcoma of the base of the tongue and free edge of the epiglottis: a case report. *J Med Case Rep* 2012; 6:400.

[9] Takehara K, Aoki H, Takehara Y, et al. Primary hepatic leiomyosarcoma with liver metastasis of rectal cancer. *World J Gastroenterol* 2012; 18:5479–84.

[10] Elouazzani H, Zouaidia F, Jahid A, et al. Primary endobronchial leiomyosarcoma of the lung: clinical, gross and microscopic findings of two cases. *J Clin Imaging Sci* 2012; 2:35.

[11] Yodonawa S, Ogawa I, Yoshida S, et al. Gastric metastasis from a primary renal leiomyosarcoma. *Case Rep Gastroenterol* 2012; 6:314–18.

[12] Moletta L, Sperti C, Beltrame V, et al. Leiomyosarcoma of the pancreas with liver metastases as a paradigm of multimodality treatment: case report and review of the literature. *J Gastrointest Cancer* 2012; 43:246.

[13] Miller RW, Young JL Jr, Novakovic B. Childhood cancer. *Cancer* 1995; 75:395.

[14] Hashimoto H, Tsuneyoshi M, Enjoji M. Malignant smooth muscle tumors of the retroperitoneum and mesentery: a clinicopathologic analysis of 44 cases. *J Surg Oncol* 1985; 28:177–86.

[15] Dahl I, Angervall L. Cutaneous and subcutaneous leiomyosarcoma: a clinicopathologic study of 47 patients. *Pathol Eur*. 1974; 9(4):307-15.

[16] Robinson E, Neugut AI, Wylie P. Clinical aspects of postirradiation sarcomas. *J Natl Cancer Inst* 1988; 80:233–40.

[17] Dalal KM, Antonescu CR, DeMatteo RP, et al. EBV-associated smooth muscle neoplasms: solid tumors arising in the presence of immunosuppression and autoimmune diseases. *Sarcoma* 2008; 2008:1-7.

[18] Purgina B, Rao U, Miettinen M, et al. AIDS-related EBV-associated smooth muscle tumors: a review of 64 published cases. *Patholog Res Int* 2011; 2011:1-10.

[19] Kleinerman RA, Tucker MA, Abramson DH, et al. Risk of soft tissue sarcomas by individual subtype in survivors of hereditary retinoblastoma. *J Natl Cancer Inst* 2007; 99:24–31.

[20] Ognjanovic S, Olivier M, Bergemann TL, et al. Sarcomas in TP53 germline mutation carriers. *Cancer* 2012; 118: 1387–96.

[21] Çiğdem UA, İsmail OK, Banu KK, et al. Neurofibromatosis type 1, gastrointestinal stromal tumor, leiomyosarcoma and osteosarcoma: Four cases of rare tumors and a review of the literature. *Crit Rev Oncol Hematol* 2013; 2(1): 191-99.

[22] Serrano C, George S. Leiomyosarcoma. *Hematol Oncol Clin North Am* 2013; 27(5):957-74.

[23] Coindre JM, Terrier P, Guillou L, et al. Predictive value of grade for metastasis development in the main histologic types of adult soft tissue sarcomas: a study of 1240 patients from the French Federation of Cancer Centers Sarcoma Group. *Cancer* 2001; 91(10):1914-26.

[24] Gladdy RA, Qin LX, Moraco N, Agaram NP, Brennan MF, Signer S. Predictors of survival and recurrence in primary leiomyosarcoma. *Ann Surg Oncol.* 2013 Jun; 20(6):1851-7.

[25] Zagars GK, Ballo MT, Pisters PW, et al. Prognostic factors for patients with localized soft-tissue sarcoma treated with conservation surgery and radiation therapy: an analysis of 1225 patients. *Cancer* 2003; 97(10):2530-43.

[26] Deneve JL, Messina JL, Bui MM, Marzban SS, Letson GD, Cheong D, Gonzalez RJ, Sondak VK, Zager JS. "Cutaneous leiomyosarcoma: treatment and outcomes with a standard margin of resection." *Cancer Control*. 2013 Oct; 20(4):307-12.

[27] European Sarcoma Network Working Group. Soft tissue and visceral sarcomas: ESMO Clinical Practice Guidelines for diagnosis treatment and follow-up. *Ann Oncol*. 2012 Oct;23 Suppl 7:vii92-9.

[28] Paryani NN, Zlotecki RA, Swanson EL. Multimodality local therapy for retroperitoneal sarcoma. *Int J Radiat Oncol Biol Phys*. 2012; 82:1128.

[29] Netter, F. H. *Atlas of Human Anatomy*. Summit, N.J.: Ciba-Geigy, 1989.

[30] Rozen WM, Ashton MW, Taylor GI. Reviewing the Vascular Supply of the Anterior Abdominal Wall: Redefining Anatomy for Increasingly Refined Surgery. *Clinical Anatomy*. 2008; 21 (89-98).

[31] Ramirez O, Ruas E, Dellon A. Components separation method for closure of abdominal-wall defects: an anatomic and clinical study. *Plastic and Reconstructive Surgery*. 1990; 86:519-526.

[32] Echo A, Otake L, Talley J, Satterwhite T, Norton J, Lee GK. "The Use of Permacol for the reconstruction of a complex thoraoabdominal wall defect from a recurrent leiomyosarcoma." *Eur J Plast Surg*. Published Online Feb 24, 2013.

[33] Otake LR, Satterwhite T, Echo A, Chiou G, and Lee GK. Single-Institution Financial Analysis of Biologic Versus Synthetic Mesh in Hernia Repair: A Retrospective analysis of patients readmitted for hernia repair, *Annals of Plastic Surgery*, July 2013. [Epub ahead of print]

[34] Paro J, Gupta D, Wright E, Lee G. Complex Abdominal Wall Reconstruction: Comparing Primary Closure, Biologic and Synthetic Meshes. From *Abdominal Wall Defects: Prevalence, Surgical Management Strategies and Clinical Care Outcomes*. Nova Science Publishers, Inc. 2014. Jose Diaz, editor.

[35] Singh NK, Khalifeh MR, Bank J. Abdominal Wall Reconstruction, in Nelligan Plastic Surgery, 3rd Edition.

[36] Kroll, S. S., Walsh, G., Ryan, B., et al. Risks and benefits of using Marlex mesh in chest wall reconstruction. *Annals of plastic surgery* 31: 303-306, 1993.

[37] Losken, A., Thourani, V. H., Carlson, G. W., et al. A reconstructive algorithm for plastic surgery following extensive chest wall resection. *British journal of plastic surgery* 57: 295-302, 2004.

[38] McCormack, P. M. Use of prosthetic materials in chest-wall reconstruction. Assets and liabilities. *The Surgical clinics of North America* 69: 965-976, 1989.

[39] Mahabir, R. C., Butler, C. E. Stabilization of the chest wall: autologous and alloplastic reconstructions. *Seminars in plastic surgery* 25: 34-42, 2011.

[40] Leber, G. E., Garb, J. L., Alexander, A. I., et al. Long-term complications associated with prosthetic repair of incisional hernias. *Archives of surgery* 133: 378-382, 1998.

[41] Cothren, C. C., Gallego, K., Anderson, E. D., et al. Chest wall reconstruction with acellular dermal matrix (AlloDerm) and a latissimus muscle flap. *Plastic and reconstructive surgery* 114: 1015-1017, 2004.

[42] Holton, L. H., 3rd, Chung, T., Silverman, R. P., et al. Comparison of acellular dermal matrix and synthetic mesh for lateral chest wall reconstruction in a rabbit model. *Plastic and reconstructive surgery* 119: 1238-1246, 2007.

[43] Lin, S. R., Kastenberg, Z. J., Bruzoni, M., et al. Chest wall reconstruction using implantable cross-linked porcine dermal collagen matrix (Permacol). *Journal of pediatric surgery* 47: 1472-1475, 2012.

[44] Sodha, N. R., Azoury, S. C., Sciortino, C., et al. The use of acellular dermal matrices in chest wall reconstruction. *Plastic and reconstructive surgery* 130: 175S-182S, 2012.

[45] Forthomme, B., Heymans, O., Jacquemin, D., et al. Shoulder function after latissimus dorsi transfer in breast reconstruction. *Clinical physiology and functional imaging* 30: 406-412, 2010.

[46] Heitmann, C., Guerra, A., Metzinger, S. W., et al. The thoracodorsal artery perforator flap: anatomic basis and clinical application. *Annals of plastic surgery* 51: 23-29, 2003.

[47] Cordeiro, P. G., Santamaria, E., Hidalgo, D. The role of microsurgery in reconstruction of oncologic chest wall defects. *Plastic and reconstructive surgery* 108: 1924-1930, 2001.

[48] Press, B. H., Colen, S. R., Boyd, A., et al. Reconstruction of a large chest wall defect with a musculocutaneous free flap using anterolateral thigh musculature. *Annals of plastic surgery* 20: 238-241, 1988.

[49] Tran PH, Lemaine V. *Reconstruction of the Perineum,* in Grabb & Smith, 7th Edition, Editor Charles Thorne, et al., Lippinoctt, Williams, & Wilkins Publishers, 2013. Nelson RA, Butler CE.

[50] Surgical outcomes of VRAM versus thigh flaps for immediate reconstruction of pelvic and perineal cancer resection defects. *Plast Reconst Surg*. 2011; 127:200-209.

In: Leiomyosarcoma
Editor: Rosemary H. Leach
ISBN: 978-1-63117-940-2

Chapter 4

Diagnosis and Treatment of Leiomyosarcomas

Meena Bedi, M.D.[1,*], David M. King, M.D.[2] and Eduardo Zambrano, M.D.[3]

[1]Department of Radiation Oncology, Medical College of Wisconsin, Milwaukee, WI, US
[2]Department of Orthopaedic Surgery, Medical College of Wisconsin, Milwaukee, WI, US
[3]Department of Pathology, Medical College of Wisconsin, Milwaukee, WI, US

Abstract

Leiomyosarcomas are rare and often aggressive forms of sarcoma that arise from various anatomic locations. Leiomyosarcomas commonly originate from the smooth muscle of the soft tissues, gastrointestinal tract and uterus and account for approximately 5% to 10% of all soft tissue sarcomas. Diagnosis and treatment of leiomyosarcomas involves a multimodality approach; however, even with aggressive treatment, survival and prognosis of this disease is relatively poor. This chapter highlights the risk factors, diagnosis, and treatment options for localized and metastatic leiomyosarcomas.

Clinical Characteristics

Leiomyosarcomas occur in the 5th and 6th decade of life and are rarely seen in the pediatric population [1, 2]. Most leiomyosarcomas are sporadic, but may develop in the setting of genetic syndomes such as hereditary retinoblastoma and Li-Fraumeni syndrome. Leiomyosarcomas may also be a result of radiation exposure; however, radiation-induced

[*] Corresponding author: Meena Bedi, MD, Department of Radiation Oncology, Medical College of Wisconsin, 8701 Watertown Plank Rd, Milwaukee, WI 53045. Tel: (414) 805-4496, Fax: (414) 805-4405, E-mail: mbedi@mcw.edu.

sarcomas are typically undifferentiated, fibrosarcomas or malignant peripheral nerve sheath tumors.

Fifty to 60% of all leiomyosarcomas arise from the uterus and retroperitoneum. Although leiomyosarcomas may be localized at presentation, the development of metastases is common and the site of origin may influence the location and rate of metastases.

Cutaneous leiomyosarcomas rarely metastasize, however, intra-abdominal and extremity tumors have a high propensity to metastasize to the liver and lung, respectively. Thus, the prognosis and treatment of histologically similar leiomyosarcomas may differ depending on the location of disease.

Leiomyosarcoma of Soft Tissue

Soft tissue leiomyosarcomas typically arise from the smooth muscle layer of small blood vessels in the retroperitoneum [2]. Retroperitoneal leiomyosarcomas initially may be asymptomatic until they become large enough to compress adjacent structures leading to symptoms such as pain, nausea, lower extremity edema and weight loss. Thus, most retroperitoneal leiomyosarcomas are locally advanced at presentation, with a median size of 15 cm [3].

Rarely, leiomyosarcomas may arise from the smooth muscle layer of low pressure, large blood vessels such as the inferior vena cava and pulmonary artery. Patients diagnosed with vascular leiomyosarcomas, like all leiomyosarcomas, have a poor prognosis, as treatments may be limited due to the challenging location of the disease [4].

Uterine Leiomyosarcoma

Uterine leiomyosarcomas arise from the smooth muscle of the uterine wall (i.e the myometrium) and occur in women between 40 and 60 years of age. The estimated incidence of uterine leiomyosarcomas is 0.64 per 100,000. They account for less than 5% of all uterine malignant tumors, and 25-30% of all uterine sarcomas [5, 6]. Patients may present with vaginal bleeding, pelvic pressure or pain prior to their diagnosis.

Histologic features such as grade determine treatment options, however, the propensity for hematogenous spread in uterine leiomyosarcomas portends a poor prognosis and survival rate in patients diagnosed with this disease [7-9].

Cutaneous Leiomyosarcoma

Cutaneous leiomyosarcomas are poorly defined because of their relative paucity compared to their soft tissue counterparts. Cutaneous leiomyosarcomas arise from the pilar erector muscle of the dermis or small vessels of the subcutaneous tissue [10] (Figure 1).

As opposed to other subtypes of leiomyosarcomas, cutaneous and subcutaneous leiomyosarcomas are more commonly seen in males and have a better prognosis compared to soft tissue leiomyosarcomas.

Although this malignancy has a much lower risk of spread, deep lesions that extend beyond the dermal layer have a 30% to 40% rate of metastasis to the lung [11-14].

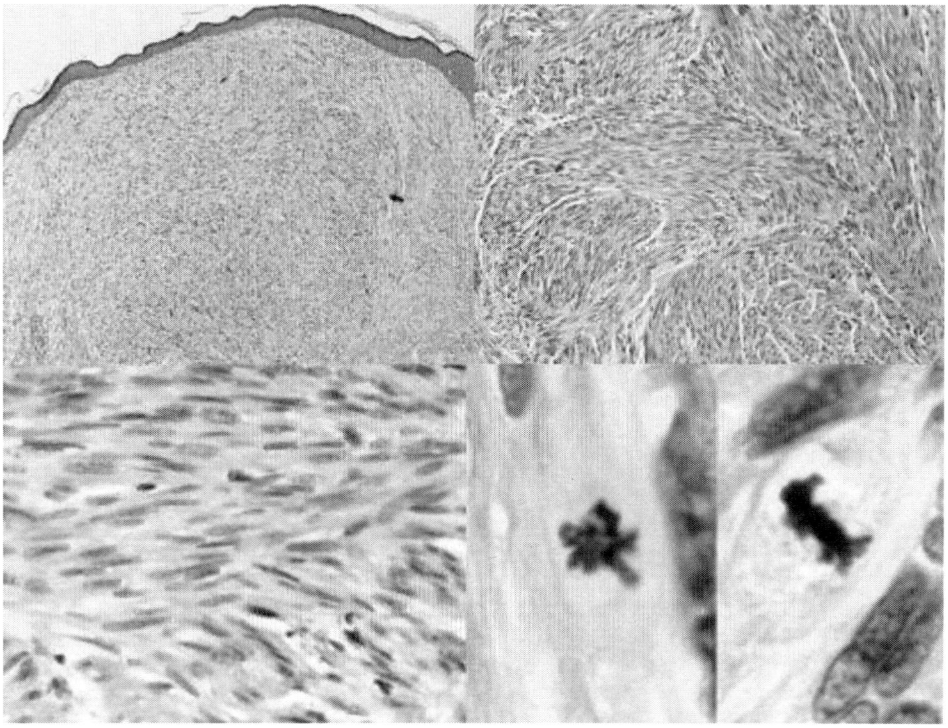

Figure 1. Cutaneous leiomyosarcoma: Highly cellular proliferation of spindle cells containing cigar-shaped nuclei within dermis.

Bone Leiomyosarcoma

Leiomyosarcomas of the bone are extremely rare and develop from the smooth muscle lining of the intraosseous vessels or from pluripotent mesenchymal cells. This subtype of leiomyosarcoma occurs in the metaphysis of the long bone, or more commonly as metastasis from soft tissue leiomyosarcomas [15, 16].

Diagnosis

Imaging

Radiographic imaging is imperative in the diagnosis of leiomyosarcomas and will often delineate the extent of disease. In the extremity, magnetic resonance imaging (MRI) is acquired to assess soft tissue extent and tumor characteristics such as swelling. Leiomyosarcomas are often seen as a poorly defined soft tissue mass which is dark on T1 and bright on T2-weighted images. Typical characteristics of leiomyosarcomas on MRI are seen in figures 2A and 2B. CT (Figure 3) and MRI both are useful in retroperitoneal and uterine leiomyosarcomas, as they assess vascular invasion and metastatic disease. The role of PET/ CT imaging is not well defined, but may be used to evaluate patients with metastatic disease or loco-regional recurrences after definitive therapy has been completed (Figure 4).

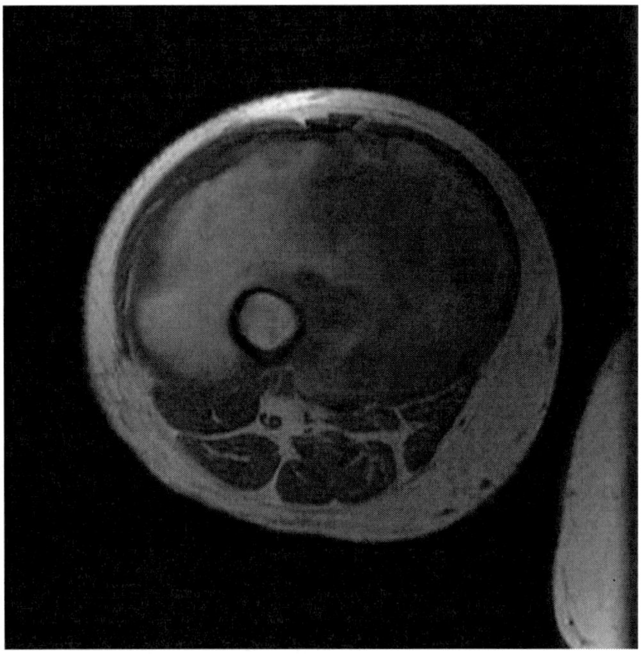

Figure 2A. Axial T1-weighted MRI-Leiomyosarcoma of the Right Thigh.

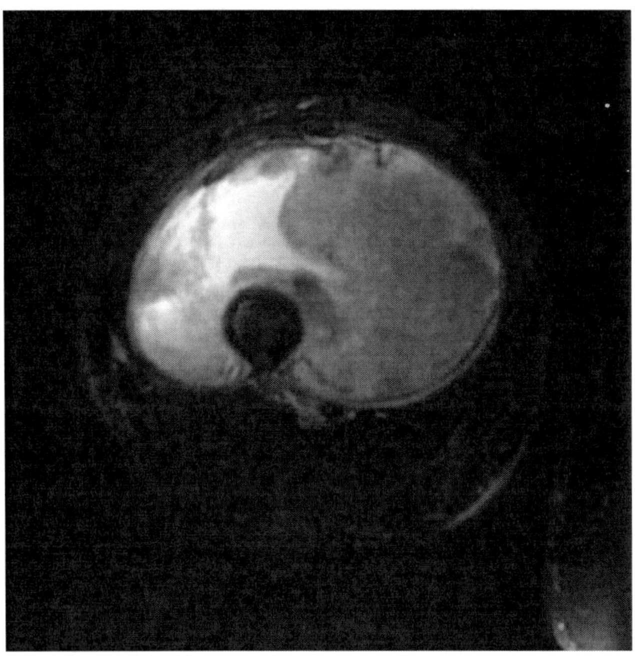

Figure 2B. Axial T2-weighted MRI-Leiomyosarcoma of the Right Thigh.

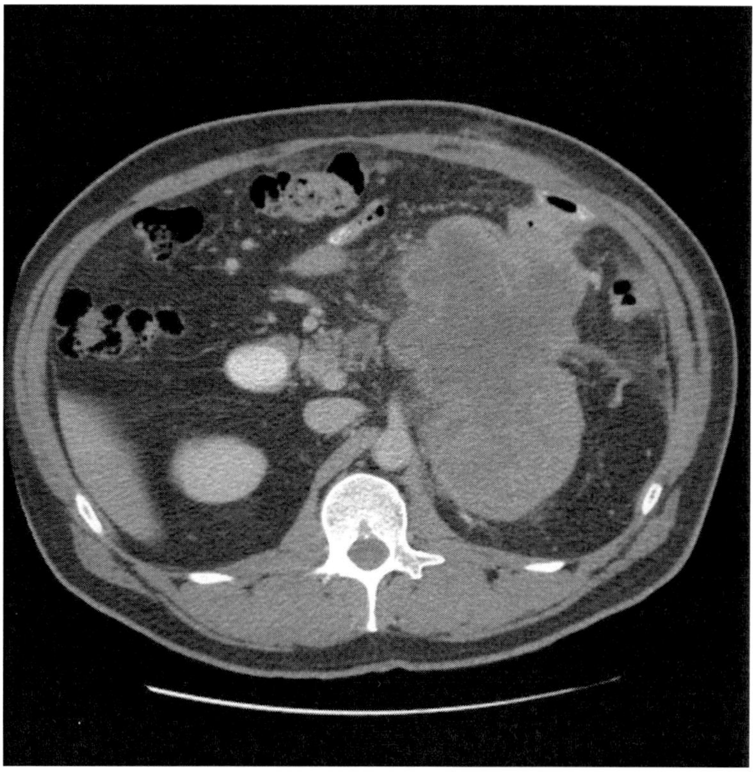

Figure 3. Retroperitoneal Leiomyosarcoma on CT with Contrast.

Biopsy

The method of biopsy in leiomyosarcomas depends on the location of primary disease. In the extremity, including bone, CT guided core biopsy is a reliable tool for the identification of sarcomas when compared to traditional open biopsy [17-21]. Advantages of an image-guided core biopsy include decreased cost and lower complications compared to open biopsy [21, 22]. In addition, percutaneous biopsy for sarcoma significantly minimizes the amount of tissue that warrants excision during resection of the biopsy tract at the time of surgical management. Retroperitoneal leiomyosarcomas are also pathologically confirmed with image-guided biopsies, as many times their appearance on CT or MRI reveals characteristics of a sarcoma. However, if biopsy or imaging findings are inconclusive, surgical resection is then performed to acquire final pathologic diagnosis. Uterine leiomyosarcomas may be diagnosed following hysterectomy or myomectomy for presumed benign leiomyomas.

However, women with abnormal or post-menopausal vaginal bleeding should undergo an endometrial biopsy to further characterize the disease [23, 24].

Pathology

Leiomyosarcomas are, in general, highly cellular neoplasms composed of elongated, spindled cells arranged in long, perpendicularly oriented, intersecting fascicles.

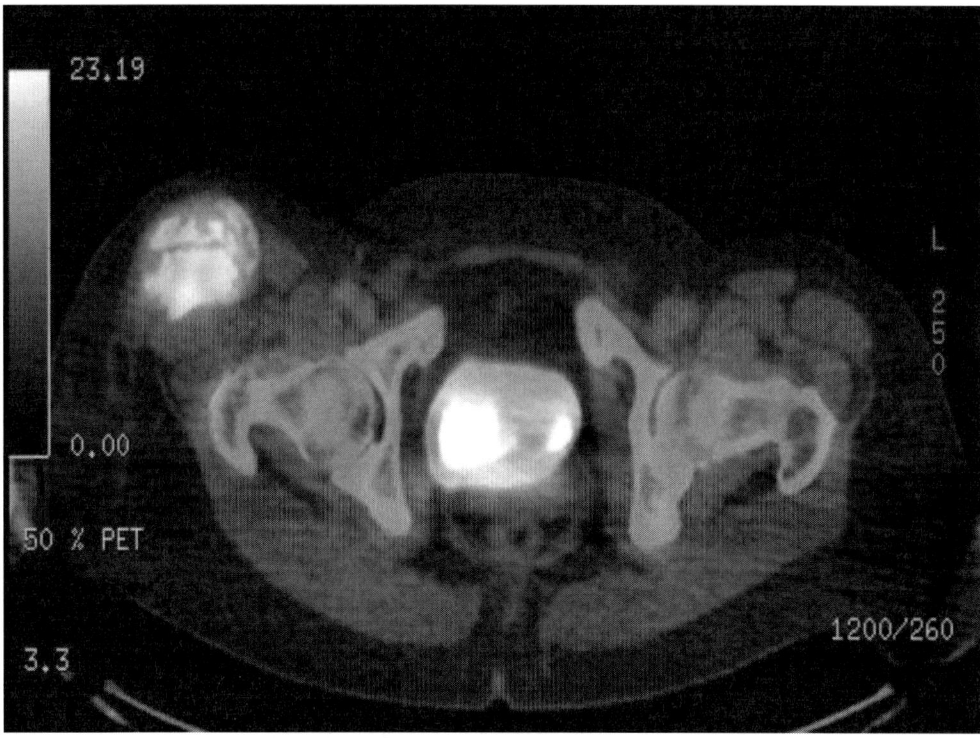

Figure 4. FDG-AVID Right Thigh Leiomyosarcoma on PET/CT.

The cells contain pale, fibrillary to brightly eosinophilic (pink) cytoplasm and elongated, blunt-ended, "cigar-shaped" nuclei (Figure 5). Clear paranuclear vacuoles may be observed. Occasionally, malignant cells can have a predominantly epitheliod appearance.

It is imperative to distinguish between benign and malignant tumors of smooth muscle, which is delineated by the degree of cellular differentiation, the presence of necrosis, mitotic activity and atypical appearing cells.

Malignant tumors of smooth muscle (i.e., leiomyosarcomas) usually contain areas of necrosis and atypical cells and have higher mitotic rates (Figures 6 & 7) [25]. Also depending on the extent of these features, leiomyosarcomas may be subcategorized as low, intermediate and high grades.

Smooth muscle cells typically express one or more of the following histologic markers: desmin, h-caldesmon, calponin, vimentin, smooth muscle actin and muscle specific actin [26]. Cytokeratins are usually negative, but may rarely be observed.

Staging

Size, depth of tumor, location, grade, nodal status and systemic disease are the variables used to stage patients with soft tissue sarcomas, including leiomyosarcomas. (Table 1).

Tumor grade is founded on a three-tiered French (FNCLCC) system which reflects differentiation, mitotic activity and the degree of necrosis [27].

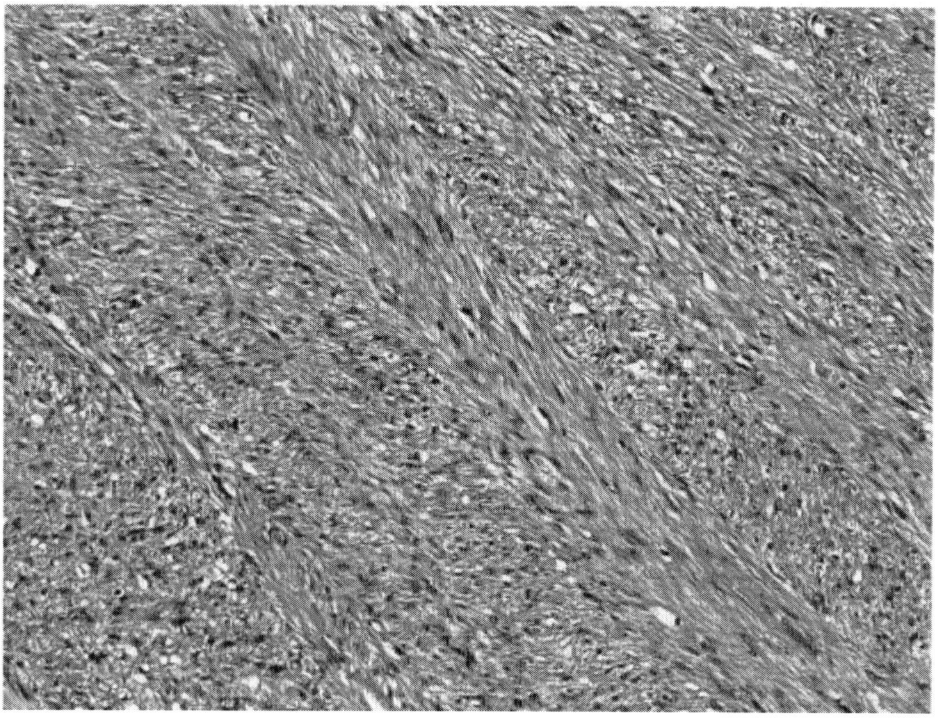

Figure 5. Low-grade leiomyosarcoma composed of long intersecting fascicles of spindle cells with brightly eosinophilic cytoplasm and elongated nuclei.

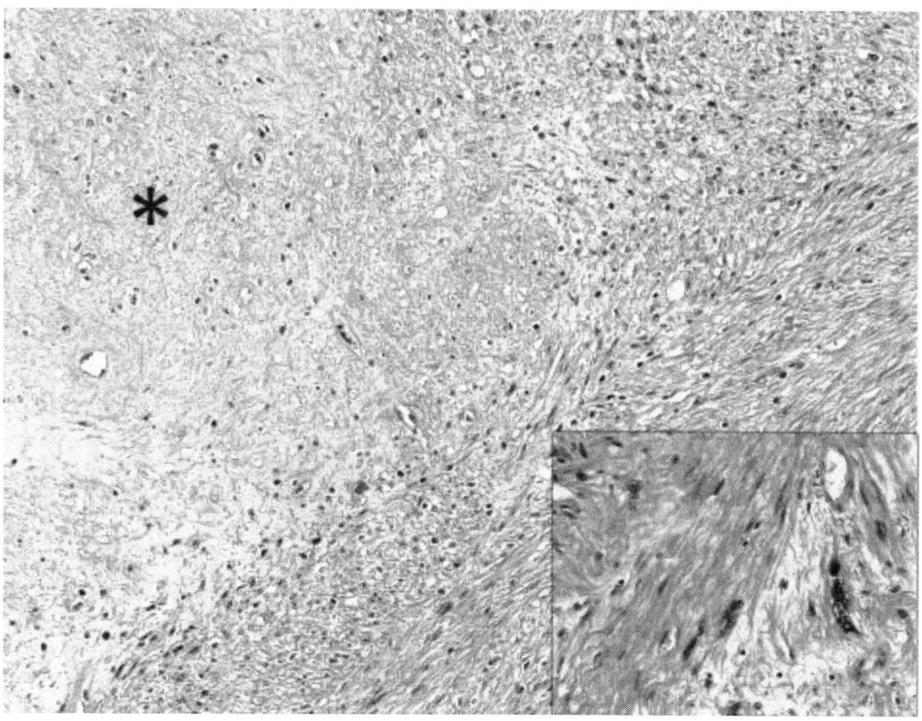

Figure 6. Areas of coagulative necrosis (asterisk) and atypical nuclei (inset) present in Leiomyosarcoma.

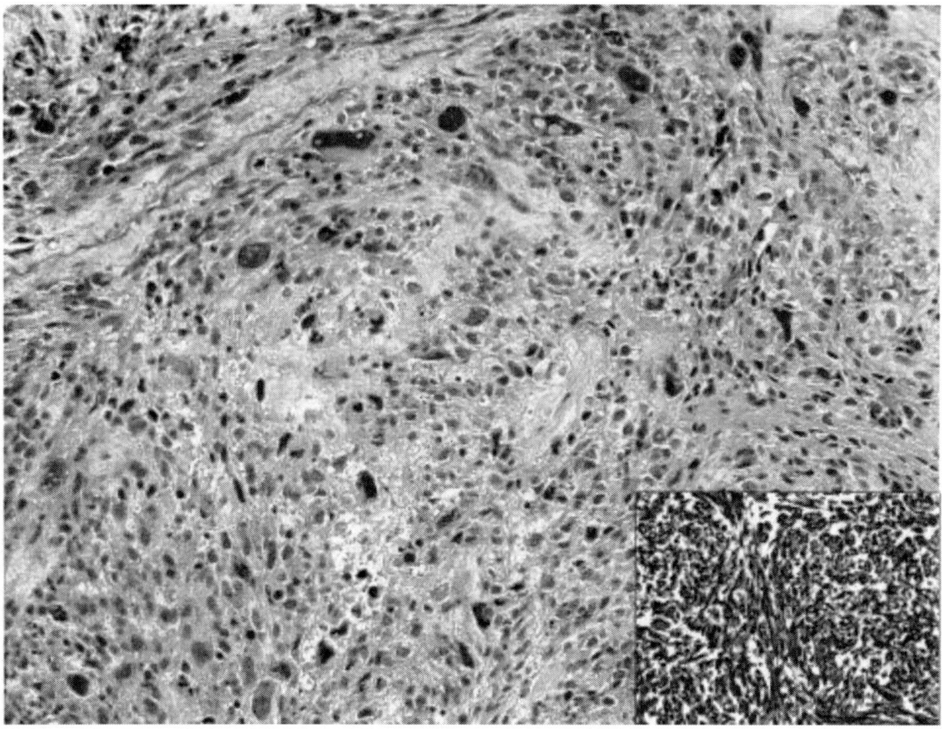

Figure 7. High-grade leiomyosarcoma containing highly pleomorphic cells. Immunohistochemical staining (e.g., desmin; inset) may be crucial to identify the tumor histologic type.

Table 1. Sarcoma Staging-AJCC 7th Edition

Stage Group	Tumor Size	Deep or Superficial to Fascia	Nodal Involvement	Grade	Metastasis
IA	≤5 cm	Superficial or Deep	-	1	-
IB	>5 cm	Superficial or Deep	-	1	-
IIA	≤5 cm	Superficial or Deep	-	2-3	-
IIB	>5 cm	Superficial or Deep	-	2	-
III	>5 cm	Superficial or Deep	+/-	3	-
IV	N/A	N/A	N/A	N/A	+

As opposed to soft tissue sarcomas, uterine sarcomas are surgically staged with the International Federation of Gynecology and Oncology (FIGO) system, which implements size, location, nodal status and systemic disease to categorize patients (Table 2) [28].

Treatment

Due to the complex nature of leiomyosarcomas as well as the rarity of this disease, multi-disciplinary evaluation and management should be completed at a center that treats a high volume of sarcoma cases.

Table 2. FIGO Staging of Uterine Sarcoma

Stage Group	T Stage	Tumor Size	Location	Nodal Involvement	Metastasis?
IA	T1a	≤5 cm	Confined to uterus	-	-
IB	T1b	>5 cm	Confined to uterus	-	-
IIA	T2a	N/A	Involvement of Adnexa	-	-
IIB	T2b	N/A	Involvement of other pelvic tissues	-	-
IIIA	T3a	N/A	Infiltration of one abdominal site	-	-
IIIB	T3b	N/A	Infiltration of more than one abdominal site	-	+
IIIC	N/A	N/A		+	-
IVA	T4	N/A	Invades bladder or rectum	-	-
IVB	N/A	N/A		-	-

Dedicated musculoskeletal orthopaedic, surgical, medical and radiation oncologists, pathologists and radiologists should be involved to optimize staging, diagnosis and treatment of these high risk patients, which leads to improvement in outcomes.

Surgery

Surgery is the mainstay of treatment for all sarcomas, including leiomyosarcomas. Operative planning is determined by preoperative imaging, neoadjuvant therapy and location of disease. Outcomes, including local control and survival are dictated by the quality of the surgical resection. Complete wide resection with negative margins (R0) has been shown to improve disease control.

Leiomyosarcomas of the extremity are managed with limb-sparing techniques. Historically, amputation was the mainstay of treatment; however, a multimodality approach with radiation therapy and surgery has been shown to yield equivalent outcomes compared to amputation, and thus is the current standard of practice when patients are deemed appropriate candidates for this approach [29].

Surgical management is also the foundation of treatment of retroperitoneal leiomyosarcomas. Similarly to extremity leiomyosarcomas, the ability to perform an R0 resection is the most important factor in locoregional control and survival [3, 30-33].

However, due to the large nature of retroperitoneal leiomyosarcomas and compression of adjacent critical tissues, R0 resections may be difficult to achieve and often require removal of normal structures such as the kidney, small and large bowel, pancreas, spleen and other intra-abdominal organs [32, 33]. Distant metastases, peritoneal implants, involvement of the aorta, portions of the vena cava, iliac and superior mesenteric vessels may make reteroperitoneal leiomyosarcomas unresectable, and thus likely incurable [34].

Resection of vascular leiomyosarcomas, particularly from the vena cava, may require vascular reconstruction, although this is controversial and subject to the location of disease [35-37].

The standard surgery for uterine leiomyosarcomas is a total abdominal hysterectomy with pelvic washings. Oophorectomy may be omitted in premenopausal women who have normal appearing ovaries on inspection at the time of surgery [38]. Lymph node dissection may provide information on prognosis, but has not been determined to improve survival [39, 40]. Thus, lymphadenectomy is reserved for patients whose nodes appear abnormal during surgery or on imaging [41].

The treatment for cutaneous leiomyosarcomas is wide local excision with negative margins. Tumors that have deep invasion into the subcutaneous tissue and positive margins have rates of local recurrence up to 40% [12].

Moreover, these extensive cases have a higher rate of distant recurrence. Adjuvant therapy for cutaneous leiomysarcoma is administered on a case-by-case basis and should be recommended after discussion in a multidisciplinary setting [12, 14].

Radiation

Radiation therapy is often delivered in conjunction with surgery to improve local control in all soft tissue sarcomas, especially in disease locations where abutment of critical structures exists. Radiation may be delivered either pre-operatively or post-operatively. The advantages of pre-operative radiation therapy includes the facilitation of surgical resection, reduction of radiation fields, lower dose, and improved tissue oxygenation preoperatively.

The NCI Canadian multicenter trial randomized patients with extremity soft tissue sarcomas to pre-operative versus post-operative radiation therapy. Eighteen of the 270 (6.7%) patients enrolled had leiomyosarcomas. At 3 years, local control was equivalent, however, there was an increased risk of wound complications in patients who underwent pre-operative compared to those that underwent post-operative radiation therapy (35% versus 17%, p=0.01). However, there was a higher risk of grade 2 or above fibrosis when radiation was delivered post-operatively compared to pre-operatively (31% versus 48%, p=0.07) [42].

A large meta-analysis also reviewed five studies comparing pre-operative to post-operative radiation therapy in resectable soft tissue sarcomas. The risk of local recurrence was lower in the patients that received pre-operative (OR 0.61, 95% CI 0.42-0.89) compared to those that underwent post-operative radiation therapy (OR 0.67 95% CI 0.39-1.15). Survival was also improved in the pre-operative radiation group (76%, range: 62%-88%) versus the post-operative radiation group (67%, range: 41%-83%) [43].

In retroperitoneal sarcomas, the tolerance of adjacent vital structures to the radiation field may limit the dose that can be administered. Thus, high doses that are required for local control of sarcomas of the retroperitoneum may not be achieved. Intraoperative radiation therapy (IORT) is a form of radiation that is delivered in conjunction with external beam radiation to improve local control of the disease, while respecting normal tissue structures such as the spinal cord, kidney, liver, and bowel. IORT delivers radiation at the time of surgery, which may be through an electron beam or high dose rate brachytherapy. IORT allows additional dose to the resection cavity while limiting the dose to adjacent normal tissues [44-46].

As opposed to leiomyosarcomas of the extremity and retroperitoneum, the advantage of adjuvant radiation in uterine leiomyosarcomas is uncertain. A phase III randomized study evaluated the role of pelvic radiation in patients with stage I to II uterine sarcomas after total abdominal hysterectomy, bilateral salpingo-oophorectomy and pelvic lymph node washings. Forty-six percent of patients had leiomyosarcomas of the uterus. Radiation was delivered to a total dose was 51 Gy in 28 fractions. Radiation improved local control in leiomyosarcomas, 2% versus 14% (p-value NR), but had no impact on progression-free or overall survival in all subtypes of sarcoma [47].

Ferrer et al., analyzed the impact of radiation therapy with or without brachytherapy in 103 patients with sarcoma (42% leiomyosarcoma) of the uterus. Patients were treated with radiation at their physician's discretion. Those that underwent radiation for management had a five-year loco-regional free interval of 76% versus 36.4% ($p<0.0001$) in the patients who did not receive radiation. Five-year survival was also improved in patients who received radiation compared to those that did not receive radiation, 73% versus 37% ($p=0.003$), respectively. On multivariate analysis, radiation therapy predicted for improved locoregional disease-free interval, disease-free interval and overall survival [48].

Chemotherapy

The role of chemotherapy in a non-metastatic setting, for all soft tissue sarcomas, including leiomyosarcomas is controversial. The Sarcoma Meta-analysis Collaboration reviewed 14 randomized trials of patients who underwent local therapy for soft tissue sarcomas with or without adjuvant doxorubicin-based chemotherapy. The addition of adjuvant chemotherapy was found to improve local recurrence-free survival by 6%, distant recurrence-free survival by 10% as well as overall recurrence-free survival by 10% [49].

As part of pre-operative management, neoadjuvant chemotherapy may provide a similar role to radiation in terms of facilitation of surgical resection. Proponents for neoadjuvant chemotherapy argue that disease reponse may be monitored and treatment may be altered based on an individual's response.

Gortzac, et *al.* reported results of a phase II study that examined patients with high-risk sarcomas who were randomized to surgery alone or three cycles of doxorubicin and ifosfamide prior to surgery. After a median follow-up of 7.3 years, the addition of chemotherapy failed to show any benefit in disease-free or overall survival [50].

Although local control in uterine leiomyosarcomas is integral in the outcome of this disease, extra-abdominal metastasis dictates survival. Moreover, while the rate of distant disease is high, the role for chemotherapy remains undetermined. Doxorubicin-based chemotherapy may have some benefit, but there has been no prospective data to show that chemotherapy leads to improved outcomes [51]. Thus, the recommendation of chemotherapy in uterine leiomyosarcomas should be made on a case-by-case basis after discussion in a multi-disciplinary setting.

Most of the studies on chemotherapy in sarcoma include all histologic types and locations of disease. However, there are currently ongoing trials investigating the use of chemotherapy specifically in leiomyosarcomas. The results of these trials may help to elucidate the optimal therapeutic algorithm for these patients.

Metastatic Disease

Chemotherapy is the mainstay of treatment for metastatic leiomyosarcoma. Doxorubicin-based chemotherapy alone or in combination with ifosfamide, as well as gemcitabine-based regimens have been shown to have sensitivity in metastatic leiomyosarcomas, especially those of uterine origin (Table 3).

The EORTC compared doxorubicin to docetaxel in patients with locally advanced soft tissue sarcomas. Thirty of the 85 (35%) patients enrolled were diagnosed with leiomyosarcoma. The response rate was 30% in doxorubicin group compared to 0% in the docetaxel group [52].

Doxorubicin in combination with other chemotherapeutic regimens has also been shown to be more effective that single-agent doxorubicin. Unfortunately, response to treatment is transient and is approximately a median of 8 months. Furthermore, although response rates may be improved with combination therapy, survival is not impacted [53].

Gemcitabine in conjunction with docetaxel has shown efficacy in patients with leiomyosarcoma of the uterus and gastrointestinal tract, with objective response rates of approximately 50% [54, 55]. Gemcitabine-based regimens with dacarbazine and vinorebline has also shown to be effective in small clinical trials in patients with metastatic leiomyosarcomas [56, 57].

Several other investigational drugs in the metastatic setting have shown promising results in leiomyosarcomas and are either being evaluated or recently approved for patients as second or third line chemotherapy. Trabectin is a drug that is derived from marine organisms. Although the exact mechanism of action is not known, it is thought to cleave DNA and result in apoptosis [58]. Response rates are promising in leiomyosarcomas. The EORTC Soft Tissue and Bone Sarcoma Phase II Trial evaluated Trabectin as second or third-line therapy in 104 patients with advanced soft tissue sarcoma. Fifty-six percent of patients with leiomyosarcoma histology had arrest of their disease [59, 60]. Trabectin is still investigational in the United States, but has been approved in Europe, Russia and South Korea.

Pazopanib is a multi-targeted tyrosine kinase inhibitor that has also shown promising results in leiomyosarcomas. The PALLETTE trial was a phase III double-blind trial that randomized patients with metastatic soft tissue sarcomas to pazopanib or placebo. Forty-five percent of patients randomized had leiomyosarcoma. Three month progression free survival was 44% for patients with leiomyosarcoma. There was no difference in overall survival, however [61]. Due to the results of this study, pazopanib has been approved for use in patients with soft tissue sarcomas who have progressed on other forms of chemotherapy.

Table 3. Chemotherapy Used in Metastatic Leiomyosarcoma

Drug	Mechanism of Action
Doxorubicin	Anthracycline
Gemcitabine	Nucleoside Analog
Trabectin	Direct DNA Damage
Pazopanib	Multi-targeted receptor tyrosine kinase inhibitor
Bendamustine	Alkylating agent

Bendamustine is an alkylating agent that has exhibited activity against metastatic leiomyosarcomas refractory to other chemotherapeutic regimens. A phase II trial enrolling 36 patients investigating bendamustine revealed stability of disease without progression in 40% of patients with leiomyosarcomas [62].

Prognostic Indicators and Outcomes

Factors associated with poor overall, disease-specific and distant-metastasis free survival include grade, size and depth of the tumor. Five-year overall survival for extremity and bone leiomyosarcomas is approximately 60 to 70% and 50-60% in retroperitoneal sarcomas.

Patients who do succumb to leiomyosarcoma, is often due to metastatic disease.

Conclusion

Leiomyosarcomas are a rare and heterogeneous histologic type of sarcoma that has a poor prognosis. Due to the aggressive nature of this disease and locations in which they may arise, leiomysarcomas can be challenging to treat. Thus, these tumors should be discussed and managed in a multi-disciplinary setting at a designated sarcoma center.

Surgical management is the mainstay of treatment for all leiomyosarcomas. Pre-operative or post-operative radiation therapy may be employed in extremity and retroperitoneal leiomyosarcomas to improve locoregional control. Pre-operative radiation therapy may also help facilitate surgical resection.

Chemotherapy as part of definitive management for localized disease is controversial in leiomyosarcomas, however, it is standard in the metastatic setting with doxorubicin-based regimens used as first-line therapy. Although there have been many studies assessing combination and substitute therapy, these have failed to lead to improvement in outcomes. Current trials enrolling patients with leiomyosarcoma are attempting to identify systemic therapies that may improve the control and survival for this rare disease.

Conflicts of interest: The authors have no conflicts of interest.

References

[1] Mankin, H. J., Casas-Ganem, J., Kim, J. I., et al. Leiomyosarcoma of somatic soft tissues. *Clin. Orthop. Relat. Res.* 2004:225-231.

[2] Gustafson, P., Willen, H., Baldetorp, B., et al. Soft tissue leiomyosarcoma. A population-based epidemiologic and prognostic study of 48 patients, including cellular DNA content. *Cancer* 1992;70:114-119.

[3] Stoeckle, E., Coindre, J. M., Bonvalot, S., et al. Prognostic factors in retroperitoneal sarcoma: a multivariate analysis of a series of 165 patients of the French Cancer Center Federation Sarcoma Group. *Cancer* 2001;92:359-368.

[4] Kevorkian, J., Cento, D. P. Leiomyosarcoma of large arteries and veins. *Surgery* 1973; 73:390-400.

[5] Harlow, B. L., Weiss, N. S., Lofton, S. The epidemiology of sarcomas of the uterus. *J. Natl. Cancer Inst.* 1986;76:399-402.

[6] Bartsich, E. G., Bowe, E. T., Moore, J. G. Leiomyosarcoma of the uterus. A 50-year review of 42 cases. *Obstet. Gynecol.* 1968;32:101-106.

[7] Gadducci, A., Landoni, F., Sartori, E., et al. Uterine leiomyosarcoma: analysis of treatment failures and survival. *Gynecol. Oncol.* 1996;62:25-32.

[8] Salazar, O. M., Bonfiglio, T. A., Patten, S. F., et al. Uterine sarcomas: natural history, treatment and prognosis. *Cancer* 1978;42:1152-1160.

[9] Berchuck, A., Rubin, S. C., Hoskins, W. J., et al. Treatment of uterine leiomyosarcoma. *Obstet. Gynecol.* 1988;71:845-850.

[10] Hashimoto, H., Daimaru, Y., Tsuneyoshi, M., et al. Leiomyosarcoma of the external soft tissues. A clinicopathologic, immunohistochemical, and electron microscopic study. *Cancer* 1986;57:2077-2088.

[11] Fields, J. P., Helwig, E. B. Leiomyosarcoma of the skin and subcutaneous tissue. *Cancer* 1981;47:156-169.

[12] Jensen, M. L., Jensen, O. M., Michalski, W., et al. Intradermal and subcutaneous leiomyosarcoma: a clinicopathological and immunohistochemical study of 41 cases. *J. Cutan. Pathol.* 1996;23:458-463.

[13] Massi, D., Franchi, A., Alos, L., et al. Primary cutaneous leiomyosarcoma: clinicopathological analysis of 36 cases. *Histopathology* 2010;56:251-262.

[14] Deneve, J. L., Messina, J. L., Bui, M. M., et al. Cutaneous leiomyosarcoma: treatment and outcomes with a standardized margin of resection. *Cancer Control* 2013;20:307-312.

[15] Brewer, P., Sumathi, V., Grimer, R. J., et al. Primary leiomyosarcoma of bone: analysis of prognosis. *Sarcoma* 2012;2012:636849.

[16] Berlin, O., Angervall, L., Kindblom, L. G., et al. Primary leiomyosarcoma of bone. A clinical, radiographic, pathologic-anatomic, and prognostic study of 16 cases. *Skeletal Radiol.* 1987;16:364-376.

[17] Shin, H. J., Amaral, J. G., Armstrong, D., et al. Image-guided percutaneous biopsy of musculoskeletal lesions in children. *Pediatr. Radiol.* 2007;37:362-369.

[18] Soudack, M., Nachtigal, A., Vladovski, E., et al. Sonographically guided percutaneous needle biopsy of soft tissue masses with histopathologic correlation. *J. Ultrasound Med.* 2006;25:1271-1277; quiz 1278-1279.

[19] Tsukushi, S., Katagiri, H., Nakashima, H., et al. Application and utility of computed tomography-guided needle biopsy with musculoskeletal lesions. *J. Orthop. Sci.* 2004;9: 122-125.

[20] Tsukushi, S., Nishida, Y., Yamada, Y., et al. CT-guided needle biopsy for musculoskeletal lesions. *Arch. Orthop. Trauma Surg.* 2010;130:699-703.

[21] Wu, J. S., Goldsmith, J. D., Horwich, P. J., et al. Bone and soft-tissue lesions: what factors affect diagnostic yield of image-guided core-needle biopsy? *Radiology* 2008; 248:962-970.

[22] Skrzynski, M. C., Biermann, J. S., Montag, A., et al. Diagnostic accuracy and charge-savings of outpatient core needle biopsy compared with open biopsy of musculoskeletal tumors. *J. Bone Joint Surg. Am.* 1996;78:644-649.

[23] Nassar, O. A., Abdul Moaty, S. B., Khalil el, S. A., et al. Outcome and prognostic factors of uterine sarcoma in 59 patients: single institutional results. *J. Egypt. Natl. Canc. Inst.* 2010;22:113-122.
[24] Park, J. Y., Kim, D. Y., Suh, D. S., et al. Prognostic factors and treatment outcomes of patients with uterine sarcoma: analysis of 127 patients at a single institution, 1989-2007. *J. Cancer Res. Clin. Oncol.* 2008;134:1277-1287.
[25] Billings, S. D., Folpe, A. L., Weiss, S. W. Do leiomyomas of deep soft tissue exist? An analysis of highly differentiated smooth muscle tumors of deep soft tissue supporting two distinct subtypes. *Am. J. Surg. Pathol.* 2001;25:1134-1142.
[26] Sakamoto, A., Oda, Y., Yamamoto, H., et al. Calponin and h-caldesmon expression in atypical fibroxanthoma and superficial leiomyosarcoma. *Virchows Arch.* 2002;440:404-409.
[27] Edge, S. B., Compton, C. C. The American Joint Committee on Cancer: the 7th edition of the AJCC cancer staging manual and the future of TNM. *Ann. Surg. Oncol.* 2010;17: 1471-1474.
[28] Prat, J. FIGO staging for uterine sarcomas. *Int. J. Gynaecol. Obstet.* 2009;104:177-178.
[29] Rosenberg, S. A., Tepper, J., Glatstein, E., et al. The treatment of soft-tissue sarcomas of the extremities: prospective randomized evaluations of (1) limb-sparing surgery plus radiation therapy compared with amputation and (2) the role of adjuvant chemotherapy. *Ann. Surg.* 1982;196:305-315.
[30] Lewis, J. J., Leung, D., Woodruff, J. M., et al. Retroperitoneal soft-tissue sarcoma: analysis of 500 patients treated and followed at a single institution. *Ann. Surg.* 1998; 228:355-365.
[31] Storm, F. K., Mahvi, D. M. Diagnosis and management of retroperitoneal soft-tissue sarcoma. *Ann. Surg.* 1991;214:2-10.
[32] Hassan, I., Park, S. Z., Donohue, J. H., et al. Operative management of primary retroperitoneal sarcomas: a reappraisal of an institutional experience. *Ann. Surg.* 2004; 239: 244-250.
[33] Catton, C. N., O'Sullivan, B., Kotwall, C., et al. Outcome and prognosis in retroperitoneal soft tissue sarcoma. *Int. J. Radiat. Oncol. Biol. Phys.* 1994;29:1005-1010.
[34] Jaques, D. P., Coit, D. G., Hajdu, S. I., et al. Management of primary and recurrent soft-tissue sarcoma of the retroperitoneum. *Ann. Surg.* 1990;212:51-59.
[35] Daylami, R., Amiri, A., Goldsmith, B., et al. Inferior vena cava leiomyosarcoma: is reconstruction necessary after resection? *J. Am. Coll. Surg.* 2010;210:185-190.
[36] Hollenbeck, S. T., Grobmyer, S. R., Kent, K. C., et al. Surgical treatment and outcomes of patients with primary inferior vena cava leiomyosarcoma. *J. Am. Coll. Surg.* 2003; 197:575-579.
[37] Fiore, M., Colombo, C., Locati, P., et al. Surgical technique, morbidity, and outcome of primary retroperitoneal sarcoma involving inferior vena cava. *Ann. Surg. Oncol.* 2012; 19:511-518.
[38] Giuntoli, R. L., 2nd, Metzinger, D. S., DiMarco, C. S., et al. Retrospective review of 208 patients with leiomyosarcoma of the uterus: prognostic indicators, surgical management, and adjuvant therapy. *Gynecol. Oncol.* 2003;89:460-469.
[39] Leitao, M. M., Sonoda, Y., Brennan, M. F., et al. Incidence of lymph node and ovarian metastases in leiomyosarcoma of the uterus. *Gynecol. Oncol.* 2003;91:209-212.

[40] Major, F. J., Blessing, J. A., Silverberg, S. G., et al. Prognostic factors in early-stage uterine sarcoma. A Gynecologic Oncology Group study. *Cancer* 1993;71:1702-1709.

[41] Goff, B. A., Rice, L. W., Fleischhacker, D., et al. Uterine leiomyosarcoma and endometrial stromal sarcoma: lymph node metastases and sites of recurrence. *Gynecol. Oncol.* 1993;50:105-109.

[42] O'Sullivan, B., Davis, A. M., Turcotte, R., et al. Preoperative versus postoperative radiotherapy in soft-tissue sarcoma of the limbs: a randomised trial. *Lancet* 2002; 359: 2235-2241.

[43] Al-Absi, E., Farrokhyar, F., Sharma, R., et al. A systematic review and meta-analysis of oncologic outcomes of pre- versus postoperative radiation in localized resectable soft-tissue sarcoma. *Ann. Surg. Oncol.* 2010;17:1367-1374.

[44] Willett, C. G., Suit, H. D., Tepper, J. E., et al. Intraoperative electron beam radiation therapy for retroperitoneal soft tissue sarcoma. *Cancer* 1991;68:278-283.

[45] Gunderson, L. L., Nagorney, D. M., McIlrath, D. C., et al. External beam and intra-operative electron irradiation for locally advanced soft tissue sarcomas. *Int. J. Radiat. Oncol. Biol. Phys.* 1993;25:647-656.

[46] Petersen, I. A., Haddock, M. G., Donohue, J. H., et al. Use of intraoperative electron beam radiotherapy in the management of retroperitoneal soft tissue sarcomas. *Int. J. Radiat. Oncol. Biol. Phys.* 2002;52:469-475.

[47] Reed, N. S., Mangioni, C., Malmstrom, H., et al. Phase III randomised study to evaluate the role of adjuvant pelvic radiotherapy in the treatment of uterine sarcomas stages I and II: an European Organisation for Research and Treatment of Cancer Gynaecological Cancer Group Study (protocol 55874). *Eur. J. Cancer* 2008;44:808-818.

[48] Ferrer, F., Sabater, S., Farrus, B., et al. Impact of radiotherapy on local control and survival in uterine sarcomas: a retrospective study from the Grup Oncologic Catala-Occita. *Int. J. Radiat. Oncol. Biol. Phys.* 1999;44:47-52.

[49] Adjuvant chemotherapy for localised resectable soft tissue sarcoma in adults. Sarcoma Meta-analysis Collaboration (SMAC). *Cochrane Database Syst. Rev.* 2000:CD001419.

[50] Gortzak, E., Azzarelli, A., Buesa, J., et al. A randomised phase II study on neo-adjuvant chemotherapy for 'high-risk' adult soft-tissue sarcoma. *Eur. J. Cancer* 2001;37:1096-1103.

[51] Wu, T. I., Chang, T. C., Hsueh, S., et al. Prognostic factors and impact of adjuvant chemotherapy for uterine leiomyosarcoma. *Gynecol. Oncol.* 2006;100:166-172.

[52] Verweij, J., Lee, S. M., Ruka, W., et al. Randomized phase II study of docetaxel versus doxorubicin in first- and second-line chemotherapy for locally advanced or metastatic soft tissue sarcomas in adults: a study of the european organization for research and treatment of cancer soft tissue and bone sarcoma group. *J. Clin. Oncol.* 2000;18:2081-2086.

[53] Bramwell, V. H., Anderson, D., Charette, M. L. Doxorubicin-based chemotherapy for the palliative treatment of adult patients with locally advanced or metastatic soft-tissue sarcoma: a meta-analysis and clinical practice guideline. *Sarcoma* 2000;4:103-112.

[54] Bay, J. O., Ray-Coquard, I., Fayette, J., et al. Docetaxel and gemcitabine combination in 133 advanced soft-tissue sarcomas: a retrospective analysis. *Int. J. Cancer* 2006;119: 706-711.

[55] Leu, K. M., Ostruszka, L. J., Shewach, D., et al. Laboratory and clinical evidence of synergistic cytotoxicity of sequential treatment with gemcitabine followed by docetaxel in the treatment of sarcoma. *J. Clin. Oncol.* 2004;22:1706-1712.

[56] Dileo, P., Morgan, J. A., Zahrieh, D., et al. Gemcitabine and vinorelbine combination chemotherapy for patients with advanced soft tissue sarcomas: results of a phase II trial. *Cancer* 2007;109:1863-1869.

[57] Garcia-Del-Muro, X., Lopez-Pousa, A., Maurel, J., et al. Randomized phase II study comparing gemcitabine plus dacarbazine versus dacarbazine alone in patients with previously treated soft tissue sarcoma: a Spanish Group for Research on Sarcomas study. *J. Clin. Oncol.* 2011;29:2528-2533.

[58] D'Incalci, M. Trabectedin mechanism of action: what's new? *Future Oncol.* 2013;9:5-10.

[59] Garcia-Carbonero, R., Supko, J. G., Maki, R. G., et al. Ecteinascidin-743 (ET-743) for chemotherapy-naive patients with advanced soft tissue sarcomas: multicenter phase II and pharmacokinetic study. *J. Clin. Oncol.* 2005;23:5484-5492.

[60] Le Cesne, A., Blay, J. Y., Judson, I., et al. Phase II study of ET-743 in advanced soft tissue sarcomas: a European Organisation for the Research and Treatment of Cancer (EORTC) soft tissue and bone sarcoma group trial. *J. Clin. Oncol.* 2005;23:576-584.

[61] Van der Graaf, W. T., Blay, J. Y., Chawla, S. P., et al. Pazopanib for metastatic soft-tissue sarcoma (PALETTE): a randomised, double-blind, placebo-controlled phase 3 trial. *Lancet* 2012;379:1879-1886.

[62] Hartmann, J. T., Mayer, F., Schleicher, J., et al. Bendamustine hydrochloride in patients with refractory soft tissue sarcoma: a noncomparative multicenter phase 2 study of the German sarcoma group (AIO-001). *Cancer* 2007;110:861-866.

In: Leiomyosarcoma
Editor: Rosemary H. Leach

ISBN: 978-1-63117-940-2

Chapter 5

Primary Intracranial Leiomyosarcoma

Zhenggang Xiong, M.D.
Department of Pathology, Tulane University School of Medicine,
New Orleans, LA, US

Abstract

Primary intracranial leiomyosarcoma is a malignant intracranial tumor of smooth muscle origin. Limited literature data suggest that it may have unique pathogenesis, which raises the possibility of special treatment and different prognosis from conventional extracranial leiomyosarcomas. This chapter discusses the epidemiology, pathology, and treatment of this tumor.

Epidemiology

Primary intracranial leiomyosarcoma is an uncommon neoplasm. There are 40 cases reported in the literature so far. This neoplasm is more common in male than female patients with a male to female ratio of approximate 3:1.

Patient's age at diagnosis ranges from 2 to 73 years. From the limited data, it appears that there is no peak patient's age for this neoplasm. 40-45% of tumors occur in immunocompromised individuals with or without Epstein-Barr virus infection [1-13]. 10-11% of patients have previous exposure to radiation [15-17]. Primary intracranial leiomyosarcoma occurred in patients with neurofibromatosis type 1 [18] and teratoma of pineal region [19]. Intraparenchymal leiomyosarcoma secondary to the adjacent chronic subdural hematoma were also reported [20]. Approximately 20% of cases have no specific medical history [21-27].

Pathology

Pathogenesis

The cellular origin and oncogenesis of primary intracranial leiomyosarcoma are largely unclear. Most of the cases are dura-based, which suggests that these tumors may develop from smooth muscle cells of vasculature or embryonic pluripotent mesenchymal cells of arachnoid membrane or pia [21, 28-29]. This tumor is seen in almost half of the reported cases with immunosuppression, in some of which Epstein-Barr virus infection is present. Epstein-Barr virus is a well-known carcinogen, and it is believed that Epstein-Barr virus may play an important role in the development of primary intracranial leiomyosarcoma in these cases [1-2, 4-6, 12, 14]. Identification of intracranial leiomyosarcoma in patients with neurofibromatosis type 1 [18] and teratoma [19] indicates that genetic factors may contribute to this tumor. Association with radiation suggests that acquired molecular alterations may promote the tumor formation [15-17]. It is worth to note that intracranial and extracranial leiomyosarcomas have been associated with chronic inflammation and hematoma [20, 30-31] and the pathogenic relation between these chronic conditions and leiomyosarcoma is not yet clear.

Morphology

Primary intracranial leiomyosarcomas are usually dura-based masses, although they can be seen in other intracranial locations such as sellar and suprasellar region, pineal region [32], ventricular cavity, and within brain parenchyma [20, 33]. They can infiltrate their adjacent tissues such as brain parenchyma and skull bone. As their counterparts in other human organ systems, leiomyosarcomas have a spectrum of macroscopic and microscopic pathological changes, and, based on these changes, they can be divided into two groups, low grade and high grade.

Macroscopically, low grade leiomyosarcomas usually exhibit as firm masses. Sectioning through the mass reveals white whorled surface, sometimes resembling a benign leiomyoma. High grade tumors tend to be soft. Necrosis and hemorrhage are often present.

Microscopically, low grade leiomyosarcomas show fascicular growth pattern with intersecting neoplastic cell bundles at right angles. Sometimes, tumor merges with blood vessel wall, indicating vascular wall origination. Tumor cells are more or less spindle-shaped with eosinophilic fibrillary cytoplasm and sometimes focal granularity. Nuclei are cigar-shaped and blunt-ended with low grade of pleomorphism. Intracytoplasmic vacuoles at both ends of nuclei are often seen. Mitotic figures are common. High grade leiomyosarcomas tend to be more infiltrative into adjacent tissue. Areas of necrosis are commonly present, especially in the central portion of the tumor. Hemorrhage is frequent. The neoplastic cells show more pleomorphism than low grade, sometimes mimicking malignant fibrous histiocytoma. Apoptosis is often seen in the high grade tumors. Leiomyosarcomas may exhibit different morphologic features. Epithelioid cells, rhabdoid cells, osteoclast-like giant cells, nuclear palisading, and myxoid change have been documented.

Ultrastructurally, the neoplastic cells remain some smooth muscle features that include thick basal lamina, cytoplasmic filaments with focal densities, and pinocytotic vesicles [30].

Immunohistochemistry

Leiomyosarcoma expresses several proteins that can be highlighted by immunohistochemical staining. Most of these tumors are positive for alpha-smooth muscle actin (SMA), muscle-specific actin (MSA), desmin, and vimentin. Some of these tumors are also positive for h-caldesmon [34] and cytokeratin. Occasionally, S100 protein is focally or weakly expressed in the tumor. In contrast to other intracranial tumors, leiomyosarcoma is negative for epithelial membrane antigen (EMA), Glial fibrillary acidic protein (GFAP), neurofilament, CD34, and CD68.

Diagnosis

Primary intracranial leiomyosarcoma can be diagnosed when the tumor is located in the cranial cavity and the tumor shows the morphological changes and immunohistochemical characters of smooth muscle cells, while the possibility of extracranial primary leiomyosarcoma is excluded. The following criteria are used: 1) smooth muscle tumor with atypia plus either mitotic activity or tumor cell necrosis, 2) intracranial location, 3) no extracranial counterpart in the same patient. It is proposed that a minimum of 1 to 2 mitotic figures per 10 high power field should be met to establish the pathologic diagnosis.

Primary intracranial leiomyosarcoma should be distinguished from other intracranial tumors that have similar pathological changes. The most common mimics are fibrosarcoma, myofibrosarcoma, malignant meningioma, malignant peripheral nerve sheath tumor (MPNST), and malignant fibrous histiocytoma (MFH). Fibrosarcoma derives from fibroblasts and can occur in the cranial cavity. In addition to vimentin, it expresses phosphotungstic acid-hematoxylin, type 1 collagen, and p53. Reticulin stain shows characteristic positivity in fibers surrounding each cell. The specific ultrastructures of smooth muscle cells are not seen in this tumor. Intracranial myofibrosarcoma is also dura-based, but the tumor expresses CD34 and S100, although it share some protein expression profile with leiomyosarcoma, such as vimentin, desmin, and SMA. Ultrastructural changes in myofibrosarcoma including subplasmalemmal aggregates of myofilaments continuous with extracellular fibronectin fibrils through the fibronexus junction are diagnostic. Malignant meningioma is a common dura-based arachnoid malignancy. Some of the tumors are morphologically similar to leiomyosarcoma. However, meningioma originates from arachnoid cells and is usually positive for epithelial markers like EMA and cytokeratin in addition to the expression of vimentin. Malignant meningioma can also be positive for claudin-1, CD99, and Bcl-2. Myofilaments are not seen in this tumor under electron microscope [35]. MPNST is a malignant neoplasm of peripheral nerve sheath. It expresses S-100 protein more diffusely than leiomyosarcoma and is negative for SMA [36]. MFH has mixed fibroblastic and histiocytic components. Although it is occasionally positive for SMA or desmin, its expression of histiocytic markers such as CD68 is characteristic.

Treatment

Surgery, radiotherapy, and chemotherapy are current choices of treatment for primary intracranial leiomyosarcoma. Radiation therapy after radical resection for the tumor has been performed widely [18, 20, 27-28, 31]. Specific regimen of chemotherapy for this tumor has not yet been established. Promising agents are doxorubicin, procarbazine, vincristine, ifosfamide, etoposide, gemcitabine, docetaxel, dacarbazine, temozolomide, and carboplatin. These drugs have been used in different combinations. Pediatric cases appear to be more sensitive to chemotherapy than adult cases. It is too early to tell whether multidrug regimens are more effective than single agent. Immunotherapy with antibody is also under investigation. Among those, bevacizumab, an antibody against vascular endothelial growth factor, has good potential [37].

Prognosis

With currently available treatment, the prognosis of primary intracranial leiomyosarcoma is generally poor. Limited literature reported that the majority of patients survived for a half to two years, except that one patient with radiation-induced intracranial leiomyosarcoma lived for eight years following the diagnosis.

References

[1] Gupta S, Havens PL, Southern JF, Firat SY, Jogal SS. Epstein-Barr virus-associated intracranial leiomyosarcoma in an HIV-positive adolescent. *J. Pediatr Hematol Oncol.* 2010; 32(4): e144-147.

[2] Suankratay C, Shuangshoti S, Mutirangura A, Prasanthai V, Lerdlum S, Shuangshoti S, Pintong J, Wilde H. Epstein-Barr virus infection-associated smooth-muscle tumors in patients with AIDS. *Clin. Infect Dis.* 2005; 40(10): 1521-1528.

[3] Bejjani GK, Stopak B, Schwartz A, Santi R. Primary dural leiomyosarcoma in a patient infected with human immunodeficiency virus: case report. *J. Neurosurgery.* 1999; 44(1): 199–202.

[4] Deyrup AT, Lee VK, Hill CE, et al. Epstein-Barr virus-associated smooth muscle tumors are distinctive mesenchymal tumors reflecting multiple infection events: a clinicopathologic and molecular analysis of 29 tumors from 19 patients. *Am. J. Surg. Pathol.* 2006; 30:75–82.

[5] Lee ES, Locker J, Nalesnik M, et al. The association of Epstein-Barr virus with smooth-muscle tumors occurring after organ transplantation. *N Engl. J. Med.* 1995; 332:19–25.

[6] McClain KL, Leach CT, Jenson HB, et al. Association of Epstein-Barr virus with leiomyosarcomas in children with AIDS. *N. Engl. J. Med.* 1995; 332:12–18.

[7] Sivendran S, Vidal CI, Barginear MF. Primary intracranial leiomyosarcoma in an HIV-infected patient. *Int. J. Clin. Oncol.* 2011; 16:63–66.

[8] Brown HG, Burger PC, Olivi A, Sills AK, Barditch-Crovo PA, Lee RR. Intracranial leiomyosarcoma in a patient with AIDS. *Neuroradiology.* 1999; 41:35–39.

[9] Lerdlum S, Lalitanantpong S, Numkarunarunrote N, Chaowanapanja P, Suankratay C, Shuangshoti S. MR imaging of CNS leiomyosarcoma in AIDS patients. *J. Med. Assoc Thai.* 2004; 87: Suppl 2S152–S160.

[10] Litofsky NS, Pihan G, Corvi F, Smith TW. Intracranial leiomyosarcoma: a neuro-oncological consequence of acquired immunodeficiency syndrome. *J. Neurooncol.* 1998; 40:179–183.

[11] Brown HG, Burger PC, Olivi A, et al. Intracranial leiomyosarcoma in a patient with AIDS. *Neuroradiology.* 1999; 41:35–39.

[12] Wong KH, Chan KC, Lee SS, et al. Epstein-Barr virus-associated smooth muscle tumor in patients with acquired immunodeficiency syndrome. *J. Microbiol Immunol Infect.* 2007; 40:173–177.

[13] Ritter AM, Amaker BH, Graham RS, Broaddus WC, Ward JD. Central nervous system leiomyosarcoma in the patients with acquired immunodeficiency syndrome. *J. Neurosurg.* 2000; 92:688–692.

[14] Takei H, Powell S, Rivera A. Concurrent occurrence of primary intracranial Epstein-Barr virus-associated leiomyosarcoma and Hodgkin lymphoma in a young adult. *J Neurosurg.* 2013; 119(2):499-503.

[15] Niwa J, Hashi K, Minase T. Radiation induced intracranial leiomyosarcoma: its histopathological features. *Acta Neurochir.* 1996; 138(12): 470–471.

[16] Toh CH, Wong HF, Jung SM, et al. Radiation-induced skull base leiomyosarcoma presenting with intracerebral hemorrhage. *Br. J. Radiol.* 2007; 80:e212–e215.

[17] Virtanen A, Pukkala E, Auvinen A. Incidence of bone and soft tissue sarcoma after radiotherapy: A cohort study of 295,712 Finnish cancer patients. *Int. J. Cancer.* 2006; 118:1017–1021.

[18] Jhas S, Henriques L, Hawkins C, Bouffet E, Rutka JT. An intracranial leiomyosarcoma in a child with neurofibromatosis type 1. *Can. J. Neurol. Sci.* 2009; 36(4): 491-495.

[19] Skullerud K, Stenwig AE, Brandtzaeg P, Nesland JM, Kerty E, Langmoen I, Saeter G. Intracranial primary leiomyosarcoma arising in a teratoma of the pineal area. *Clin. Neuropathol.* 1995; 14(4): 245–248.

[20] Mathieson CS, St George EJ, Stewart W, Sastry J, Jamal S. Primary intracranial leiomyosarcoma: a case report and review of the literature. *Childs Nerv Syst.* 2009; 25:1013–1017.

[21] Almubaslat M, Stone JC, Liu L, Xiong Z. Primary intracranial leiomyosarcoma in an immunocompetent patient. *Clin. Neuropathol.* 2011; 30:154–157.

[22] Aeddula NR, Pathireddy S, Samaha T, Ukena T, Hosseinnezhad A. Primary intracranial leiomyosarcoma in an immunocompetent adult. *J. Clin. Oncol.* 2011; 29:e407–e410.

[23] Fujimoto Y, Hirato J, Wakayama A, Yoshimine T. Primary intracranial leiomyosarcoma in an immunocompetent patient: case report. *J. Neurooncol.* 2011; 103:785–790.

[24] Kelley BC, Arnold PM, Grant JA, Newell KL. Primary intracranial β-human chorionic gonadotropin-producing leiomyosarcoma in a 2-year-old immunocompetent child. *J. Neurosurg Pediatr.* 2012; 10(2):121-125.

[25] Hussain S, Nanda A, Fowler M, Ampil FL, Burton GV. Primary intracranial leiomyosarcoma: report of a case and review of the literature. *Sarcoma.* 2006; 2006:52140.

[26] Lee TT, Page LK. Primary cerebral leiomyosarcoma. *Clin. Neurol. Neurosurg.* 1997; 99:210–212.

[27] Asai A, Yamada H, Murata S, Matsuno A, Tsutsumi K, Takemura T, Matsutani M, Takakura K. Primary leiomyosarcoma of the dura mater. Case report. *J. Neurosurg.* 1988; 68: 308–311.

[28] Louis DN, Richardson EP Jr, Dickersin GR, Petrucci DA, Rosenberg AE, Ojemann RG. Primary intracranial leiomyosarcoma. Case report. *J. Neurosurg.*1989; 71(2): 279–282.

[29] Anderson WR, Cameron JD, Tsai SH. Primary intracranial leiomyosarcoma. Case report with ultrastructural study. *J. Neurosurg.* 1980; 53: 401–405.

[30] Ali Y, Kehinde EO, Makar R, Al-Awadi KA, Anim JT. Leiomyosarcoma complicating chronic inflammation of the testis. *Med. Princ Pract.* 2002; 11: 157–160.

[31] Myoui A, Aozasa K, Iuchi K, Mori T, Yamamoto S, Kuratsu S, Ohsawa M, Ono K, Matsumoto K. Soft tissue sarcoma of the pleural cavity. *Cancer.* 1991; 68: 1550–1554.

[32] Li NY. Primary leiomyosarcoma of the pineal gland - a case report. *Zhonghua Zhong Liu Za Zhi.* 1987; 9:463–464.

[33] Eckhardt BP, Brandner S, Zollikofer CL, Wentz KU. Primary cerebral leiomyosarcoma in a child. *Pediatr. Radiol.* 2004; 34:495–498.

[34] Ceballos KM, Nielsen GP, Selig MK, O'Connell JX. Is anti-hcaldesmon useful for distinguishing smooth muscle and myofibroblastic tumors? An immunohistochemical study. *Am. J. Clin. Pathol.* 2000; 114:746–753.

[35] Sugita Y, Shigemori M, Harada H, et al. Primary meningeal sarcoma with leiomyoblastic differentiation: a proposal for a new subtype of primary meningeal sarcoma. *Am. J. Surg. Pathol.* 2000; 24:1273–1278.

[36] Rodriguez FJ, Scheithauer BW, Abell-Aleff PC, Elamin E, Erlandson RA. Low grade malignant peripheral nerve sheath tumor with smooth muscle differentiation. *Acta Neuropathol.* 2007; 113:705–709.

[37] Jain A, Sajeevan KV, Babu KG, Lakshmaiah KC. Chemotherapy in adult soft tissue sarcoma. *Indian J. Cancer.* 2009; 46:274–287.

In: Leiomyosarcoma
Editor: Rosemary H. Leach
ISBN: 978-1-63117-940-2

Chapter 6

Adult Urologic Leiomyosarcomas

Manuel Soto-Delgado, M.D.[1,*], Pastora Beardo-Villar, M.D.[1], David Corrales-Mateo, M.D.[2] and Álvaro Juárez-Soto, M.D.[1]

[1]Department of Urology of the Jerez Hospital, Spain
[2]Department of Pathology of the Virgen del Rocío Hospital, Spain

Abstract

Sarcomas represent a rare class of soft tissue cancers that can occur anywhere in the body. Soft tissue sarcomas represent 0.7% of all malignant tumors. Urologic primary sarcomas are extremely rare. They can arise from the testes, paratesticular tissues, penis, bladder, prostate, kidneys and retroperitoneal tissue. The most common type is a leiomyosarcoma (LMS), but other types of sarcomas can occur including liposarcomas, rhabdomyosarcomas, and fibrosarcomas. The purpose of this review is to present the epidemiology and possible risk factors in each of the urogenital sites, together with clinical presentation and imaging modalities that can assist in diagnosing LMS. Also presented are histological diagnosis and the immunohistochemical use of myogenic markers (h-caldesmon, desmin and muscle-specific actin) to help define smooth or skeletal muscle differentiation in soft tissue tumors (skeletal alpha actin, myogenin, MyoD1 and myoglobin). Current treatment options for genitourinary tumors are addressed: surgery, radiation therapy, chemotherapy and new targets such as antiangiogenic therapy. This review also examines the systemic approaches currently used, or which are under evaluation, to improve the outcome of patients with this disease.

Introduction

Soft tissue sarcomas represent 0.7% of the malignant tumors. Primary urologic sarcomas are extremely rare. In a series considered by the authors as the biggest in Europe at the time

[*] Email: sotodelgadomanuel@gmail.com.

of its publication in 2005, 8 institutions in Italy had collected 22 cases over a period of 19 years. However, a larger series containing 131 cases treated over a period of 26 years have been collected in the Memorial Sloan-Kettering Cancer Center of New York [1].

Due to the rarity of these tumors, it is difficult to obtain clinical experience with this type of neoplasia, even in the large Centers [1].

Of all the soft tissue sarcomas, approximately 5-10% are leiomyosarcomas which is the sub-type most commonly observed among the urologic sarcomas.

Whether because of its origin in the cells of organs or by direct spread from tumors originating in adjacent structures, leiomyosarcoma is a disease of rare occurrence in urology.

The urologic sarcomas can proceed from the testicles, paratesticular tissue, penis, bladder, prostate, kidney, seminal vesicles, or retroperitoneal soft tissue.

In this chapter we describe the different urologic leiomyosarcomas.

Renal and Retroperitoneal Leiomyosarcoma

Primary sarcomas constitute from 0.8 to 2.7% of all renal tumors in adults [2]. Amongst the renal sarcomas, leiomyosarcoma is the most common histological subtype, accounting for 50–60% of all cases [3]. Renal sarcomas may arise from the smooth muscle fibers of renal parenchyma, renal capsule, renal pelvis, or renal vessels [4]. It is essentially a tumor of adults, or the elderly, but cases have also been reported in children [5].

Clinical presentation is very similar to more common renal malignancies, and consists of flank pain and mass with or without hematuria, weight loss, and an abdominal mass [6]. It can sometimes present as spontaneous rupture of the kidney [7]. Originally, the differential diagnosis included renal cell carcinoma and, sometimes, invasive transitional cell carcinoma.

The radiologic assessments-of-choice are computerized axial thoraco-abdominal tomography and nuclear magnetic resonance [8].

They have a tendency to re-occur locally and to metastasize early via the hematogenous route [8]. Leiomyosarcomas, metastasizing to lungs, liver, small intestine, and colon have been discussed in the literature. However, renal leiomyosarcomas with colon segment adhesion, but without any microscopic evidence of metastases, are rare.

Treatment of leiomyosarcoma consists of radical nephrectomy. Surgery, followed by chemotherapy and radiation therapy, has been recommended and, considering the aggressive nature of the neoplasm, the success achieved has been limited.

Macroscopically, the tumors resemble leiomyomas, with their well-circumscribed margins. However, in the neighboring areas there are signs of necrosis, hemorrhagia and cystic degeneration. Microscopically, characteristics of smooth muscle tumor with spindle-form cells, blunt without apparent nucleus and moderate eosinophilic cytoplasm are described together with indicators of non-necrotic malignancy, such as nuclear pleomorphism and elevated mitotic index.

Immunohistochemically, the tumor cells show positivity to muscle actin (SMA) desmin and vimentin. The epithelial membrane antigen (EMA) is positive, while the pancytokeratin and high molecular weight cytokeratin (34b E12) are negative [9] (Figures 1 and 2).

The surgical strategy in renal and retroperitoneal leiomyosarcoma involves, in the first place, assessing the resectability of the tumor. To obtain a margin that is free of disease it may be necessary to resect parts of neighboring organs, with an important intra-operative margin of safety i.e., being aware at all times of the vascular structures in the resection. According to the classification of Mingoli, the origin of the inferior vena cava (IVC) is further divided into three levels, with respect to hepatic and renal veins: Level I, lower level (IVC below the renal veins); Level II, middle level (renal veins to hepatic veins, most frequently affected); Level III, upper level (entry of hepatic veins up to the level of the diaphragm); and level IV (extends inwards to right atrium) [10].

In renal, or in retroperitoneal leiomyosarcoma, the middle portion of the IVC (level II) is most frequently involved. Leiomyosarcomas of the IVC are extremely rare and, usually, they have a slow growth so symptoms may be absent in early stages of the disease.

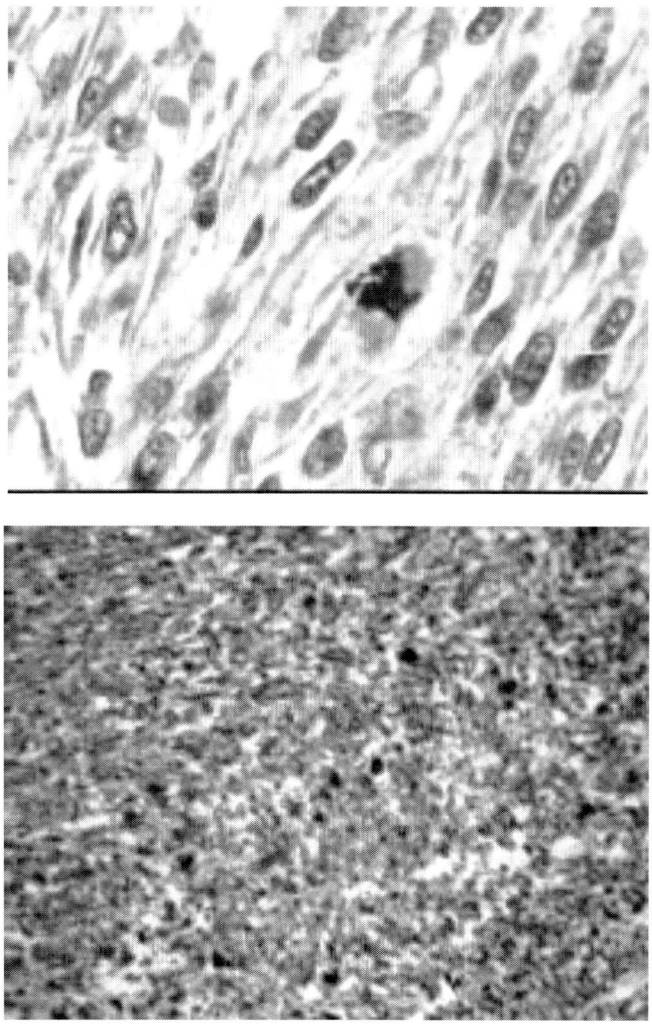

Figures 1 and 2. Renal leiomyosarcoma.

However, even with extensive IVC involvement, severe venous obstructive symptoms are not often seen, probably because of the development of extensive venous collaterals, which maintain adequate blood flow around the obstruction [11].

The reconstructive regimen depends on the affected IVC segment, the availability of retroperitoneal collateral circulation, and the invasion of adjacent structures which are especially dictated by the involvement of unilateral or bilateral renal veins. There are several options available for the management of Level II IVC including primary repair, autologous patching, ligation, or reconstruction with a prosthetic graft. Extensive venous involvement and large tumor size often preclude short segment resection with simple repair or patching. Daylami et al. suggested that the resection of IVC below the hepatic veins should require no IVC reconstruction due to the abundant collateral circulation; the secondary lower extremity edema could be transitory, well tolerated, and generally safe, especially in those with pre-operative IVC thrombosis. The advantage is that the IVC ligation can reduce surgical operation time, graft infection, high output cardiac failure by creating a fistula, and the need for long-term anticoagulation [12]. However, the majority of research groups prefer to perform vascular reconstruction. Kieffer et al. [13] used a proximal pressure reading of 30 mm Hg (or more) in the IVC as an indication for caval reconstruction; and found reconstruction to be necessary in most cases. Polytetrafluoroethylene (PTFE) patch is the most commonly used prosthetic material, and which has been shown to be a suitable replacement for the IVC. Infections and graft thrombosis are the 2 major complications of this type of reconstruction, but both are rare. Graft thrombosis may or may not have any clinical importance. Methods used to decrease its incidence include the use of ring-reinforced PTFE to prevent compression, short-term anticoagulation, and placement of an arterio-venous fistula to augment flow. PTFE graft infection after IVC replacement has been shown to occur, but rarely. The treatment is usually conservative but, in some cases, the graft must be removed.

Vascular prostheses have been recommended to replace the affected renal vessels; the objective being to minimize the post-operative occurrence of acute renal failure [14]. If this option is not feasible, restoration of flow to the right renal vein by re-implantation (or pelvic kidney autologous transplantation) is mandatory to maintain right kidney function. But, this is optional for the left renal vein because of the left kidney's considerable collateral drainage through the adrenal, inferior phrenic, gonadal and paravertebral vessels.

Peri- and post-operative complications associated with resection and reconstruction of the IVC also include general complications such as pneumonia, pleural effusion and cardiac arrest. Published mortality rates are extremely variable (0-11.1%). However, the need for extensive surgery, with relatively good outcomes, has been proposed by various groups. According to Tanaka et al. [15] and Yazici et al. [16], the extent of tumor length is not an increased risk factor for adverse survival potential. Likewise, Chiappini et al. [17] state that tumor extension into the IVC, to whatever degree, is not associated with an adverse prognosis, provided a complete resection is undertaken.

The reported comparative survival of renal LMS is about 25% (5-year overall survival) to 60% (5-year cause-specific survival) with a median overall survival of 25 months. Radical resections, tumor size < 5 cm, low histologic grade, and negative lymph node metastasis are all associated with better prognoses.

Emerging therapies: Pazopanib is a multi-targeted inhibitor of tyrosine kinase which has been approved for use in renal cell carcinoma, ovarian cancer and, more recently, soft tissue sarcomas (STS) [18]. It was shown, initially, to have significant responses in the phase II setting in the treatment of leiomyosarcoma, synovial sarcoma and other STS [19]. As a result of a recently concluded phase III study, STS has become an approved indication [20]. Its indication for leiomyosarcoma, synovial sarcoma and other non-GIST sarcomas has provided a new treatment option for this group of rare tumors.

Bladder Leiomyosarcoma

The sarcoma is a mesenchymatous tumor of the bladder, and is the histologic type that is the most frequent leiomyosarcoma, and which represents 0.1% of bladder cancers. Around 100 cases have been published in the literature on vesicle leiomyosarcoma. This type of tumor is more frequent in males (2:1 with females) and the majority of cases are aged between 60 and 80 years [21]. In relation to its localization, 50% are encountered in the bladder dome and 25% in the lateral sides [22].

There have not been any risk factors identified specifically for this type of tumor. In revising the literature, the possible risk factors for vesicle leiomyosarcoma we identified were: mutations in the retinoblastoma gene (10 cases published) [23], the use of immunosuppressant treatment with cyclophosphamide and pelvic radiotherapy. Von Recklinghausen neurofibromatosis has been related to the presence of leiomyosarcomas, as well [24].

Many authors have proposed that the most frequent presentation symptom is macroscopic hematuria. Other symptoms and signs that we have encountered on physical examination are dysuria, polakiuria, abdominal pain, obstruction of the upper urinary tract, and pelvic mass [24].

Diagnosis is with the usual techniques (echography, cystoscopy), although none of these indicate the presence of leiomyosarcoma. Cystoscopy shows a tumor with the form of a fungus, with areas of central shedding and calcified encrustation [25].

The definitive diagnosis can only be done using surgical exploration and the subsequent histopathology evaluation following the excision of the lesion using transurethral resection [26].

As occurs with all transurethral excisions of vesicular tumors, it is important to confirm that the biopsies are wide and deep, given that multiple and superficial biopsies are very low sensitivity in the anatomo-pathologic diagnosis of vesicle leiomyosarcoma. Histologically, it consists of spindle cells with anaplastic characteristics, and elevated mitosis number [27].

Differential diagnosis of leiomyosarcoma of the bladder includes the inflamed myofibroblastic tumor, the urothelial sarcomatoid carcinoma, leiomyoma, and inflamed pseudo-tumor [28].

Immunohistochemical diagnosis confirms muscular origin, the use of immunohistochemistry methods being necessary when dealing with very non-differentiated tumor. In these, the presence of specific muscle desmin, vimentin and actin confirm the diagnosis of leiomyosarcoma. Also, positivity to these epithelial membrane antigens and to cytokeratin has been described. For some authors immunohistochemistry staining is necessary. Electron microscopy shows a prominent rough endoplasmic reticulum and abundant intra-cytoplasmic filaments [27]. (Figures 3 and 4).

Once the diagnosis of leiomyosarcoma has been established, it is important to segregate this type of tumor into 2 distinct prognostic sub-types according to the mitotic activity, the nuclear atypia, and the grade of tumor necrosis [28].

The two largest series of patients with extensive follow-up are that of Mills et al. and Martin et al., who proposed to differentiate between leiomyosarcomas of high- and low-risk as a function of the number of mitoses per 10 high-power fields (HPF) and nuclear atypia. If the presentation is of <5 mitoses per 10 HPF and slight-to-moderate nuclear atypia, the tumor is low-risk and if, on the contrary, there are >5 mitoses per 10HPF, this is considered high-risk. The mean survival is of 7 months for high-risk, and 65 months for low-risk tumors [29, 30].

The study at the Mayo Clinic defined tumors of low risk as those with slight-moderate nuclear atypia, <5 mitoses per 10 HPF and <25% tumor necrosis. Low-risk leiomyosarcomas that infiltrate the muscle cap of the bladder, have an increased risk of metastases and of local relapse [28].

Nevertheless, the most important diagnostic factor appears to be the absence of positive surgical margins [31].

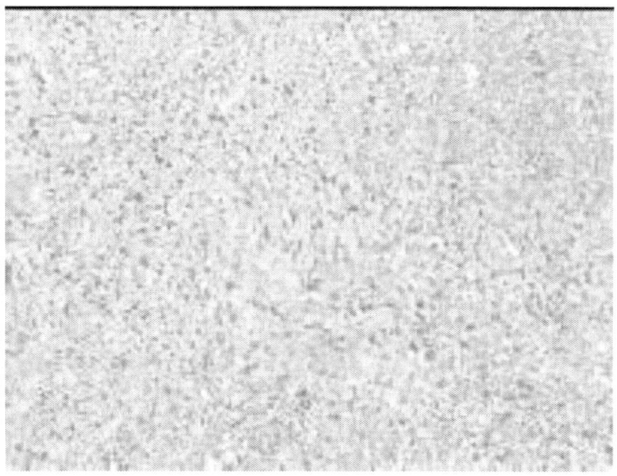

Figures 3 and 4. Vesicle leiomyosarcoma.

According to the large series published to date, local recurrence of vesicle leiomyosarcomas is around 16%; most frequently detected in the pelvis. The appearance of distant metastases is around 53%; the most common sites being lung, liver, bone and brain [32]. In imaging studies, positron emission tomography (PET/CAT) with

^{18}fluordeoxyglucose is routinely used in the staging and evaluation of response to treatment of the leiomyosarcomas. However, the urinary bladder is in an anatomically difficult site to evaluate using this technique because of the urinary excretion of the ^{18}fluordeoxyglucose. There has been only one case described in the literature in which this technique was useful in evaluating the loco-regional spread of the tumor, or distant metastases [21].

Due to the low incidence of cases, there is no consensus regarding treatment options for patients affected by vesicle leiomyosarcoma. Minimally-invasive treatments such as transurethral resection, or laser fulguration, followed by chemotherapy or adjuvant radiotherapy, have been used for patients with small lesions. Some authors propose partial cystectomy in those cases in which tumor site enables excision of the tumor with appropriate surgical margins of at least 2 cm of healthy tissue. Because of the potential invasiveness of these lesions, the treatment-of-choice for this type of tumor is radical cystectomy (including extirpation of the uterus and vaginal segment) [31].

There is no consensus regarding complementary therapy, with or without adjuvant therapy. It is considered that they are not radiosensitive. Hence, only in cases of positive surgical margins is adjuvant radiotherapy indicated. Chemotherapy (such as polychemotherapy with doxorubicin, cyclophosphamide, cisplatin, docetaxel) is reserved for cases of metastatic disease [27, 31].

Local recurrences need to be treated with systemic chemotherapy and/or external pelvic radiotherapy because salvage surgery in these cases have proved to be ineffective, with a mean survival of 20 months post-surgery [32].

In general, the behavior of these tumors is very aggressive, with <40% of patients tumor-free after resection.

Prostate Leiomyosarcoma

Prostate sarcoma is an extremely rare and highly aggressive neoplasm that is responsible for <1% (0.7%) of primary prostate malignancies in adults [33]. Owing to its rarity, knowledge of the clinical features, management, and prognosis has been derived, primarily, from case reports, small single-institution case series, and of assessments of other genitourinary sites [34-36].

In studies with large numbers of cases [37-39], prostate sarcoma in adults presents in relatively young males of between 40-70 years of age, with a large tumor size at the time of diagnosis. Leiomyosarcoma is the predominant sub-type, and with a high percentage of high-grade sarcoma. In these series, the symptoms resulting from obstruction of the lower urinary tract are the predominant clinical presentation.

In contrast to prostate adenocarcinoma, the prostate-specific antigen level is generally not elevated in patients with prostate sarcoma. This can be explained by the non-epithelial origin of the sarcoma. Initial diagnosis can be established, in most patients, pre-operatively using image-guided needle biopsy [37, 39].

Generally, prostate leiomyosarcomas in adults follow a very aggressive course, with a variable survival time and poor prognosis [39]. This is associated with a high incidence of local relapse and development of metastases, located essentially in lung, liver and bone [40].

Once prostate leiomyosarcoma is diagnosed, and due to the high incidence of metastases, it is mandatory to perform CAT scan of the thorax-abdomen-pelvis and bone scintigraphy in the pre-operative staging, and post-operative follow-up.

Only a few studies have examined the predictors of outcome for adult prostate sarcoma. Sexton et al. [37] concluded that negative surgical margins and the absence of metastatic disease at presentation were predictive of favorable survival. This conclusion was also supported by Vandoros et al. [40].

Several studies have confirmed that surgery of curative intent offers the best chance of survival in patients presenting with non-metastatic disease. However, a high percentage of patients with non-metastatic disease have cancer that is deemed non-resectable at presentation. Surgical resection with negative margins should be the goal of surgery, even if it is sometimes difficult to achieve. One of the essential challenges facing urologic oncologists is radical resection with organ preservation because prostate sarcoma is prone to adjacent organ invasion; the bladder being the most common organ. Hence, radical cystoprostatectomy is the most-used technique by those authors with the most experience of prostate leiomyosarcoma [37, 38, 41].

Sexton et al. [37] suggested a survival advantage for patients treated with a combined multimodal approach, even if surgery had been the mainstay of treatment. Hence, the application of aggressive chemotherapy and radiotherapy should be considered [42]. The rarity of adult prostate sarcoma has hindered the critical evolution of treatment modalities, and differences of opinions regarding standard treatment recommendations remain unresolved. We believe that surgical resection with negative margins, when feasible, plays the leading role in the management of prostate leiomyosarcoma and should be attempted in all adult patients with non-metastatic disease. A prospective, randomized comparison of a large patient series is necessary to clarify the contribution of chemotherapy and radiotherapy in conjunction with surgery, on the outcomes of these patients [39].

Paratesticular Leiomyosarcoma

Paratesticular leiomyosarcoma in the adult is very rare, but is the most frequent histologic type of paratesticular sarcoma. The mean of the few cases published on paratesticular leiomyosarcoma was 60 years and, in the majority of cases, the age ranged between 40 and 70 years [43]. The etiology of paratesticular leiomyosarcoma is uncertain, although some authors suggest that local irradiation in infancy could be a potential cause [44].

The vast majority occur in the spermatic cord, while epididymal location is extremely rare [45]. Clinically, the majority of the paratesticular leiomyosarcomas present as a scrotal or inguino-scrotal mass of slow growth, solid, irregular, negative to trans-illumination, and can be accompanied by pain, and occasionally accompanied by a small hydrocele. Echography is the most-used diagnostic method, and which shows a solid mass but with blood flow (Figure 5). The studies of spread include thoraco-abdomino-pelvic computerized axial tomography (CAT) and magnetic resonance (MR) of the inguinal-scrotal region [46]. Paratesticular leiomyosarcoma is difficult to diagnose pre-operatively, and the definitive diagnosis requires histologic examination of extirpated tissue to observe the differentiation of smooth muscle morphology, and immunohistochemistry [45] (Figures 6 and 7).

Other rare tumors, such as leiomyoma, fibrous mesothelioma, various fibrous tumors and pseudotumors need to be considered in the differential diagnosis of paratesticular leiomyosarcomas.

Histologically, leiomyosarcoma is characterized by typical features of spindle cell neoplasm with a fascicular architecture, atypical cytology foci, and mitoses. A considerable level of necrosis is generally observed in high-grade tumors. Neoplastic cells inmunostain for smooth muscle actin, muscle-specific actin, and desmin. Further, h-caldesmon may be used to confirm smooth muscle differentiation, and myogenicity to exclude spindle cell rhabdomyosarcoma. The diagnosis of malignancy is made mainly on the basis of mitosis number. Generally, in this site, any mitotic activity with nuclear atypia is considered a marker of malignancy [47-49]. The clinical and biological behavior of paratesticular leiomyosarcoma is generally unpredictable. The main prognostic factors of leiomyosarcoma are site, size, the grade of primitive tumors, and nodal or distant metastasis.

The optimum local and systemic treatment of these tumors is controversial, but radical inguinal orchiectomy with a high ligation of the spermatic cord is the standard surgical treatment.

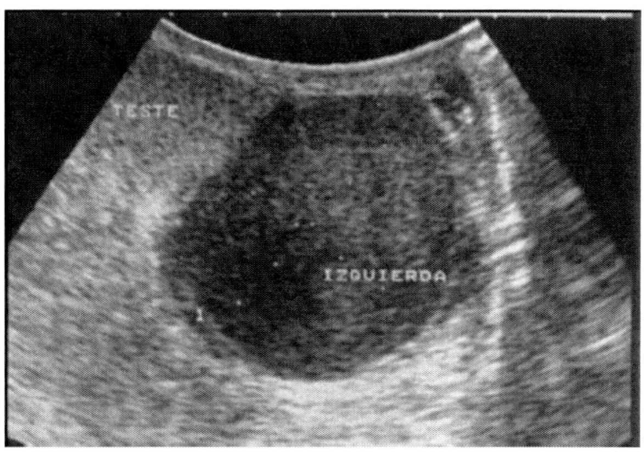

Figure 5. Echography image of paratesticular leiomyosarcoma displacing the left testicle upwards.

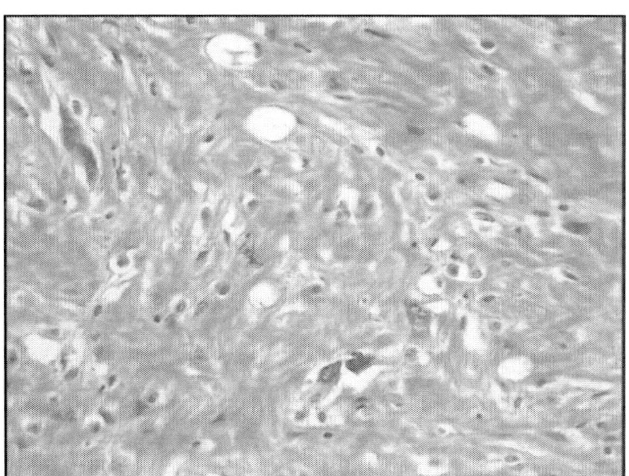

Figure 6. Proliferation of sarcoma cells with marked atypia and differentiation towards smooth muscle.

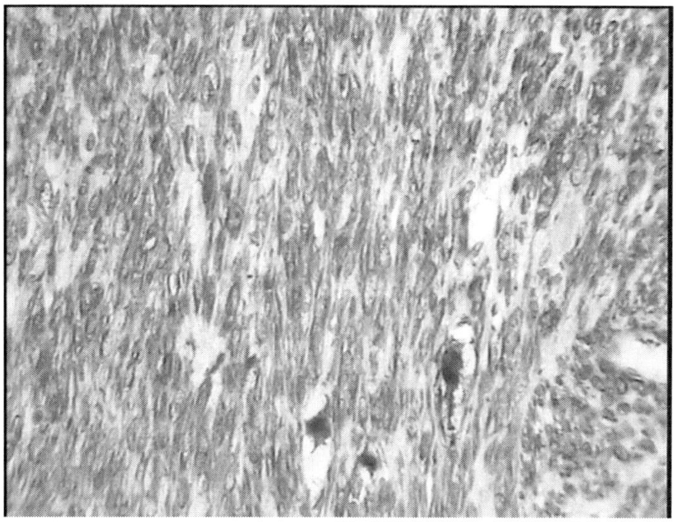

Figure 7. Intense positivity of sarcoma cells against smooth muscle-actin.

However, even after appropriate surgery with negative margins, between 25 and 37% have microscopic persistence of the disease, and recurrence [46].

Fagundes et al. communicated the absence of local recurrence in patients receiving adjuvant radiotherapy after orchiectomy, compared to those who were treated with orchiectomy alone. These results indicated that a simple excision is inadequate and that adjuvant loco-regional radiotherapy after surgery should be recommended. Despite these findings, the benefits of post-operative radiotherapy with or without chemotherapy are not conclusive, due to the small number of cases [Author: reference #50 is missing from the sequence] [50].

The principal pattern of spread of paratesticular leiomyosarcomas is by continuity across the inguinal canal and, from this, to the abdominal cavity. Less frequent are the hematogenous and/or lymphatic routes. This can explain why retroperitoneal lymphadectomy has not demonstrated changes in the prognosis, nor survival to date [46].

Intra-Testicular Primary Leiomyosarcoma

Intra-testicular leiomyosarcoma is an extremely rare tumor; only 10 adult cases having been described in the literature. The age range in the patients varies between 30 and 76 years, with a mean age of 50 years [51]. The etiology of testicular leiomyosarcoma is not known. However, risk factors such as high doses of anabolic steroids, chronic inflammation of the testes, and irradiation of the testicular field have been described in the few cases that have been collected [52-54]. Assessment of tumor markers (alfaproteín, chorionic gonadotropin beta, and lactate dehydrogenase) for paratesticular leiomyosarcoma, especially in the evaluation of metastatic disease, is limited [51]. Based on a review of the literature, the treatment for intra-testicular leiomyosarcoma is radical orchiectomy, with a follow-up using radiologic examination in case of stage I. There are no data on treatment of tumors in stages

II-III. Radiotherapy is not effective for the leiomyosarcomas, although additional chemotherapy is required in advanced cases [51].

Recently, gemcitabine and docetaxel have been used as chemotherapy agents in the treatment of metastatic uterine leiomyosarcoma, with high levels of response [55].

It is necessary to explore the use of new agents for the treatment of metastatic testicular leiomyosarcomas. New clinical investigations are required to establish the treatment of intra-testicular leiomyosarcoma [50-52].

Leiomyosarcoma of the Seminal Vesicles

Pelvic sarcomas in males are infrequent, and the most common site is the prostate; representing 0.1-0.2% of all prostate tumors [56].

Primary tumors of the seminal vesicles are rare, and the majority of cases described correspond to carcinomas; the exceptions being malignant mesenchymal tumors. Many of the cases described have been questioned with respect to their origin. The tendency of the neoplasias to invade neighboring structures, places in doubt whether it is the seminal vesicle primary tumor invading neighboring structures that is being treated, or whether it is malignant mesenchymal tumor of the retro-vesicle space surrounding and growing into the seminal vesicles [56-58]. Given that primary malignant tumors of the seminal vesicle end by infiltrating the adjacent structures (prostate, bladder, ureter, large intestine), and taking into account that the pathologic process in these structures are more frequent than those in the seminal vesicle, there appears to be a consensus in the literature to label as retro-vesicle mass all large-sized new formations located in the posterior aspect of the bladder [59].

These retro-vesicle masses not only represent specific symptomatology, but these symptoms appear when the lesion reaches a large size (pelvic pain, and symptoms of urinary or rectal obstruction) [56, 57]. Leiomyosarcomas represent 5-10% of soft tissue sarcomas, and their localization in seminal vesicle is exceptional. They are tumors of adult life and, in general, more frequent in females. The criteria used for the diagnosis of malignancy in smooth muscle are size, cellularity, nuclear atypia, necrosis and mitotic activity. Given the few cases described of leiomyosarcoma in the seminal vesicle, the mitosis number from which smooth muscles tumor is considered malignant, is uncertain. Retroperitoneal leiomyosarcomas are considered very aggressive tumors which cause death not only by metastatic spread to the lung and liver, but also by its loco-regional spread [60]. In the few cases of seminal vesicle leiomyosarcoma described in the literature, complete surgical extirpation had been performed, and the patients described as free of disease for periods varying between 1 and 2 years following surgery [56-58].

Leiomyosarcoma are malignant tumors with poor prognosis and complete surgical excision is the treatment of choice.

Leiomyosarcoma of the Penis

Tumors of the penis represent 0.4% to 0.6% of the total malignant neoplasias in the USA, Europe, Africa, and in some countries of South America. From these, sarcoma of the penis represents 5% of the total. Primary leiomyosarcoma of the penis is an extremely rare tumor. There have been only 47 cases reported in the worldwide literature [61-63].

The age range is very variable between 6 and 80 years, and only 3 cases have been described in young people; the majority between the 3rd and 5th decade of life. The clinical picture is one of indolence. It presents as a nodule in the majority of cases and, depending on the site, as superficial or profound [63, 64].

Mc Kenzie et al. [65] were the first in recognizing 2 types of leiomyosarcoma, the superficial and the profound. The former, developed from smooth muscle cells from glandular surface dermal layers and/or distal third of the penis, are generally asymptomatic and have a lower grade of malignancy, with a slight tendency to invade more profound structures, and with urethral involvement specific to the exploration. With the latter, it is argued that they develop from smooth muscle cells from the cavernous and/or spongy bodies, advancing from the base of the penis up to the perineum, in the majority of reported cases. With a very aggressive behavior and greater tendency to affect the urethra, produce symptoms and to present greater potential for metastases, a total penectomy is recommended. The procedure-of-choice involves the perineal meatus, but the percentage mortality at 2 years from the 1st consultation continues to be high (mean of 9 months), with 52% survival [65].

Ganglionar disease is very rare. Lymphadectomy is not recommended. Case presentation is only of concomitant indication of disease at distance, principally the lung. Other metastatic sites are liver and head. Recurrences are treatment with excision or amputation, and can be accompanied with adjuvant chemotherapy or radiotherapy [66].

The most important prognosis factor is the form of initial presentation; superficial or profound [67].

Those that are superficial are treated with local excision, with disease-free margins. Those that are profound are treated by total or partial amputation of distal lesions, and radical penectomy in proximal lesions [68].

Patients with profound lesions have a greater tendency to relapse, and to develop metastatic disease (ganglion or distant) and, as such, radical penectomy is recommended.

Radiotherapy of the sarcomas has not shown improvement in survival in the few cases studied. There have not been clinical studies carried-out in which benefit of radiotherapy in leiomyosarcoma of the penis is demonstrated. Brachytherapy is being used in superficial lesions, but the results have not been described, as yet [69].

Chemotherapies with anthracyclines and etoposide have demonstrated slight-moderate benefit. However these last two modalities had been applied as palliative care in patients that could not be referred to surgery [70]. Due to the high incidence of recurrence with local excision, adjuvant radiotherapy and chemotherapy are recommended in these cases, despite there not being any increase in overall survival [71,72].

It is a disease with high recurrence and the current recommendations for these cases are to be radical and complementary with adjuvant radiotherapy, despite there not being any studies demonstrating that adjuvant radiotherapy diminishes the risk of recurrence. The follow-up should involve strict monitoring with chest x-rays because of the high recidivist index and the development of distant metastases [73-76].

References

[1] Froehner, M.; Schober, R. R.; Koch, R.; Lossnitzer, A.; Laniado, M.; Wirth, M. P. Adult urologic sarcoma: experience during 2 decades. *Urol. Oncol.*, 2013;31(7):985-989.

[2] Vogelzang, N. J.; Fremgen, A. M.; Guinan, P. D.; Chmiel, J. S.; Sylvester, J. L.; Sener, S. F. Primary renal sarcoma in adults. A natural history and management study by American Cancer Society, Illinois Division. *Cancer,* 1993;71:804-810.

[3] Srinivas, V.; Sogani, P. C.; Hajdu, S. I.; Whitmore, W. F. Jr. Sarcomas of the kidney. *J. Urol.*, 1984;132:13-16.

[4] Choudhury, M.; Singh, S. K.; Pujani, M.; Pathania, O. P. A case of leiomyosarcoma of kidney clinically and radiologically misdiagnosed as renal cell carcinoma. *Indian J. Cancer*, 2009;46:241-243.

[5] González-Crussi, F.; Baum, E. S. Renal sarcomas of childhood. A clinicopathologic and ultrastructural study. *Cancer,* 1983;51(5):898-912.

[6] Venkatesh, K.; Lamba-Saini, M.; Nivedith, S. R.; Krisnagiri C.; Babu, S. Primary Leiomyosarcoma of the kidney. *Patholog. Res. Int.,* 2010; 2010: 652398.

[7] Grasso, M.; Blanco, S.; Fortuna, F.; Crippa, S.; Di Bella, C. Spontaneous rupture of renal leiomyosarcoma in a 45-year-old woman. *Arch. Esp. Urol.*, 2004;57 (8):870–872.

[8] Martíınez-Cornelio, A.; Ramos-Salgado, F.; Hernández-Ramírez, D.; García-Álvarez, K. G.; Alvarado-Cabrero, I.; Hernández-Toriz, N. Leiomyosarcoma of the kidney: case report. *Cir. Cir.,* 2011;79 (3):282–285.

[9] Zamora-Varela, F. R.; Ponce-de León Ballesteros, F. Leiomiosarcoma renal. *Rev. Mex. Urol.,* 2012; 72 (6): 297-300.

[10] Mingoli, A.; Sapienza, P.; Cavallaro, A.; Di Marzo, L.; Burchi, C.; Giannarelli, D.; Feldhaus, R. J. The effect of extend of caval resection in the treatment of inferior vena cava leiomyosarcoma. *Anticancer Res.,* 1997;17:3877–3881.

[11] Dzsinich, C.; Gloviczki, P.; van Heerden, J. A.; Nagorney, D. M.; Pairolero, P. C.; Johnson, C. M.; Hallett, J. W. Jr.; Bower, T. C.; Cherry, K. J. Jr. Primary venous leiomyosarcoma: a rare but lethal disease. *J. Vasc. Surg.,* 1992; 15: 595-603.

[12] Daylami, R.; Amiri, A.; Goldsmith, B.; Troppmann, C.; Schneider, P. D.; Khatri, V. P. Inferior vena cava leiomyosarcoma: Is reconstruction necessary after resection. *J. Am. Coll. Surg.*, 2010;210:185–190.

[13] Kieffer, E.; Alaoui, M.; Piette, J. C.; Cacoub, P.; Chiche, L. Leiomyosarcoma of the inferior vena cava: experience in 22 cases. *Ann. Surg.*, 2006;244:289-295.

[14] Angiletta, D.; Fullone, M.; Greco, L.; Marinazzo, D.; Frontino, P.; Regina, G. Leiomyosarcoma of the inferior vena cava: resection and vascular reconstruction using a dacron graft and an Adam De Weese clip. Three-year follow-up. *Ann. Vasc. Surg.*, 2011;25:557. e5-9.

[15] Tanaka, M.; Fujimoto, K.; Okajima, E.; Tanaka, N.; Yoshida, K.; Hirao, Y. Prognostic factors of renal cell carcinoma with extension into inferior vena cava. *Int. J. Urol.*, 2008;15:394-398.

[16] Yazici, S.; Inci, K.; Bilen, C. Y.; Gudeloglu, A.; Akdogan, B.; Ertoy, D.; Kaynaroglu, V.; Demircin, M.; Ozen, H. Renal cell carcinoma with inferior vena cava thrombus: The Hacettepe experience. *Urol. Oncol.*, 2010;28:603-609.

[17] Chiappini, B.; Savini, C.; Marinelli, G.; Suárez, S. M.; Di Eusanio, M.; Fiorani, V.; Pierangeli, A. Cavoatrial tumor thrombus: single-stage surgical approach with profound hypothermia and circulatory arrest, including a review of the literature. *J. Thorac. Surg.*, 2002;124:684-688.

[18] Schutz, F. A.; Choueiri, T. K.; Sternberg, C. N. Pazopanib: Clinical development of a potent anti-angiogenic drug. *Crit. Rev. Oncol. Hematol.*, 2011;77:163-171.

[19] Deeks, E. D. Pazopanib: in advanced soft tissue sarcoma. *Drugs,* 2012;72:2129-2140.

[20] Van der Graaf, W. T.; Blay, J. Y.; Chawla, S. P.; Dong-Wan, K.; Bui-Nguygen, B.; Casali, P. G. Pazopanib for metastatic soft-tissue sarcoma (PALETTE): a randomised, double-blind, placebo-controlled phase 3 trial. *Lancet,* 2012;379:1879-1886.

[21] Makis, W.; Rakheja, R.; Nahal, A.; Hickeson, M.; Lisbona, R. Urinary bladder leiomyosarcoma. Staging with F-FDG PET/TC. *Clinical Nuclear Medicine,* 2013;38(5):218-222.

[22] Cruz-Guerra, N. A.; Fradejas-Rodríguez, A.; del Valle-Manteca, A.; Ursúa-Sarmiento, I.; Tarroc- Blanco, A. Bladder leiomyosarcoma: case report. *Arch. Esp. Urol.,* 2006;59(2):198-201.

[23] Minagawa, T.; Okaneya, T.; Kamigaito, M.; Nishizawa, S.; Ogawa, T.; Kawakami, M. Leiomyosarcoma of the urinary bladder in a patient with bilateral retinoblastoma. *Int. J. Urol.*, 2008;15:548-550.

[24] Gil-Fabra, J.; Fernández-Fernández, A.; Gracía-Marzo, A.; Soria-Ruiz, S.; Otero-Mauricio, G. Bladder leiomyosarcoma. Report of two cases. *Arch. Esp. Urol.,* 1996;49(1):59-62.

[25] Begara-Morillas, F.; Luengo-Alpuente, S.; Salinas-Casado, J.; Rapariz-González, M.; Hernandez- Villaverde, A.; Esteban-Fuertes, M.; Remezal M.; Sanz-Esponera J.; Resel-Estevez L. Leiomyosarcoma within a bladder diverticulum. *Actas Urol. Esp.,* 1995;19(4):337-340.

[26] Ataus, S.; Yaycioglu, O.; Demirkesen, O.; Uygun, N.; Yalcin, V.; Solok, V. Retrovesical Leiomyosarcoma. *Int. J. Urol.,* 2000;7(12):467-469.

[27] Rioja, J.; Rosell Costa, D.; Rincón Mayans, A.; Saiz Sansi, A.; Panizo Santos, A.; Berian Polo, J. M. Leiomiosarcoma vesical. Presentación de un nuevo caso y revisión de la literatura. *Actas Urol. Esp.,* 2009; 33(7): 816-821.

[28] Lee, T. K.; Miyamoto, H.; Osunkoya, A. O.; Guo, C. C.; Weiss, S. W.; Epstein, J. I. Smooth muscle neoplasms of the urinary bladder: A Clinicopathologic Study of 51 Cases. *Am. J. Surg. Pathol.,* 2010:34(4): 502-509.

[29] Mills, S. E.; Bova, G. S.; Wick, M. R.; Young, R. H. Leiomyosarcoma of the urinary bladder. A clinicopathologic and immunohistochemical study of 15 cases. *Am. J. Surg. Pathol.*, 1989;13:480–489.

[30] Martin, S. A.; Sears, D. L.; Sebo, T. J.; Lohse, C. M.; Cheville, J. C. Smooth muscle neoplasms of the urinary bladder: a clinicopathologic comparison of leiomyoma and leiomyosarcoma. *Am. J. Surg. Pathol.,* 2002; 26:292–300.

[31] Ricciardi, E.; Maniglio, P.; Schimberni, M.; Moscarini, M. A case of high-grade leiomyosarcoma of the bladder with delayed onset and very poor prognosis. *World J. Surg. Oncol.,* 2010;19(8):16. doi: 10.1186/ 1477-7819-8-16.

[32] Spiess, P. E.; Kassouf, W.; Steinberg, J. R.; Tuziak, T.; Hernandez, M.; Tibbs, R. F.; Czerniak, B.; Kamat, A. M.; Dinney, C. P.; Grossman, H. B. Review of the M. D. Anderson experience in the treatment of bladder sarcoma. *Urol. Oncol.*, 2007;25:38-45.

[33] Janet, N. L.; May, A. W.; Akins, R. S. Sarcoma of the prostate: a single institutional review. *Am. J. Clin. Oncol.*, 2009;32:27-29.

[34] Humphrey, P. A. Angiosarcoma of the prostate. *J. Urol.*, 2012; 187: 684-685.

[35] Ren, F. Y.; Lu, J. P.; Wang J., Ye J. J., Shao; C. W.; Wang, M. J. Adult prostate sarcoma: radiological clinical correlation. *Clin. Radiol.*, 2009;64:171-177.

[36] Boyle, H.; Flechon, A.; Droz, J. P. Treatment of uncommon malignant tumours of the bladder. *Curr. Opin. Urol.*, 2011;21:309-314.

[37] Sexton, W. J.; Lance, R. E.; Reyes, A. O.; Pisters, P. W.; Tu, S. M.; Pisters, L. L. Adult prostate sarcoma: the M. D. Anderson Cancer Center experience. *J. Urol.*, 2001;166:521-525.

[38] Dotan, Z. A.; Tal, R.; Golijanin, D.; Snyder, M. E.; Antonescu, C.; Brennan, M. F.; Russo, P. Adult genitourinary sarcoma: the 25-year Memorial Sloan-Kettering experience. *J. Urol.*, 2006;176:2033-2038.

[39] Wang, X.; Liu, L.; Tang, H.; Rao, Z.; Zhan, W.; Li, X.; Zeng, H.; Zhang, P.; Wei, B.; Lin, T.: Wei, Q.; Lu, Y.; Li, X. Twenty-five cases of adult prostate sarcoma treated at a high-volume institution from 1989 to 2009. *Urology,* 2013;82(1):160-165.

[40] Vandoros, G. P.; Manolidis, T.; Karamouzis, M. V.; Gkermpesi, M.; Lambropoulou, M.; Papatsoris, A. G.; Zachos, I.; Konstantinopulos, P. A. Leiomyosarcoma of the prostate: case report and review of 54 previously published cases. *Sarcoma,* 2008;2008:458709. doi: 10.1155/ 2008/458709. Epub 2008 Nov 18.

[41] Cheville, J. C.; Dundore, P. A.; Nascimento, A. G.; Meneses, M.; Kleer, E.; Farrow, G. M.; Bostwic, D. G. Leiomyosarcoma of the prostate: report of 23 cases. *Cancer,* 1995;76:1422-1427.

[42] Aragon-Ching, J. B.; Maki, R. G. Treatment of adult soft tissue sarcoma: old concepts, new insights, and potential for drug discovery. *Cancer Invest.*, 2012;30:300-308.

[43] Astigueta-Pérez, J. C.; Abad-Licham, M.; Pow-Sang Godoy, M.; Destefano-Urrutia, V.; Sánchez -Lihon, J. Adult paratesticular sarcomas. Management and evolution of the disease. *Actas Urol. Esp.*, 2009; 33(6): 639-645.

[44] Dalton, D. P.; Rushovich, A. M.; Victor, T. A.; Larson, R. Leiomyosarcoma of the scrotum in a man who had received scrotal irradiation as a child. *J. Urol.*, 1988;139;136-138.

[45] Evans, H. L.; Shipley, J. Smooth muscle tumors. In: Fletcher C. D. M., Unni K. K., and Mertens F., (Eds). Pathology and genetics of tumours of soft tissue and bone. Lyon: World Health Organization; 2002; pp. 131–134.

[46] Gigantito, V.; La Mantia, E.; Franco, R.; Cecere, S.; Rossetti, S.; Di Napoli, M.; Pisano, C.; Berretta, M.; Galzerano, A.; Botti, G.; Pignata, S.; Facchini, G. Testicular and testicular adnexa tumors in the elderly. *Anti-Cancer Drugs*, 2013;24:228–236.

[47] Hashimoto, H.; Daimaru, Y.; Tsuneyoshi, M.; Enjoji, M. Leiomyosarcoma of the external soft tissues. A clinicopathologic, immunohistochemical, and electron microscopic study. *Cancer,* 1986;57:2077–2088.

[48] Wile, A. G.; Evans, H. L.; Romsdahl, M. M. Leiomyosarcoma of soft tissue: a clinicopathologic study. *Cancer*, 1981;48:1022–1032.

[49] Folpe, A. L.; Weiss, S. W. Paratesticular soft tissue neoplasms. *Semin. Diagn. Pathol.*, 2000;17:307–318.

[50] Fagundes, M. A.; Zietman, A. L.; Althausen, A. F.; Coen, J. J.; Shipley, W. U.; The management of spermatic cord sarcoma. *Cancer,* 1996; 77: 1873–1876.

[51] Yoshimine, S.; Kono, H.; Nakagawa, K.: Kikuchi, E.; Miyajima, A.; Kameyama, K.; Mukai, M.; Oya, M. Primary intratesticular leiomyosarcoma. *CUAJ,* 2009;3(6):E74-E76.

[52] Froehner, M.; Fischer, R.; Leike, S.; Hakenberg, O. W.; Noack, B.; Wirth, M. P. Intratesticular leiomyosarcoma in a young man after high dose doping with Oral-Turinabol: a case report. *Cancer,* 1999;86:1571-1575.

[53] Ali, Y.; Kehinde, E. O.; Makar, R.; Al-Awadi, K. A.; Anim, J. T. Leiomyosarcoma complicating chronic inflammation of the testis. *Med. Princ. Pract.,* 2002;11:157-160.

[54] Canales, B. K.; Lukasewycz, S. J.; Manivel, J. C.; Pryor J. L. Postradiotherapy intratesticular leiomyosarcoma. *Urology*, 2005;66:657.

[55] Hensley, M. L.; Blessing, J. A.; Mannel, R.; Rose, P. G. Fixed-dose rate gemcitabine plus docetaxel as first-line therapy for metastatic uterine leiomyosarcoma: a Gynecologic Oncology Group phase II trial. *Gynecol. Oncol.*, 2008;109:329-334.

[56] Algaba, F.; Moreno, A.; Trias, I. Uropathology tumor. In: Tumors of the testis and its annexed, Chapter V. Barcelona: Grafos Press; 1996. P. 350-351.

[57] Agrawal, V.; Kumar, S.; Sharma, D.; Singh, U. R.; Gupta, A. Primary leiomyosarcoma of the seminal vesicle. *Int. J. Urol.,* 2004;11:253-255.

[58] Upreti, I., Bhargava, S. K.; Kumar, A. Imaging of primary leiomyosarcoma of the seminal vesicle. *Australas. Radiol.*, 2003;47: 70-72.

[59] Muentener, M.; Hailemariam, S.; Dubs, M.; Hauri, D.; Sulser, T. Primary leiomyosarcoma of the seminal vesicle. *J. Urol.,* 2000;164: 2027.

[60] Cauvin, C.; Moureau-Zabotto, L.; Chetaille, B.; Hilgers, W.; Denoux, Y.; Jacquemier, J.; Guiramand, J.; Sarran, A.; Bertucci F. Primary leiomyosarcoma of the seminal vesicle: case report and review of the literature. *BMC Cancer*, 2011 Jul 29;11:323. doi: 10.1186/1471-2407-11-323.

[61] Lucia, M. S.; Miller, G. J. Histopathology of the malignant lesion of the penis. In Crawford E. D., Das S. (Eds). Philadelphia: The urologic clinics of North America W. B. Sauders;1992. pp. 227-238.

[62] Dehner, L. P.; Smith, B. H. Soft tissue tumors of the penis. A clinicopathologic study of 46 cases. *Cancer,* 1970;25:1431-1447.

[63] Pratt, R. M.; Ross, R. T. Leiomyosarcoma of the penis. A report of a case. *Br. J. Surg.*, 1969;56:870-872.

[64] Nkposong, E. O.; Osunkoya, B. O. Leiomyosarcoma of the penis. Report of a case. *West Afr. Med. J. Niger. Pract.,* 1972;21(2):34-36.

[65] Mckenzie Pratt, R.; Ross, R. Leiomyosarcoma of the penis: a report of a case. *Br. J. Surg.,* 1968;56:870-872.

[66] Srivinas, V.; Morse, M. J.; Herr, H. W.; Sogani, P. C.; Whitmore, W. F. Jr. Penile cancer: relation of extent of nodal metastasis to survival. *J. Urol.*, 1987;137:880-882.

[67] Centeno-Flores, M.; García-Rodríguez, F.; Gil, R.; Padrón-Rivera, L. H. Primary leiomyosarcoma of the penis. *Rev. Mex. Urol.*, 2013;73(1):46-49.

[68] Pow-Sang, M. R.; Orihuela, E. Leiomyosarcoma of the penis. *J. Urol.,* 1994;151:1643-1645.

[69] Greenwood, N.; Fox, H.; Edwards, E. C. Leiomyosarcoma of the penis. *Cancer,* 1972;29:481-483.

[70] Sutton, G.; Blessing, J. A.; Ball, H. Phase II trial of paclitaxel in leiomyosarcoma of the uterus: a gynecological oncology group study. *Gynecol. Oncol.*, 1999;74:346-349.

[71] Antunes, A. A.; Nesrallah, L. J. Deep seated sarcoma of the penis. *Clinical Urology,* 2005;31:245-250.
[72] Piana, M.; Martínez, R.; Codone, J.; Elizalde, F.; Diez, M.; Reyes, E.; Pipaón, F.; Villeta, M,. Solano, F.; Lioy-Lupis, M.; Amante, M. Penile leiomyosarcoma: case report and bibliographic review. *Arch. Esp. Urol.,* 2006;59:728-731.
[73] Valadez, R. A.; Waters, W. B. Leiomyosarcoma of penis. *Urology,* 1986;27:265-267.
[74] Isa, S. S.; Almaraz, R.; Magovern, J. Leiomyosarcoma of the penis. Case report and review of the literature. *Cancer*, 1984;54 (5):939-942.
[75] Nanri, M.; Kondo, T.; Okuda, H.; Tanabe, K.; Toma, H. A case of leiomyosarcoma of the penis. *Int. J. Urol.*, 2006;13:655-658.
[76] Katsikas, V. S.; Kalyvas, K. D.; Ioannidis, S. S.; Papathanasiou, M. V.; Panagiotopoulou, K. P.; Hitiroglou, P. M.; Yannakoyorgos, K. Leiomyosarcoma of the penis. *Sarcoma,* 2002;6:75-77.

In: Leiomyosarcoma
Editor: Rosemary H. Leach
ISBN: 978-1-63117-940-2

Chapter 7

Cardiac Leiomyosarcoma

***Nedal Omran**, M.D.*[1], *Jan Laco, M.D., Ph.D.*[2], *Petr Habal, M.D., Ph.D*[1] *and Jan Harrer, M.D., Ph.D*[1].**

[1]Department of Cardiac Surgery and [2]The Fingerland Department of Pathology, Charles University in Prague, Faculty of Medicine and Faculty Hospital, Hradec Kralove, Czech Republic

Abstract

Leiomyosarcoma is an aggressive mesenchymal tumor derived from smooth muscle cells accounting for up to 30% of all sarcomas. Cardiac impairment is often a character of its metastatic involvement or, less likely, the heart can be the only organ targeted by this rare tumor disease.

Patients with established diagnosis of cardiac leiomyosarcoma present with various symptoms relating to the tumor disease itself or may have symptoms associated with the location and extent of the tumor mass in the heart. Imaging modalities used in routine practice are of great importance in establishing diagnosis, assessing tumor disease staging and in evaluating the response to the selected therapeutic modality.

Unfortunately, the long asymptomatic course of cardiac leiomyosarcoma and the aggressive behavior of this tumor have made available therapeutic interventions at presentation of limited efficacy. While the role of chemotherapy is not well established and considering that leiomyosarcoma is known to have a low radiosensitivity, surgical resection of the tumor mass is the treatment option with proven positive impact on patient's survival, symptoms and quality of life. In general, leiomyosarcoma is difficult to treat and has a poor prognosis.

In this article we review cardiac leiomyosarcoma, its prevalence, clinical manifestation, the diagnostic modalities used for establishing the diagnosis of leiomyosarcoma, current treatment options available for the management of this disease and patient prognosis and outcomes.

* Corresponding author: Nedal Omran, M.D., Department of Cardiac Surgery, Charles University Hospital, Sokolska 581, 500 05 Hradec Kralove, Czech Republic. Tel.: +420 495 833 277. Fax: +420 495 833 026. E-mail: nidal81@gmail.com.

Introduction

Primary cardiac neoplasms are rare entities and thus represent a topic of little investigation [1]. They could be divided into benign and malignant tumors contributing to 75% and 25% of all primary cardiac tumors, respectively [2]. However, even a small benign fibroelastoma can cause obstruction to coronary blood flow leading to sudden cardiac death.

Metastatic heart involvement is more frequent and can be witnessed in up to 20% of patients with generalized malignancy [3].

Cardiac myxoma, which is extensively described in the literature, is considered as the representative of primary benign tumors. While sarcomas, which arise from pluripotent mesenchymal cells, are the most common primary malignant tumors [4] and form about 90% of all primary cardiac malignancies [5,6]. Leiomyosarcoma, which is an aggressive mesenchymal tumor with differentiation toward smooth muscle tissue, represents up to 9% of all primary malignant cardiac tumors [7]. On the other hand, leiomyosarcoma is the most common sarcoma involving great vessels with tendency for local and invasive spread [8-11]. Furthermore, 25% of patients with soft tissue sarcoma have cardiac metastasis [12], with leiomyosarcoma being the most commonly detected histological subtype [13].

Patients with an established diagnosis of cardiac leiomyosarcoma, regardless of the origin, present with various symptoms relating to the tumor itself or may have symptoms associated with the location and extent of the tumor mass in the heart, i.e., valvular dysfunction, pericardial syndromes, obstruction to blood flow, arrhythmias or tumor mass embolization [14].

Imaging modalities used in routine practice, such as echocardiography, computed tomography, magnetic resonance and positron emission tomography are of great importance in establishing diagnosis and thus establishing the relationship between tumor mass and surrounding structures. Evaluation of appropriate response to selected therapeutic modality can also be assessed. Before recent advances in diagnostic modalities leading to its wide application in daily routine practice, the diagnosis of cardiac leiomyosarcoma was established only in post mortem studies [15]. Despite this fact, the prognosis of cardiac leiomyosarcoma and sarcomas in general is still dismal mainly due to its invasive growth to the surrounding tissues, which makes surgical removal of the tumor mass often impossible, and even in case of successful tumor removal, leiomyosarcoma tends to relapse locally or metastasize elsewhere over a variable period of time [16, 17].

In addition, the role of chemotherapy is not well established and leiomyosarcoma is considered to have a low radiosensitivity [18].

From the literature review, aggressive and extended surgical resection of the tumor mass is the therapeutic option with proven positive impact on the patient's survival, symptoms and quality of life [19].

Prevelence and Demographic Features

Cardiac and great vessel sarcomas contribute only 1% of all sarcomas [20]. Considering the rarity of cardiac leiomyosarcoma and the fact that metastatic heart involvement prevails upon primary cardiac leiomyosarcoma impairment, the true incidence of this entity is not well established. Reports about primary cardiac involvement consist of isolated case reports and few observational retrospective studies with low number of analyzed cases [20]. As for several types of sarcomas age related incidence shows two peaks. The first minor peak is between the age of 0 and 5 years with rhabdomyosarcoma being the leading diagnosis among the detected sarcomas. The second major peak is between the 5th and 6th decade with leiomyosarcoma being the prevailing subtype of diagnosed sarcomas [21-26].

The incidence of leiomyosarcoma according to many national registers is consistently up to 30% of all detected sarcomas, which is not seen in other histological types of sarcomas. In other types of sarcomas the incidence could vary between two neighboring countries [21].

Leiomoyosarcoma is diagnosed much more frequently in females than in males [2, 4] suggesting the role of hormonal signalization that may take part in tumor proliferation [27]. Leiomyosarcoma can be diagnosed at any anatomical site, but the uterus and the retroperitoneum are the most affected sites [26]. There are no well-established risk factors for leiomyosarcoma and little is known about the etiology of sarcomas per se. Association between increased incidence of sarcomas and hereditary syndromes, such as Li–Fraumeni and Werner syndromes, has been reported [22]. A possible relationship between radiation and herbicides exposure has been pronounced as well [28-32].

Multifocal leiomyosarcomas in a transplanted heart associated with Ebstein-Barr virus infection have been reported as well [33].

Cinical Manifestation

Leiomyosarcoma, like other cardiac sarcomas, can have an asymptomatic course over a long period of time. In advanced stages of disease with invasive growth into surrounding tissues or metastatic involvement may provoke symptoms leading to its late diagnosis. An incidental finding of leiomyosarcoma when using a diagnostic method for another purpose is not uncommon.

Fatigue, fever, weight loss, malaise and other non-specific symptoms can be the first manifestation of this disease making diagnosis of leiomyosarcoma a difficult task. Symptoms associated with local tumor growth, such as dyspnea, chest pain and syncope, are seen in advanced tumor stages [34]. These symptoms are related to obstruction of blood flow due to valvular dysfunction, pericardial syndromes such as pericardial effusion and constrictive peircariditis, and arrhythmias [14]. Emboligennic events caused by tumor mass embolization [34] or by thromboembolism due to tumor-induced thrombophilia can be noticed as well.

At presentation the tumor mass can be mistaken with myxoma due to the fact that leiomyosarcoma commonly has a myxoid appearance and like myxoma arises preferably from the left atrium (in about half of the cases) [35, 1]. Unlike myxoma, leiomyosarcoma do not have the typical relationship with the mid-portion of the interatrial septum [18] and often presents with diffuse thickening of the atrial wall and valvular leaflets [36].

The second most frequent site for cardiac leiomyosarcoma is the right atrium accounting for 26% of all reported cardiac leiomyosarcomas [1]. In this particular location metastatic involvement by clear cell carcinoma of kidney and inferior vena cava sarcomas must be excluded.

Furthermore, angiosarcoma, which is an aggressive mesenchymal tumor of vascular origin, not rarely occurs in the right atrium [37, 38] but unlike lieomyosarcoma is much more common in males than in females [4]. Leiomyosarcoma involves the ventricles less frequently than atria. It is diagnosed in the right and the left ventricle in 16% and 0.1% of cases, respectively [1].

With regard to great vessel involvement, the inferior vena cava and pulmonary veins are the most often involved sites by sarcomas and leiomyosarcoma is the most commonly diagnosed histological subtype [20].

In a clinical setting of 150 patients who underwent pulmonary thrombendarterectomy, pulmonary artery sarcomas were diagnosed in 6 cases, with leiomyosarcoma being among the diagnosed histological subtypes [39].

Histopathology

Leiomyosarcoma is defined as malignant tumor with smooth muscle differentiation [40]. It may arise from soft tissues, skin and various internal organs, including the female genital tract and gastrointestinal tract.

Grossly, leiomyosarcoma usually appears as a fleshy greyish sessile mass. Cystic degeneration and areas of hemorrhage and necrosis are frequently found particularly in larger tumors. Due to its most common localization in the left atrium, leiomyosarcoma is not rarely misdiagnosed as myxoma [41]. But unlike myxoma, leiomyosarcoma shows an infiltrative growth pattern with invasion of pulmonary veins and mitral valve and arises rather from the posterior wall of the left atrium in most cases [42].

Microscopically, leiomyosarcoma is a highly cellular tumor, composed of spindle-shaped cells with variable cytologic atypia frequently arranged in intersecting, sharply marginated fascicles and bundles (Figure 1).

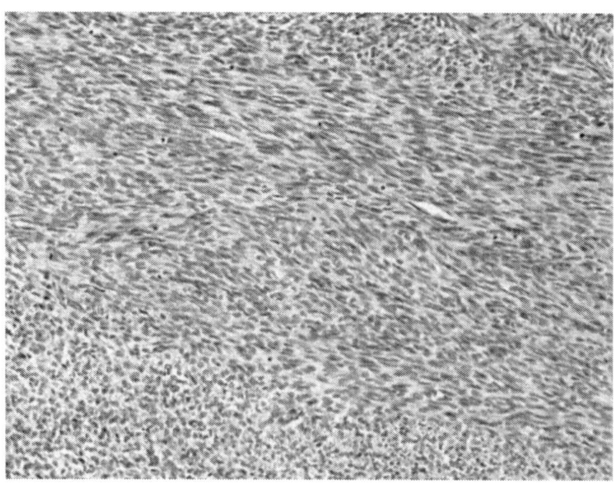

Figure 1. Leiomyosarcoma as highly cellular tumor, consisting of atypical spindle cells with enlarged nuclei and pale-to-eosinophilic cytoplasm. Note fascicular growth pattern. (hematoxylin-eosin, original magnification 200x).

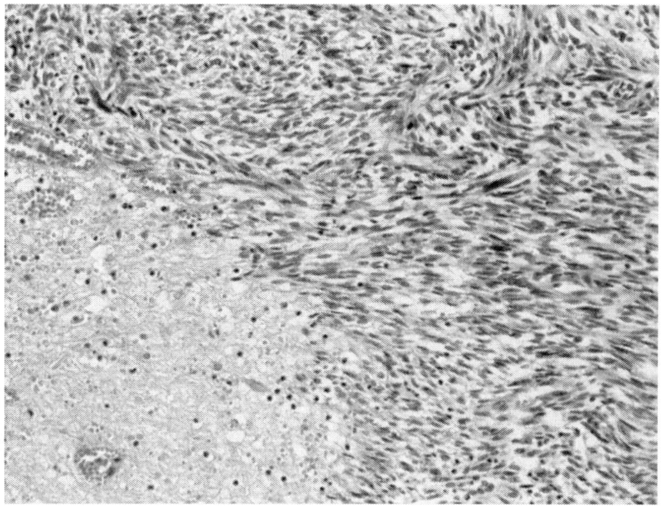

Figure 2. Abrupt transition from viable leiomyosarcoma (right) to coagulative tumor cell necrosis (left). (hematoxylin-eosin, original magnification 200x).

Zones of edema, cystic degeneration, hemorrhage, coagulative tumor necrosis (Figure 2), fibrosis and hyalinization are commonly present. Tumor margins are typically ill-defined and infiltration of the surrounding tissues is evident. Vascular invasion of tumor cells is a usual finding.

The tumor cells have elongated blunt-ended nuclei with coarse chromatin and occasional nucleoli. Nuclear hyperchromatism and pleomorphism are variable. Mitotic figures are usually plentiful (more than 10 mitoses per 10 high power fields) but may be scarce in some variants. Atypical mitoses are also found. The cytoplasm is eosinophilic-to-pale with frequent fibrillar appearance and vacuolization. Less common features includes presence of granular cytoplasmic changes, giant cells resembling osteoclasts and prominent inflammatory infiltrate with xanthoma cells. Epithelioid and myxoid leiomyosarcomas are two well-defined variants with distinctive microscopic features which represent classical diagnostic pitfalls.

As there is no special grading system for cardiac leiomyosarcomas the FNCLCC (Federation Nationale des Centres de Lutte Contre le Cancer) system which evaluates tumor differentiation, mitotic rate and amount of tumor necrosis could be used for cardiac leiomyosarcoma grading [43, 44].

In an immunohistochemical study of 78 leiomyosarcomas of different tissue origin, it was found that smooth muscle actin (Figure 3) was the most sensitive marker. It is expressed in 95 % of cases followed by muscle specific actin and calponin which were positive in 91 % and 88 % of cases respectively. Other diagnostically helpful markers included (in descending order) desmin, caldesmon and myosin which were positive in 73 %, 66 % and 64 % of the cases respectively. In this study a possible relationship between the tissue origin and expressed antigen was highlighted [45]. Importantly, the expression of markers of smooth muscle differentiation may be variably lost in high-grade or undifferentiated leiomyosarcomas. Furthermore, aberrant expression of cytokeratins or epithelial membrane antigen could be focally observed.

The differential diagnosis of low-grade leiomyosarcoma would theoretically include leiomyoma, however, this benign tumor has been not yet been described in cardiac localization. Using immunohistochemistry, high-grade leiomyosarcoma must be distinguished from other cardiac sarcomas, e.g., fibrosarcoma, liposarcoma, rhabdomyosarcoma, synovial sarcoma, angiosarcoma, and undifferentiated pleomorphic sarcoma.

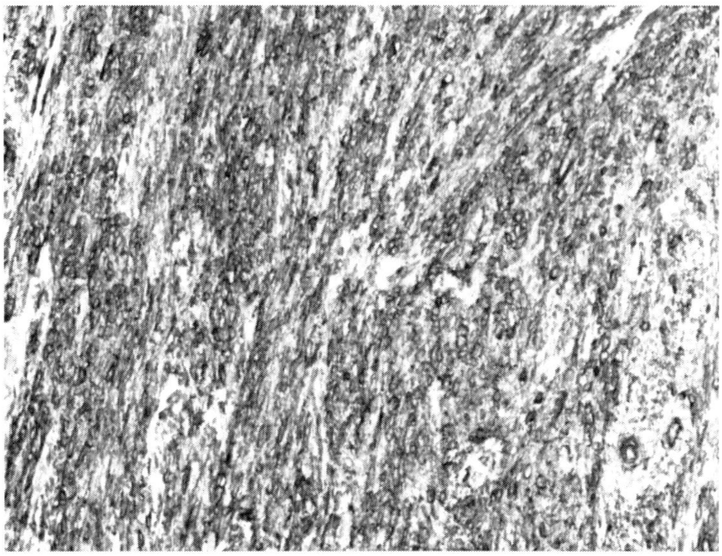

Figure 3. Diffuse cytoplasmic expression of smooth muscle actin in leiomyosarcoma. (original magnification 200x).

Imaging Modalities

Imaging modalities can be applied for establishing the diagnosis of cardiac malignancies, tumor staging assessment and to evaluate the response to selected therapeutic modalities. In routine practice, the most frequently used methods for this purpose include echocardiography, computed tomography, magnetic resonance imaging and positron emission tomography.

Regardless of the selected imaging modality, none can yield specific imaging for leiomyosarcoma or sarcomas in general. Besides, cases of leiomyosarcoma presumed to be infective endocarditis [46], pulmonary embolus [39] or cardiac myxoma [47, 48] have been reported. Thus histopathological examination of the lesion is the cornerstone in establishing the diagnosis.

Echocardiography

Echocardiography is a non-invasive, available, cost-effective and reproducible method used for the assessment of ventricular function, valvular apparatus, intracardiac masses (Figure 4 A, B) and pericardium. When performed transesophageally a better view of the interatrial septum, atria, cavo-atrial junction and the pulmonary veins can be obtained. It is necessary for the diagnosis of intracardiac masses, evaluating the efficacy of therapy (Figure 5 A, B), providing therapeutic and diagnostic pericardial drainage, navigation during transthoracic or transvenous tumor biopsy [49] and for the assessment of changes in cardiac function in patients undergoing neo/adjuvant therapy. The sensitivities of transthoracic and transesophageal echocardiography are about 93% and 96% respectively [50]. On the other hand, cases of cardiac fibrosarcoma and angiosarcoma were misdiagnosed by echocardiography and the definite diagnosis was established after tumor biopsy [51, 52].

Considering the fact that cardiac involvement can be diagnosed in up to 25% of patients with soft tissue sarcomas [12], echocardiography screening must be carried out so a secondary cardiac involvement could be confirmed or excluded.

Despite wide application of this method in clinical practice its restricted anatomic coverage and inability to demonstrate the relationship to the surrounding tissues are considered as disadvantageous.

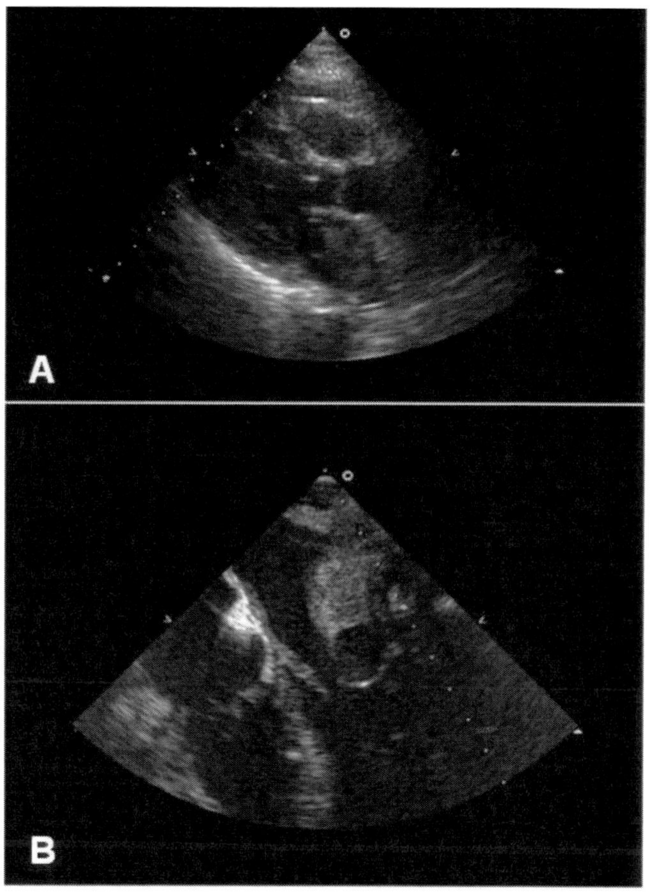

Figure 4 (A and B). Echocardiograms showing primary left atrial leiomyosarcoma prior surgical excision.

Computed Tomography (CT)

CT is a commonly available method used for the diagnosis, assessment of the relationship between tumor mass and surrounding structures and the evaluation of tumor staging. The risk of radiation and nephrotoxicity of the iodine contrast agent must be considered when applying CT. On the other hand in a report of 11 cases of cardiac sarcomas CT failed to determine the diagnosis in 4 patients and the diagnosis was established by echocardiography [13].

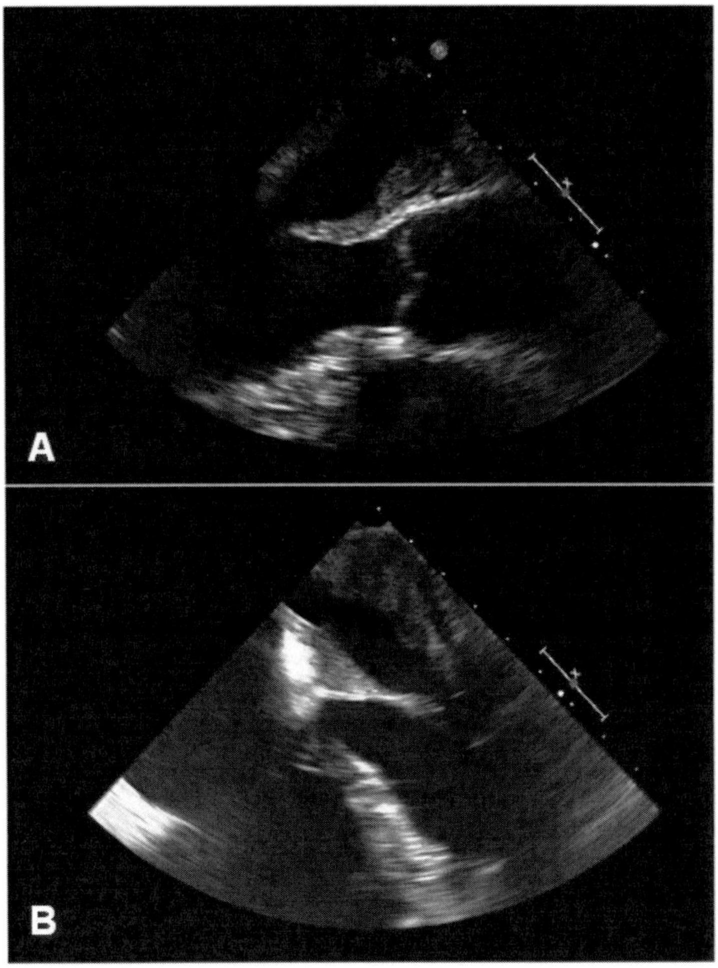

Figure 5. Echocardiograms from the same patients, obtained 10 (A) and 16 (B) months, respectivly, after the surgical resection of the primary lesion. Local tumor relaps with infiltrative growth of the posterior atrial wall and miral valve leafleats are evident.

Magnetic Resonance Imaging (MRI)

Unlike CT, the risk of radiation and the nephrotoxicity associated with iodine contrast agent application can be avoided in case of MRI use. Besides, MRI yields better results regarding the structure of the tumor mass, heart infiltration (Figure 6 A, B) and the extensity of mediastinal soft tissue infiltration. On the other hand, it is contraindicated in patients with implantable cardioverter-defibrillator and pacemakers.

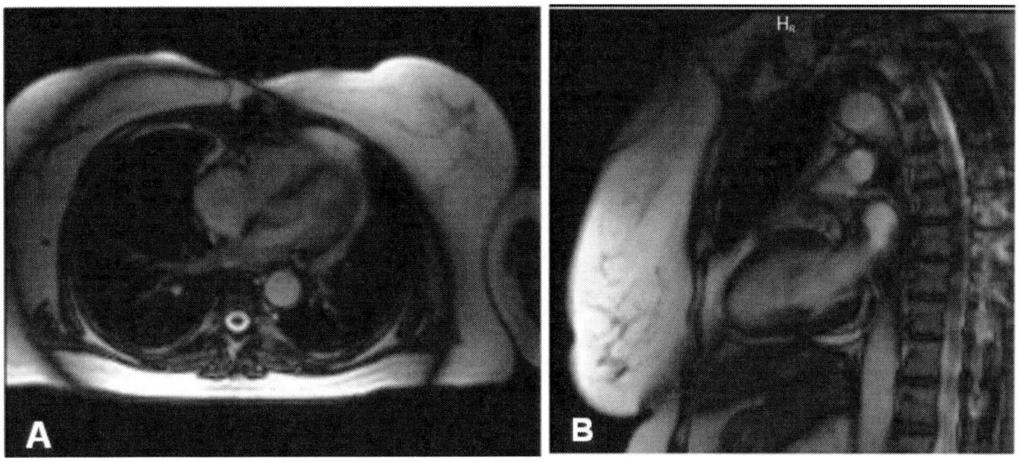

Figure 6 (A and B). Magnetic resonance imaging demonstrating the tumorous infiltration of the left atrium and the mitral valve leaflets.

Positron Emission Tomography (PET)

The high uptake of 18-fluorodeoxyglucose during PET (FDG PET) imaging is highly specific for tissues with increased metabolic activity including tumor cells. Thus, FDG PET could be applied for establishing the diagnosis of cardiac malignancy, for the assessment of therapy outcome, and for establishing disease staging in patients with cardiac tumors. When combined with CT or MRI as a hybrid modality (Figure 7), further valuable anatomical features could be obtained.

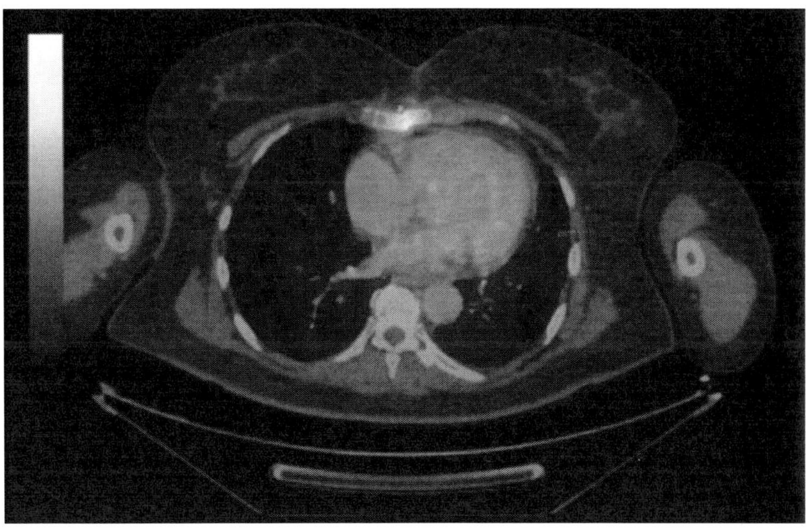

Figure 7. PET/CT demonstrating accumulation of the radioactive agent in the left atrium, reflecting leiomyosarcoma growth.

Treatment Options

Surgical Therapy

The long asymptomatic course of cardiac leiomyosarcoma and delayed diagnosis makes the curative therapeutic interventions at the time of diagnosis often limited. According to literature, aggressive surgical resection to achieve tumor free margins is the treatment of choice with proven positive impact on patient survival rate and quality of life [53]. This approach includes extensive resection of the tumor mass with subsequent reconstruction of cardiac chambers using autologous or bovine pericardium, valve replacement, heart explantation with ex vivo tumor resection and heart re-implantation. Lung resection procedures in case of pulmonary veins or lung parenchyma involvement are also recommended [18, 54-57]. This extensive surgical treatment could also be justified in case of secondary heart involvement, when the primary origin of the tumor seems to be completely treated. A case of a patient with an aggressive and inoperable sarcoma at presentation treated by heart explanation and implantation of mechanical support as a bridge to transplantation was described [58]. However, the concomitant use of adjuvant chemotherapy may manifold the risk of fatal infection [59]. Surgical procedure should be also considered even for these patients, in whom negative tissue margins could not be obtained as it may relieve the obstruction to blood flow and improve the quality of life [36].

Chemotherapy

Unlike surgical treatment, the role of neoadjuvant/adjuvant chemotherapy in the treatment of cardiac leiomyosarcoma is not well established [27, 60, 61] and only a paucity of controversial reports of small patient series is available in the literature in this regard. Furthermore, the vast majority of patients with cardiac leiomyosarcoma present with advanced tumor disease and thus the application of chemotherapy is often palliative with intention to control the tumor growth and to improve the patient's symptoms. Besides, in case of cardiac leiomyosarcoma and sarcomas in general, chemotherapy is administered almost always in combination with surgical procedure. That is why it is difficult to establish the role of chemotherapy alone in influencing the patients' outcome [60]. Another reason contributing to the uncertainty in outcomes of patients receiving chemotherapy in patients with leiomyosarcomas is that studies assessing the efficacy of applied chemotherapy regimen encounter a heterogeneous group of patients with various subtypes of sarcomas and even for the same histopathologic subtype, various organs with variable degree of chemo-sensitivity are enrolled.

Except for non-gastrointestinal stromal tumors, soft tissue sarcomas including leiomyosarcomas are often treated similarly with doxorubicin or ifofosfamide based regimen alone or in combination [62] with an efficacy rate up to 25% for both agents [63, 64].

Regarding doxorubicin, the cardiotoxicity and the narrow therapeutic index represent further obstacle to its administration [65]. Infusional administration, the use of cardioprotectant agents such as dexrazoxane and the use of liposomal encapsulated doxorubicin may increase the therapeutic index of doxorubicin [66]. Other options for enhancing doxorubicin toxicity is the use of membrane integrated efflux pump blocker responsible for chemoresistence development such as biricodar [67] and the concomitant use of cyclin-dependent kinase inhibitor roscovitine which enhances doxorubicin cytotoxicity and facilitates tumor cells autophagy [68]. However, this synergistic cytotoxicity between doxorubicin and roscovitine has been evident in only three sarcoma histological subtypes including uterine leiomyosarcoma [68]. Other chemotherapy regimens include gemcitabine and docetaxel. When given in combination they show promising response rates compared to doxorubicin alone (27-53% and 25%, respectively) [69].

Pazopanib, an inhibitor of several tyrosine kinase receptors, proved beneficial in the treatment of non-adipocyte and non-gastrointestinal sarcomas, when first line chemotherapy regimen had failed [70]. The role of estrogen receptors modulators and aromatase inhibitors was described, which render another option for the management of patients with leiomyosarcomas expressing estrogen receptors [71].

As for cardiac leiomyosarcomas the positive impact of chemotherapy on survival rate is evident in patients with obtained negative tumor resection margins [53, 19] and several reports showed that postoperative chemotherapy does not improve survival rate in patients with incomplete tumor resection [19].

Radiation Therapy

Only few reports supporting the use of radiation therapy for the treatment of sarcomas involving the cardiovascular system are on record [72,57]. As for cardiac leiomyosarcoma, it is known that leiomyosarcomas have low radio-sensitivity [18], and in case of its application the risk of radiation-induced pericarditis and myocariditis should be considered [18]. On the other hand, radiation therapy prior to chemotherapy for patients with malignant pericardial effusion reduced the need of pericaridocentesis [13] and prolongs the survival rate when compared with pericardiocentesis alone [73]. Regardless the selected modalities used for the management of cardiac malignancies a closer follow-up of patients with cardiac leiomyosarcoma must be planned considering the facts that cardiac leiomyosarcoma tend to relapse locally or metastatize over a variable period of time [16, 17].

Prognosis

The prognosis of cardiac leiomyosarcoma and cardiac sarcomas in general is dismal. The reasons for this dismal prognosis include the advanced tumor stage at presentation and the absence of tumor related specific symptoms, which lead to decrease clinical awareness of cardiac tumor involvement, which in turn lead to diagnosis in advanced stages [34]. In addition, the aggressive behavior of this tumor makes the available therapeutic options at the time of diagnosis often of limited efficacy. Even in case of obtained negative tumor resection margins the tendency for local tumor relapse or metastatic involvement may participate in further worsening of patients' prognosis.

Relatively, a better prognosis seems to be associated with left atrial tumor location, low histologic grading with low mitotic activity, absence of necrosis, myxoid appearance, and absence of metastasis at presentation [74]. The vascular origin of leiomyosarcoma is an independent adverse prognostic factor for metastatic free survival and overall survival in patients with this malignancy [75]. Complete tumor resection with negative resection margins is associated with prolonged survival period in patients with cardiac sarcomas compared to patients with palliative surgical resection (24 months vs. 10 months, respectively) [76], where the hospital mortality associated with the surgical procedure ranges between 5-22% [76].

Conclusion

Cardiac leiomyosarcoma is a rare cardiac malignancy with dismal prognosis. The non-specific symptoms, the advanced tumor stage at presentation, the aggressive biologic behavior and the tendency to local relapse and metastatic dissemination make the available arsenal of therapeutic modalities of limited efficacy. A multidisciplinary approach to patients with cardiac malignancy is unquestionable. Considering the rarity of this disease an international register of patients with cardiac sarcomas enabling experience sharing would be of great importance for future studies.

Acknowledgment

Supported by the MH CZ—DRO (UHHK, 00179906) and the research program PRVOUK P37/03.

References

[1] Yuan, SM; Shinfeld, A; Lavee, J; Kuperstein, R; Haizler, R; Raanani, E. Imaging morphology of cardiac tumours. *Cardiol J,* 2009 16, 26–35.

[2] Silverman, NA. Primary cardiac tumor. Ann Surg, 1980 1919, 127-138.

[3] Abad, C. Cardiac tumors (II). Malignant primary tumors. Metastatic tumors. Carcinoid tumor. *Rev Esp Cardiol,* 1998 2, 103-114.

[4] Hattori, Y; Iriyama, T; Watanabe, K; Negi, K; Takeda, I; Sugimura, S. Primary Cardiac sarcoma: two case reports. *Jpn Circ J,* 2000 64, 222-224.

[5] Burke, A. Primary malignant cardiac tumors. *Semin Diagn Pathol,* 2008 25, 39–46.

[6] Shapiro, LM. Cardiac tumours: diagnosis and management. *Heart* 2001 85, 218–222.

[7] Butany, J; Nair, V; Naseemuddin, A; Nair, GM; Catton, C; Yau, T. Cardiac tumours: diagnosis and management. *Lancet Oncol,* 2005 6, 219–228.

[8] Burke, AP; Virmani, R. Sarcomas of the great vessels. A clinicopathologic study. *Cancer,* 1993 71, 1761–1773.

[9] Blansfield, JA; Chung, H; Sullivan, TR Jr; Pezzi, CM. Leiomyosarcoma of the major peripheral arteries: Case report and review of the literature. *Ann Vasc Surg,* 2003 17, 565–570.

[10] Mingoli, A; Feldhaus, RJ; Cavallaro, A; Stipa, S. Leiomyosarcoma of the inferior vena cava: Analysis and search of world literature on 141 patients and report of three new cases. *J Vasc Surg,* 1991 14, 688–699.

[11] Sebenik, M; Ricci, A Jr; DiPasquale, B; Mody, K; Pytel, P; Jee, KJ; Knuutila, S; Scholes, J. Undifferentiated intimal sarcoma of large systemic blood vessels: Report of 14 cases with immunohistochemical profile and review of the literature. *Am J Surg Pathol,* 2005 29, 1184-1193.

[12] Hallahan, DE; Vogelzang, NJ; Borow, K; Bostwick, DG; Simon, MA. Cardiac metastases from soft-tissue sarcomas. *J Clin Oncol,* 1986 4, 1662–1669.

[13] Takenaka, S; Hashimoto, N; Araki, N; Hamada, K; Naka, N; Joyama, S; Kakunaga, S; Ueda, T; Myoui, A; Yoshikawa, H. Eleven Cases of Cardiac Metastases from Soft-tissue Sarcomas. *Jpn J Clin Oncol,* 2011 41, 514–518.

[14] Okby, NT; Travis, WD. Liposarcoma of the pleural cavity: clinical and pathologic features of four cases with a review of the literature. *Arch Pathol Lab Med,* 2000 1245, 699-703.

[15] Masauzi, N; Ichikawa, S; Nishimura, F; Yoshino, Y; Mihara, J; Hayama, Y; Shimazaki, E; Kawase, I; Toyama, M; Kokubo, T. Primary angiosarcoma of the right atrium detected by magnetic resonance imaging. *Intern Med,* 1992 31, 1291-1297.

[16] Thomas, CR; Johnson, GW; Stoddard, MF; Clifford, S. Primary malignant cardiac tumors: Update 1992. *Med Pediatr Oncol,* 1992 20, 519-531.

[17] Llombart-Cussac, A; Pivot, X; Contesso, G; Rhor-Alvarado, A; Delord, JP; Spielmann, M; Türsz, T; Le Cesne, A. Adjuvant chemotherapy for primary cardiac sarcomas: The IGR experience. *Br J Cancer,* 1998 78, 1624-1628.

[18] Minakata, K; Konishi, Y; Matsumoto, M; Nonaka, M; Yamada, N. Primary leiomyosarcoma of the left atrium. *Jpn Circ J,* 1999 63, 414-415.

[19] Putnam, JB Jr; Sweeney, MS; Colon, R; Lanza, LA; Frazier, OH; Cooley, DA. Primary cardiac sarcomas. *Ann Thorac Surg,* 1991 51, 906-910.

[20] Mayer, F; Aebert, H; Rudert, M; Königsrainer, A; Horger, M; Kanz, L; Bamberg, M; Ziemer, G; Hartmann, JT. Primary Malignant Sarcomas of the Heart and Great Vessels in Adult Patients -A Single-Center Experience. *Oncologist,* 2007 12, 1134-1142.

[21] Wibmer, C; Leithner, A; Zielonke, N; Sperl, M; Windhager, R. Increasing incidence rates of soft tissue sarcomas? A population-based epidemiologic study and literature review. *Ann Oncol,* 2010 21, 1106-1111.

[22] Ji, J; Eng, C; Hemminki, K. Familial risk for soft tissue tumors: a nation-wide epidemiological study from Sweden. J *Cancer Res Clin Oncol,* 2008 134, 617–624.

[23] Levi, F; La Vecchia, C; Randimbison, L; Te, VC. Descriptive epidemiology of soft tissue sarcomas in Vaud, Switzerland. *Eur J Cancer,* 1999 35, 1711–1716.

[24] Toro, JR; Travis, LB; Wu, HJ; Zhu, K; Fletcher, CD; Devesa, SS. Incidence patterns of soft tissue sarcomas, regardless of primary site, in the surveillance, epidemiology and end results program, 1978–2001: an analysis of 26,758 cases. *Int J Cancer,* 2006 119, 2922–2930.

[25] Zahm, SH; Fraumeni, JF Jr. The epidemiology of soft tissue sarcoma. *Semin Oncol,* 1997 24, 504-514.

[26] Penel, N; Italiano, A; Isambert, N; Bompas, E; Bousquet, G; Duffaud, F. French Sarcoma Group (Groupe Sarcome Français/Groupe d'Etude des Tumeurs Osseuses).

Factors affecting the outcome of patients with metastatic leiomyosarcoma treated with doxorubicin-containing chemotherapy. *Ann Oncol,* 2010 21, 1361-1365.

[27] Oliai, BR; Tazelaar, HD; Lloyd, RV; Doria, MI; Trastek, VF. Leiomyosarcoma of the pulmonary veins. *Am J Surg Pathol,* 1999 23, 1082-1088.

[28] Mikoczy, Z; Schutz, A; Hagmar, L. Cancer incidence and mortality among Swedish leather tanners. *Occup Environ Med,* 1994;51:530–535.

[29] Franceschi S, Serraino D: Risk factors for adult soft tissue sarcoma in northern Italy. *Ann Oncol,* 1992 3, 85–88.

[30] Hoppin, JA; Tolbert, PE; Flanders, WD; Zhang, RH; Daniels, DS; Ragsdale, BD; Brann, EA. Occupational risk factors for sarcoma subtypes. *Epidemiology,* 1999 10, 300–306.

[31] 31. Lampi, P; Hakulinen, T; Luostarinen, T; Pukkala, E; Teppo, L. Cancer incidence following chlorophenol exposure in a community in southern Finland. *Arch Environ Health,* 1992 47, 167–175.

[32] Hoar Zahm, S; Blair, A; Holmes, FF; Boysen, CD; Robel, RJ. A case-referent study of soft-tissue sarcoma and Hodgkin's disease. Farming and insecticide use. *Scand J Work Environ Health,* 1988 14, 224–230.

[33] Nur, S; Rosenblum, WD; Katta, UD; Islam, H; Brown, K; Ramaswamy, G. Epstein-Barr virus-associated multifocal leiomyosarcomas arising in a cardiac transplant recipient: autopsy case report and review of the literature. *J Heart Lung Transplant,* 2007 26, 944-952.

[34] Shanmugam, G: Primary cardiac sarcoma. *Eur J Cardiothorac Surg,* 2006 29, 925-932.

[35] Pérez-Díez, D; Estévez-Cid, F; Barge-Caballero, E; Pérez-López, J. Chewing Gum Inside the Heart. *Circulation,* 2009 119, 525-526.

[36] Hrdinova, M; Omran, N; Polansly, P; Vesely, J; Steiner, I; Belobradek, Z; Sorm Z. Left atrial leiomyosarcoma: A rare cause of mitral valve (pseudo)stenosis. *Cor et Vasa,* 2013 55, 457-459.

[37] Burke, AP; Tazelaar, H; Butany, J; El-Demellawy, D; Loire, R; Geva, T; Bonilla, F; Galvin, JR; Veinot, JP; Virmani, R; Kamiya, H; Watanabe, G; Grandmougin, D; Horimoto, M; Hiraga, H. Title: Cardiac sarcomas. In: Travis WD, Brambilla E, Mueller-Hermelink HK, Harris CC editors. Title: *Pathology and Genetics of Tumours of the Lung,* Pleura, Thymus and Heart. Lyon, France: IARC Press, 2004; 273–281.

[38] Majano-Lainez, RA: Cardiac tumors: A current clinical and pathological perspective. *Crit Rev Oncog,* 1997 8, 293–303.

[39] Anderson, MB; Kriett, JM; Kapelanski, DP; Tarazi, R; Jamieson, SW. Primary pulmonary artery sarcoma: a report of six cases. *Ann Thorac Surg,* 1995 59, 1487-1490.

[40] Mankin, HJ; Casas-Ganem, J; Kim, JI; Gebhardt, MC; Hornicek, FJ; Zeegen, EN. Leiomyosarcoma of somatic soft tissues. *Clin Orthop Relat Res,* 2004 421, 225-231.

[41] Morin, JE; Rahal, D; Hüttner, I. Myxoid leiomyosarcoma of the left atrium: a rare malignancy of the heart and its comparison with atrial myxoma. *Can J Cardiol,* 2001 17, 331-336.

[42] O'Donnell, DH; Abbara, S; Chaithiraphan, V; Yared, K; Killeen, RP; Cury, RC; Dodd, JD. Cardiac tumors: optimal cardiac MR sequences and spectrum of imaging appearances. *AJR Am J Roentgenol,* 2009 193, 377-387.

[43] Trojani, M; Contesso, G; Coindre, JM; Rouesse, J; Bui, NB; de Mascarel, A; Goussot, JF; David, M. Soft-tissue sarcomas of adults; study of pathological prognostic variables and definition of a histopathological grading system. *Int J Cancer,* 1984 33, 37-42.

[44] Domanski, HA; Akerman, M; Rissler, P; Gustafson, G. Fine-needle aspiration of soft tissue leiomyosarcoma: an analysis of the most common cytologic findings and the value of ancillary techniques. *Diag Cytopathol,* 2006 34, 597-604.

[45] Carvalho, JC; Thomas, DG; Lucas, DR. Cluster analysis of immunohistochemical markers in leiomyosarcoma delineates specific anatomic and gender subgroups. *Cancer,* 2009 115, 4186-4195.

[46] Jurcut, R; Savu, O; Popescu, BA; Florian, A; Herlea, V; Moldovan, H; Ginghina, C. Images in cardiovascular medicine: Primary cardiac leiomyosarcoma: when valvular disease becomes a vascular surgical emergency. *Circulation,* 2010 121, 415-418.

[47] Casselman, FP; Gillinov, AM; Kasirajan, V; Ratliff, NB; Cosgrove, DM 3rd. Primary synovial sarcoma of the left heart. *Ann Thorac Surg,* 1999 68, 2329-2331.

[48] Laroia, ST; Potti, A; Rabbani, M; Mehdi, SA; Koch, M. Unusual pulmonary lesions: pulmonary vein leiomyosarcoma presenting as a left atrial mass. *J Clin Oncol,* 2002 20, 2749-2751.

[49] Burling, F; Devlin, G; Heald, S. Primary cardiac lymphoma diagnosed with transesophageal echocardiography-guided endomyocardial biopsy. *Circulation,* 2000 101, 179-181.

[50] Meng, Q; Lai, H; Lima, J; Tong, W; Qian, Y; Lai, S. Echocardiographic and pathologic characteristics of primary cardiac tumors: a study of 149 cases. *Int J Cardiol,* 2002 84, 69-75.

[51] Seal, EC; Rutter, HR; Horrigan, MC; Britton, MG. Left atrial tumour mimicking pulmonary embolism. *Respir Med,* 1997 91, 562-564.

[52] Bic, JF; Fade-Schneller, O; Marie, B; Neimann, JL; Anthoine, D; Martinet, Y. Cardiac angiosarcoma revealed by lung metastases. *Eur Respir J,* 1994 7, 1194-1196.

[53] Oh, SJ; Yeom, SY; Kim, KH. Clinical implication of surgical resection for the rare cardiac tumors involving heart and great vessels. *J Korean Med Sci,* 2013 28, 717-724.

[54] Shimono, T; Yuasa, H; Yuasa, U; Yasuda, F; Adachi, K; Tokui, T; Takao, M; Namikawa, S; Yada, I. Pulmonary leiomyosarcoma extending into left atrium or pulmonary trunk: Complete resection with cardiopulmonary bypass. *J Thorac Cardiovasc Surg,* 1998 115, 460-461.

[55] Gyhra, AS; Santander, CK; Alarcon, EC; Mucientes, FH; Carillo H. Leiomyosarcoma of the pulmonary veins with extension to the left atrium. *Ann Thorac Surg,* 1996 61, 1840–1841.

[56] Antunes, MJ; Vanderdonck, KM; Andrade, CM; Rebelo, LS. Primary cardiac leiomyosarcomas. *Ann Thorac Surg,* 1991 51, 999–1001.

[57] Zerkowski, HR; Hofmann, HS; Gybels, I; Knolle, J. Primary sarcoma of pulmonary artery and valve: Multimodality treatment by chemotherapy and homograft replacement. *J Thorac Cardiovasc Surg,* 1996 112, 1122–1124.

[58] Pirk, J; Maly, J; Szarszoi, O; Urban, M; Kotulak, T; Riha, H; Neuzil, P; Netuka, I. Total artificial heart support with two continuous-flow ventricular assist devices in a patient with an infiltrating cardiac sarcoma. *ASAIO J,* 2013 59, 178-180.

[59] Maly, J; Szarszoi, O; Netuka, I; Dorazilova, Z; Pirk, J. Fungal infections associated with long-term mechanical circulatory support-diagnosis and management. *J Card Surg,* 2014 29, 95-100.

[60] Malyshev, M; Safuanov, A; Gladyshev, I; Trushyna, V; Abramovskaya, L; Malyshev, A. Primary left atrial leiomyosarcoma: Literature review and lessons of a case. *Asian Cardiovasc Thorac Ann,* 2006 14, 435-440.

[61] Hattori, Y; Iriyama, T; Watanabe, K; Negi, K; Takeda, I; Sugimura, S. Rapidly growing primary cardiac leiomyosarcoma. *Surg Today,* 2000 30, 838-840.

[62] Sleijfer, S; Ouali, M; van Glabbeke, M; Krarup-Hansen, A; Rodenhuis, S; Le Cesne, A; Hogendoorn, PC; Verweij, J; Blay, JY. Prognostic and predictive factors for outcome to first-line ifosfamide-containing chemotherapy for adult patients with advanced soft tissue sarcomas An exploratory, retrospective analysis on large series from the European Organization for Research and Treatment of Cancer-Soft Tissue and Bone Sarcoma Group (EORTC-STBSG) *Eur J Cancer,* 2010 46, 72-83.

[63] Verweij, J; Lee, SM; Ruka, W; Buesa, J; Coleman, R; van Hoessel, R; Seynaeve, C; di Paola, ED; van Glabbeke, M; Tonelli, D; Judson, IR. Randomized phase II study of docetaxel versus doxorubicin in first and second-line chemotherapy for locally advanced or metastatic soft tissue sarcomas in adults: a study of the european organization for research and treatment of cancer soft tissue and bone sarcoma group. *J Clin Oncol,* 2000 18, 2081–2086.

[64] Keohan, ML; Taub, RN. Chemotherapy for advanced sarcoma: therapeutic decisions and modalities. *Semin Oncol,* 1997 24, 572-579.

[65] Rubin, E; Hait, W. Title: *Drugs That Target DNA Topoisomerases.* In: Kufe D, Bast R, Hait W editors. Title: Cancer Medicine 7. Hamilton, Ontario: BC Decker, Inc., 2006; 690-693.

[66] Pfeffer, B; Tziros, C; Katz, RJ. Current concepts of anthracycline cardiotoxicity: pathogenesis, diagnosis and prevention. *Br J Cardiol,* 2009 16, 85-89.

[67] Bramwell, VH; Morris, D; Ernst, DS; Hings, I; Blackstein, M; Venner, PM; Ette, EI; Harding, MW; Waxman, A; Demetri, GD. Safety and efficacy of the multidrug-resistance inhibitor biricodar (VX-710) with concurrent doxorubicin in patients with anthracycline-resistant advanced soft tissue sarcoma. *Clin Cancer Res,* 2002 8, 383.

[68] Lambert, LA; Qiao, N; Hunt, KK; Lambert, DH; Mills, GB; Meijer, L; Keyomarsi, K. Autophagy: a novel mechanism of synergistic cytotoxicity between doxorubicin and roscovitine in a sarcoma model. *Cancer Res,* 2008 68, 7966-7974.

[69] Gupta, A; Yao, X; Verma, S; Mackay, H; Hopkins, L; Sarcoma Disease Site Group and the Gynecology Cancer Disease Site Group. Systematic chemotherapy for inoperable, locally advanced, recurrent, or metastatic uterine leiomyosarcoma: a systematic review. *Clin Oncol,* 2013 25, 346-355.

[70] Hardman, MP; Roman, JJ; Burnett, AF; Santin, AD. Metastatic uterine leiomyosarcoma regression using an aromatase inhibitor. *Obstet Gynecol,* 2007 110, 518-520.

[71] Mery GM, Reardon MJ, Haas J, Lazar J, Hindenburg A. A combined modality approach to recurrent cardiac sarcoma resulting in a prolonged remission: A case report. *Chest,* 2003 123, 766–1768.

[72] van der Graaf, WT; Blay, JY; Chawla, SP; Kim, DW; Bui-Nguyen, B; Casali, PG; Schöffski, P; Aglietta, M; Staddon, AP; Beppu, Y; Le Cesne, A; Gelderblom, H; Judson, IR; Araki, N; Ouali, M; Marreaud, S; Hodge, R; Dewji, MR; Coens, C;

Demetri, GD; Fletcher, CD; Dei Tos, AP; Hohenberger, P; EORTC Soft Tissue and Bone Sarcoma Group; PALETTE study group. Pazopanib for metastatic soft-tissue sarcoma (PALETTE): a randomised, double-blind, placebo-controlled phase 3 trial. *Lancet,* 2012 379, 1879-1886.

[73] Kralstein, J; Frishman, H. Malignant pericardial diseases: diagnosis and treatment. *Cardiol Clin,* 1987 5, 583–589.

[74] Orlandi, A; Ferlosio, A; Roselli, M; Chiariello, L; Spagnoli, LG. Cardiac sarcomas: an update. *J Thorac Oncol,* 2010 5, 1483–1489.

[75] Italiano, A; Toulmonde, M; Stoeckle, E; Kind, M; Kantor, G; Coindre, JM; Bui, B. Clinical outcome of leiomyosarcomas of vascular origin: comparison with leiomyosarcomas of other origin. *Ann Oncol,* 2010 21, 1915-1921.

[76] Bakaeen, FG; Reardon, MJ; Coselli, JS; Miller, CC; Howell, JF; Lawrie, GM; Espada, R; Ramchandani, MK; Noon, GP; Weilbaecher, DG; DeBakey, ME. Surgical outcome in 85 patients with primary cardiac tumors. *Am J Surg,* 2003 186, 641-647.

In: Leiomyosarcoma
Editor: Rosemary H. Leach

ISBN: 978-1-63117-940-2

Chapter 8

Cutaneous Leiomyosarcoma

***Sara Alcántara Luna*[1*], *Ana Delina Lozano Salazar*[2], *Lara Ferrándiz Pulido*[1] *and Juan José Ríos-Martín*[2]**

[1]Unidad de Gestión Clínica de Dermatología
del Hospital Universitario Virgen Macarena (Sevilla)
[2]Unidad de Gestión Clínica de Anatomía Patológica
del Hospital Universitario Virgen Macarena (Sevilla) Sevilla- Spain

Abstract

Atypical intradermal smooth muscle neoplasms (AISMN, formerly known as cutaneous leiomyosarcomas) are uncommon neoplasms, which seem to be remarkable for their excellent prognosis in contrast to their deeper counterparts. We evaluated the histologic and immunohistochemical features of 4 cases of AISMN.

The immunohistochemical stains such as smooth muscle actin and muscle specific actin, when are used in combination, can identify smooth muscle differentiation in 100% of the cases. With some caveats, CD34, S100, and CK 5/6 are helpful in ruling out other important cutaneous spindle cell neoplasms. Malignancy criteria established by WHO include high cellularity, nuclear atypia significantly and at least one mitosis by 10 high power fields. Actually noted the utility of immunohistochemical marker of mitosis phosphohistone H3 (phH3) in diagnostic leiomyosarcomas with mitotic activity and some degree of atypia nuclear.

AISMN can have significant morphologic variation and overlap with other spindle cell neoplasms of the skin and that a limited panel of key immunohistochemical stains should be used to distinguish this lesion.

* Corresponding author: Sara Alcántara Luna, Unidad de Gestión Clínica de Dermatología, Hospital Universitario Virgen Macarena, Avda. Dr. Fedriani s/n. 41073, Seville-Spain; Fax: +00-34-954-382763; Tel: +00-34-954-376474; Mail: alcantaralunasara@gmail.com

Introduction

Cutaneous and subcutaneous leiomyosarcomas have been traditionally regarded as a single homogeneous entity. However, there exists preliminary evidence that tumour depth may significantly influence the clinical outcome. Cutaneous leiomyosarcoma (CLM) or atypical intradermal smooth muscle neoplasm (AISMN), is a rare smooth muscle neoplasm arising in the dermis. Unlike the subcutaneous and deep counterparts, namely subcutaneous and deep leiomyosarcomas, true AISMNs are intradermal with limited extension into subcutaneous tissue and are thought to have an excellent prognosis. Although local recurrences have been repeatedly reported for the cutaneous variety, distant metastasis is generally considered so unlikely that one should reconsider the diagnosis should metastasis occur. Kraft and Fletcher [1] have proposed a change in nomenclature from cutaneous leiomyosarcoma to AISMN because of the extremely rare chance of distant metastasis. Nonetheless, there is a report of a distant metastasis 15 years after excision [2]. CLM has a characteristic demographic, it typically occurs on the upper extremities region of middle aged to elderly patients, but has also been identified in adolescents and younger adults and can occur on the trunk [3,4]. Most case series report a male predominance [3,4,5].

Although CLMs may retain smooth muscle morphology (intersecting fascicles of elongated cells with ovoid or cigar-shaped, blunt-ended nuclei, and eosinophilic cytoplasm), they are distinguished from benign leiomyomas by virtue of nuclear atypia and mitoses [6]. CLMs usually grow as a single nodule, but diffuse patterns have also been observed, mimicking desmoplastic spindle cell carcinoma or melanoma [7,8]. We present a retrospective study of 4 cases, comparing extensive histopathologic and immunohistochemical details with clinical management.

Case Reports

Case 1. A 46-year-old man presented a new lesion, which had gradually grown, on top of an epidermoid cyst scar on the left shoulder, which was removed 3 years ago. There are none pathology´s records. The patient was in apparently good health. Physical examination revealed a whitish, non-ulcerated, firm and painful nodule in the left scapular area. There were no palpable local lymph nodes. Surgical excision was performed and the histopathological study showed a malignant mesenchymal neoplasm of 0.9 cm in diameter, with nodular growth pattern, without necrosis, ulceration or pleomorphism and prominent mitotic activity.

The mitotic index was 8/10 high power fields (HPF) (Figure 1). Immunohistochemical staining was positive for Smooth Muscle Actin (SMA) and desmin, and negative for CD34. A diagnosis of cutaneous leiomyosarcoma was made. The excision had positive margins and the patient was referred for wide local excision and penetrating as deep as the underlying fascia. The tumor was definitively cleared. Metastasis work-up was negative and the patient is in follow-up every four months, without any evidence of disease recurrence or metastatsis to date of the present study.

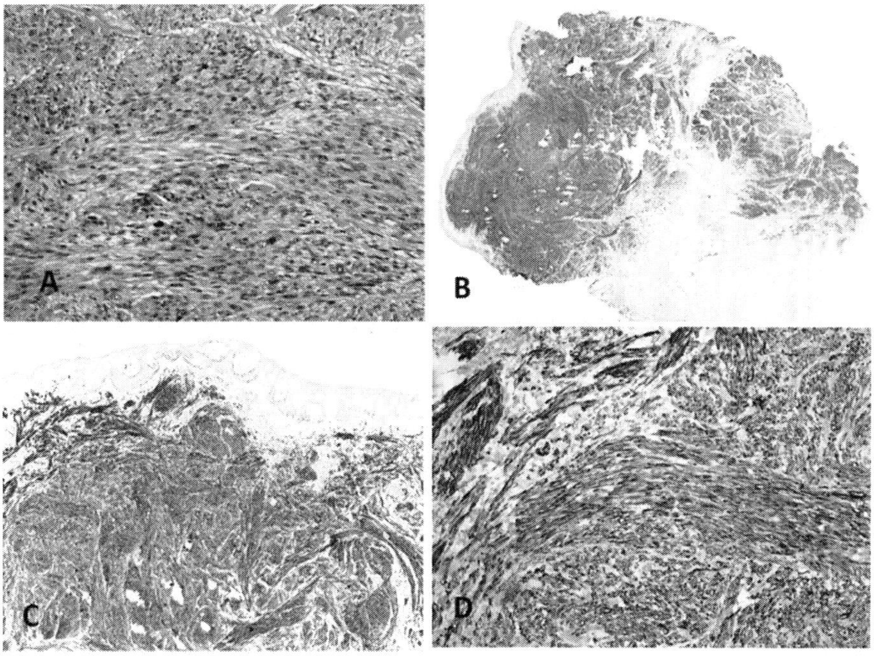

Figure 1. A. The spindle-celled neoplasm (H&E, x40). B y C. Inmunohistochemical staining positive for desmin. D. Smooth muscle actin.

Case 2. A 80-year-old man with a history of diabetes mellitus and arterial hypertension. No known allergies. He was referred to our Department of Dermatology due to a slowly progressing cutaneous tumor measuring 1cm x 0.5cm on the scalp, like a squamous cell carcinoma, for the last 8 months. On physical examination, a firm, skin-colored, ulcerated and partly covered by hyperkeratosis located on right parietal area was noted. Lateral cervical lymph nodes were not palpable. A punch biopsy was performed and the histopathological study showed a spindle-celled ulcerated neoplasm of 1.1cm in diameter without necrosis or nuclear plemorphism, but with prominent mitotic activity (9 mitosis /10HPF) (Figure 2). Inmmunohistochemical staining was positive for immunoreactivity for muscle markers (desmin and SMA), and negative for epithelial (cytokeratin), melanocytic (HMB45 and S100) and vascular (CD34). Ki67 was above 10%. The tumor involved the entire thickness of the dermis and deep edge affects resection. Wide local excision was made. Systemic examination and investigations were within normal limits. Periodic monitoring is still no evidence of recurrence to date.

Case 3. A 69-year-old man presented a one year history of a slow growing cutaneous nodule located on his left knee, to which surgical excision was performed by his primary care physician without histopathological study. The surgical wound did not heal properly, so he was treated with analgesia and antibiotic therapy without any improvement. Later, he was evaluated by dermatologists. During physical examination, a 3-cm solitary pink nodular lesion was noted on the left knee. No local adenopathies were noted. We removed the lesion with histopathological study which showed a mesenchymal, ill-defined neoplasm of 3 cm in diameter predominantly dermal location with involvement of the subcutaneous. Moreover, it was not ulcerated, without necrosis, with moderate nuclear pleomorphism and amounting to 7 mitotic figures per 10 HPF. The margins were clear, although they were adjusted to the tumor (less than 1mm). Immunohistochemistry was positive for SMA and desmin, and negative for CD34 (Figure 3). With these findings the diagnosis of leiomyosarcoma was established.

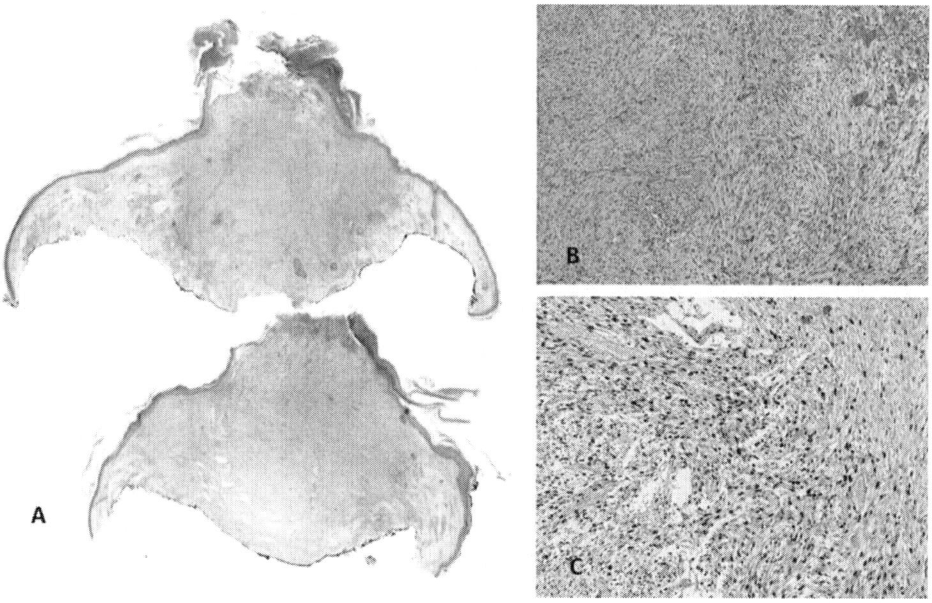

Figure 2. A. The ulcerated neoplasm (H&E, x4). B. Elongated spindle cells arranged in interlacing fascicles (H&E, x40). C. Ki67 is above 10%.

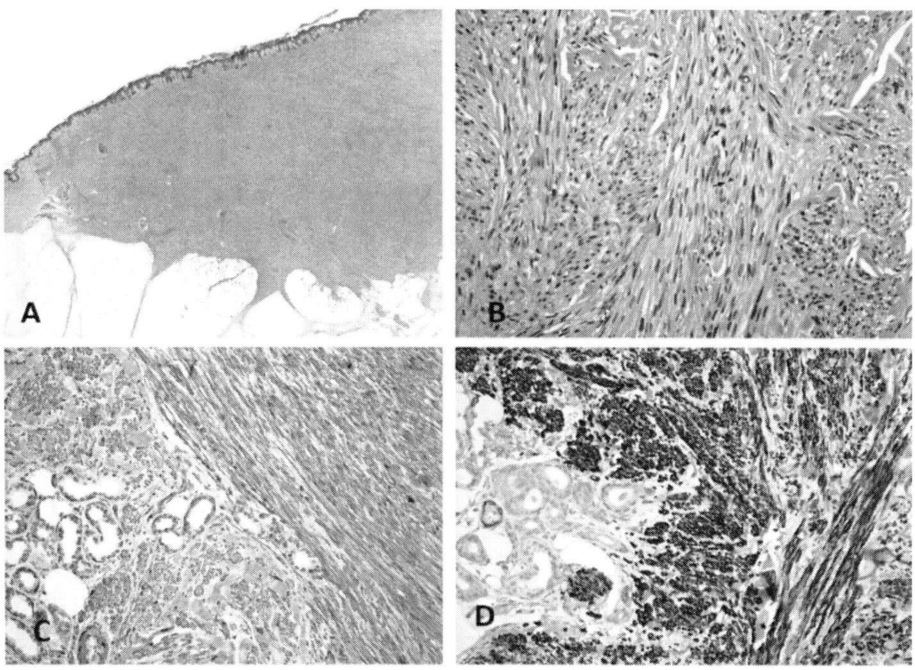

Figure 3. A. Ill-defined neoplasm predominantly dermal location with involvement of the subcutaneous (H&E, x4). B. Atypical mitotic figures (H&E, x40). C. Inmunohistochemistry is positive for SMA. D. Desmin.

The patient was surgically treated with a wide local excision with 2-cm lateral margins and the metastasis work-up was negative. Currently, he is in ongoing quarterly checks without evidence of recurrence.

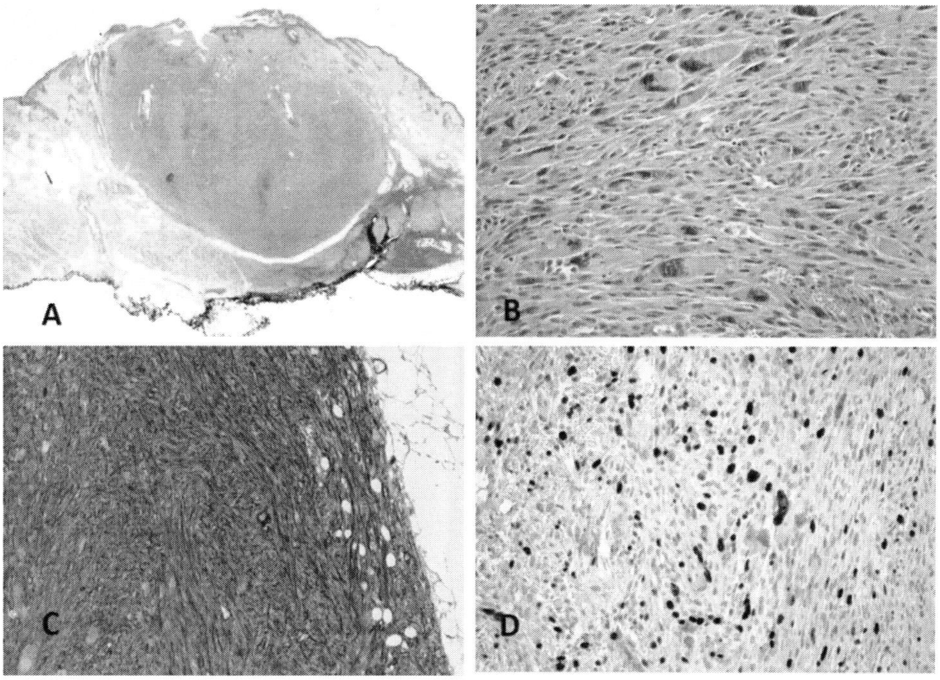

Figure 4. A. The neoplasm with expansive borders (H&E, x4). B. The neoplasm is composed of bundles of elongated spindle cells arranged in interlacing fascicles with atypical mitotic figures (H&E, x40). C. SMA. D. Ki-67 is above 20%.

Case 4. A 64-year-old man with hypertension, hyperuricemia, anticoagulated for atrial fibrillation, congestive heart failure, dilated cardiomyopathy and he had a permanent pacemaker. He had no known allergies. He presented with a asymptomatic nodule on his face which had progressively grown over the past 6 months. Physical examination revealed a firm, raised nodule of erythematous-brownish appearance, with destruction of hair follicles and surrounded by a halo of edematous skin located on the middle third of the left ciliary region. There were no palpable cervical lymph nodes. The tumor was removed. Pathologic examination revealed a malignant mesenchymal neoplasm of 7 mm in diameter, expansive borders, occupying the entire thickness of the dermis and extending into the hypodermis, located 1 mm from deep margin resection. The neoplasm was composed of bundles of elongated spindle cells arranged in interlacing fascicles. The nuclei were atypical, pleomorphic, elongated and rounded edges. The mitotic index was high (15 mitosis/10HPF). Immunohistochemistry was positive for muscle markers (SMA, desmin, caldesmon), and negative for S100 and CD34. The cell proliferation index, assessed with Ki67 was 20% (Figure 4). The diagnosis was dermal leiomyosarcoma with subcutaneous infiltration. The patient was surgically treated with a wide local excision and there was not evidence of metastasis. Twelve months after surgery, the patient is checked regularly, without evidence of recurrence.

Table 1 presents the aforementioned clinical data.

Table 1. Clinical history, type of procedure and follow-up on 4 cases of AISMN

Case	Age (years)	Sex	Location	Size (cm)	Procedure	Margin status	Wide local excision	Recurrence	Metastasis work-up	Follow_up (months)
1	46	Male	Shoulder	0.9	Excision	Positive	Yes	None	Negative	42
2	80	Male	Scalp	1.1	Biopsy	Positive	Yes	None	Negative	24
3	69	Male	Knee	3	Excision	Negative	Yes	None	Negative	6
4	64	Male	Eyebrow	0.7	Excision	Negative	Yes	None	Negative	12

Table 2. Morphologic and histologic characteristics

Case	Type	Pleomorphism	Mitoses /10HPF	Necrosis	Ulceration	Minimal subcutaneous extension
1	Nodular	No	8	No	No	No
2	Nodular	No	9	No	Yes	No
3	Diffuse	Yes	7	No	No	Yes
4	Nodular	Yes	15	No	No	Yes

Table 3. Inmunohistochemical properties

Case	Desmin	Smooth muscle actin (SMA)	h- caldesmon	CD34	S100	CK 5/6	Ki67
1	+	+		-			>20%
2	+	+		-	-	-	>10%
3	+	+		-			>20%
4	+	+	+	-	-		>20%

+ indicates positive; -, negative.

Discussion

CLMs are rare, indolent, soft tissue tumors of smooth muscle derivation. With a peak incidence in the fifth to seventh decade, these spindle-cell tumors present clinically as small, erythematous, indurated, solitary nodular lesions, commonly with overlying black, blue, or brown discoloration. When encountering a spindle cell neoplasm in the skin, a very broad differential should be considered. Entities, which may have overlapping features with CLM, include spindle cell squamous cell carcinoma, atypical fibroxanthoma, pleomorphic undifferentiated sarcoma, desmoplastic malignant melanoma, cellular neurofibroma, benign fibrous histiocytoma/dermatofibroma, cellular dermatofibroma, and leiomyoma. Definitive diagnosis usually requires immunohistochemical staining for vimentin, smooth muscle actin, caldesmon, laminin, and desmin [9]. CLMs are often asymptomatic, but symptomatic patients report associated pain, pruritus, bleeding, and burning sensation.

CLMs are thought to arise from arrector pili muscles or dermal vasculature. Differentiating CLMs from subcutaneous and deep leiomyosarcomas is important because the probability of metastasis differs greatly. Subcutaneous leiomyosarcomas have been shown to recur in up to 70% of cases and metastasize in 30% to 40% of cases [10]. To date only 1 case of distant metastasis from a primary CLM has been reported 15 years after the primary diagnosis, and there was subcutaneous involvement[2]. This difference in behavior underscores the importance of histologically differentiating CLMs as either intradermal or subcutaneous [11].

A diagnosis of CLM should be made in combination with morphologic features, such as immunohistochemical evidence of smooth muscle differentiation, diffuse or nodular growth pattern histologically, nuclear pleomorphism, presence of mitotic figures, atypical mitotic figures or necrosis [12] (these data of our patients are collected in Table 2). Malignancy criteria established by WHO include high cellularity, nuclear atypia significantly and at least one mitosis by 10 high power fields [13]. In our cases all were characterized by recognizable mitotic activity. Mitotic indices varied from 7 to 15/10 HPF.

Histologic subtype of nodular versus diffuse did not seem to correlate with degree of smooth muscle differentiation because clinicians usually took an aggressive surgical approach to excise a diffuse lesion. CLMs with a diffuse pattern of growth have been regarded as a diagnostic challenge due to their often inconspicuous mitoses and minimal cytologic atypia [14].

Immunohistochemistry can be very helpful in arriving at a correct diagnosis, but many variant staining patterns in CLMs exist and pathologists should be aware of the limitations of immunohistochemical staining [15,16]. Leiomyosarcomas are characterized by co-expression of desmin and muscle-specific actin. These four cases reported were diagnosed by the typical histological and immunohistochemical features of these tumors (Table 3). Desmin and SMA, together, were positive in 4 (100%) of the cases. With some caveats, CD34, S100, and CK 5/6 were helpful in ruling out other important cutaneous spindle cell neoplasms.

Recently, Hall and Grossman [17] have considered that PTEN staining does not add to the utility of a diagnostic immunohistochemical panel. More studies are needed to determine whether this stain can distinguish CLMs from its benign counterpart, deeply located counterparts, or other cutaneous spindle cell neoplasms [18].

Conclusion

CLM can have significant morphologic variation and overlap with other spindle cell neoplasms of the skin and that a limited panel of key immunohistochemical stains should be used to distinguish this lesion. Desmin, SMA and caldesmon staining are positive in a vast majority of cases. However, none of these markers is absolutely specific for smooth muscle, and positivity for two of these markers is more supportive of leiomyosarcoma.

References

[1] Kraft S, Fletcher CD. Atypical intradermal smooth muscle neoplasms: clinicopathologic analysis of 84 cases and a reappraisal of cutaneous "leiomyosarcoma". *Am. J. Surg. Pathol.* 2011;35: 599–607.

[2] Massi D, Franchi A, Alos L, et al. Primary cutaneous leiomyosarcoma: clinicopathological analysis of 36 cases. *Histopathology*. 2010;56:251–262.

[3] Bernstein SC, Roenigk RK. Leiomyosarcoma of the skin. Treatment of 34 cases. *Dermatol Surg*. 1996;22:631–635.

[4] Kaddu S, Beham A, Cerroni L, et al. Cutaneous leiomyosarcoma. *Am. J. Surg. Pathol.* 1997;21:979–987.

[5] Porter CJ, Januszkiewicz JS. Cutaneous leiomyosarcoma. *Plast. Reconstr Surg.* 2002;109:964–967.

[6] Holst VA, Junkins-Hopkins JM, Elenitsaset R. Cutaneous smooth muscle neoplasms: Clinical features, histologic findings, and treatment options. *J. Am. Acad. Dermatol.* 2002;46:477–90.

[7] Diaz-Cascajo C, Borghi S, Weyers W. Desmoplastic leiomyosarcoma of the skin. *Am. J. Dermatopathol.* 2000;22:251–255.

[8] Choy C, Cooper A, Kossard S. Primary cutaneous diffuse leiomyosarcoma with desmoplasia. *Australas J. Dermatol.* 2006;47:291–295.

[9] Annest NM, Grekin S, Seabury Stone M, Messingham MJ. Cutaneous leiomyosarcoma: A tumor of the head and neck. *Dermatol. Surg.* 2007;33:628–33.

[10] Fauth CT, Bruecks AK, Temple W, Arlette JP, DiFrancesco LM. Superficial leiomyosarcoma: A clinicopathologic review and update. *J. Cutan Pathol.* 2010;37:269-76.

[11] Humphreys TR, Finkelstein DH, Lee JB. Superficial leiomyosarcoma treated with Mohs micrographic surgery. *Dermatol. Surg*. 2004;30:108–12.

[12] Hornick JL, Fletcher CD. Criteria for malignancy in non- visceral smooth muscle tumors. *Ann. Diagn Pathol.* 2003;7:60–6.

[13] Weedon D, Willamson RM, Patterson JW. Smooth and skeletal muscle tumors. In LeBoit PE, BurgG, Weedon D, Sarasin A, eds. World health organization classification of tumors pathology and genetics skin tumors. Lyon: IARC Press, 2006; 251.

[14] Limaiem F, Chelly I, Bellil S, et al. Primary cutaneous leiomyosarcoma: a histological and immunohistochemical study of 4 cases. *Pathologica.* 2007;99:415–419.

[15] Idriss MH, Kazlouskaya V, Malhotra S, Andres C, Elston DM. Phosphohistone-H3 and Ki-67 immunostaining in cutaneous pilar leiomyoma and leiomyosarcoma (atypical intradermal smooth muscle neoplasm). *J. Cutan Pathol.* 2013;40:409-12.

[16] Feigenbaum L, Skinner D, Golda N. Atypical cutaneous leiomyosarcoma with skip-lesion behaviour. *Dermatol. Surg.* 2013;39:660-2.

[17] Hall B, Grossman AH, Webber NP, Ward RA, Tripp SR, Rosenthal HG et al. Atypical Intradermal Smooth Muscle Neoplasms (Formerly Cutaneous Leiomyosarcomas): Case Series, Immunohistochemical Profile and Review of the Literature. *Appl. Immunohistochem. Mol. Morphol.* 2013;21:132–38.

[18] Hernando E, Charytonowicz E, Dudas ME, et al. The AKT-mTOR pathway plays a critical role in the development of leiomyosarcomas. *Nat. Med.* 2007;13:748–753.

In: Leiomyosarcoma
Editor: Rosemary H. Leach

ISBN: 978-1-63117-940-2

Chapter 9

Diagnosis and Pitfalls of Uterine Leiomyosarcoma

Dr. Rani Kanthan* and Jenna-Lynn Senger
Department of Pathology & Laboratory Medicine,
University of Saskatchewan, Saskatoon, SK

Abstract

Uterine leiomyosarcoma, though the most common mesenchymal tumor, yet constitutes only 1-2% of all uterine malignancies [1]. This malignancy is well known for its aggressiveness and confers a poor prognosis, even if diagnosed at an early stage; once disseminated, the overall survival is usually only 2.8 years [1, 2]. The majority of these tumors are only identified at histopathological examination of hysterectomy or myomectomy specimens [1]. An increasing trend towards conservative treatment of leiomyomas such as uterine artery embolization and gonadotropin-releasing-hormone agonists, may further delay the accurate diagnosis of these tumors, posing the risk of an increased incidence of high-grade tumors at presentation [1, 3].

Etiology

These malignancies are most commonly idiopathic. They are thought to be the result of complex and unbalanced karyotypes resulting in severe genome instability with varied gene alterations and multiple genomic aberrations. However, the identity of the majority of affected genes has not yet been discovered [2]. Frequent loss of chromosomes 10 and 13q has been noted in extrauterine and uterine leiomyosarcomas [4]. Somatic mutations of the gene *MED12*, has been identified in uterine leiomyosarcoma: the role of which remains unclear.

* Contact Author: Dr. Rani Kanthan, Room 2868, G-Wing, Department of Pathology & Laboratory Medicine, Royal University Hospital, 103 Hospital Drive, Saskatoon, SK, S7N 0W8. Telephone: 306-655-2158; Fax: 306-655-2223; E-mail: rani.kanthan@saskatoonhealthregion.ca

Overexpression of proteins that regulate mitotic centrosome and spindle function (i.e., UBE2C, Aurora A and B kinase, TPX2, Polo-like kinase I) have also been reported. The role of microRNA (miRNA) has additionally been investigated, which reveals that leiomyosarcoma is related to bone marrow-derived mesenchymal cells whereas leiomyomas appear to be linked with mature smooth muscle cells of the myometrium [5].

Hereditary retinoblastoma, Li-Fraumeni syndrome, and Epstein-Barr virus in the setting of immunosuppression may predispose patients to developing leiomyosarcoma [2]. Though obesity, hypertension, and diabetes are known risk factors for endometrial carcinoma, their implications on the development of leiomyosarcoma are relatively unknown. Unopposed estrogen may play a role, as tamoxifen use and oral contraceptives have been recognized as potential risk factors. Cigarette smoking has been reported as protective against the development of uterine leiomyosarcoma [6].

Clinical Charactersitics

While uterine leiomyosarcomas arise in patients after the third decade of life, they are most common in perimenopausal women [2]. As such, these tumors typically arise 10 years later than leiomyomas. The precise etiology remains elusive, and risk factors remain ill identified. While it was once conceived that leiomyosarcomas arise from leiomyomas, less than 1% of women with a clinical uterine leiomyoma have leiomyosarcoma; the current consensus therefore is that most leiomyosarcomas arise *de novo*. A leiomyoma that doubles in size every 3-6 months should, therefore, raise the concern of an underlying malignant process; however, the accuracy of this time frame remains controversial. A recent review found that only 0.27-2.6% of women who reported a rapidly growing pelvic mass were confirmed to have a leiomyosarcoma [7].

As with other soft tissue sarcomas, leiomyosarcomas are typically nonspecific on presentation, with symptoms attributed to mass effect rather than invasion [2]. The most common symptoms at presentation are abnormal vaginal bleeding in 53%, abdominal pain in 35%, and a palpable abdominal mass in 14% [7]. “Abnormal vaginal bleeding” may include menorrhagia, metorrhagia, or postmenopausal bleeding [6]. Pain is typically colicky in nature, and is associated with the passage of blood clots [7]. A rapidly growing uterine mass is another typical presentation [3]. Other symptoms may include abdominal distension or urinary symptoms. Patients may also be asymptomatic, with the diagnosis being made only on hysterectomy specimens, typically obtained at surgery for ‘leiomyomas’ [3, 6]. Of all patients who undergo hysterectomy for a fibroid (leiomyoma), only 0.5% are subsequently diagnosed with leiomyosarcoma [3].

If a patient presents with disseminated disease, symptoms related to lung, liver, bone or brain metastases may be the presenting complaint [6]. Less common sites of metastatic spread include the skull, heart, pancreas, and thyroid [8].

As there remains no definitive pre-operative procedure to differentiate a leiomyoma from a leiomyosarcoma, any ‘myoma’ with rapid growth in a postmenopausal female not taking hormone replacement should be suspected to be a sarcoma until proven otherwise [6].

Diagnostic Workup

The preoperative diagnosis of leiomyosarcomas continues to be a challenge. Despite the availability of techniques such as radiological imaging and/or endometrial curettage/biopsy, the diagnosis of leiomyosarcoma is often only confirmed on histopathological examination of the definitive hysterectomy specimen.

Imaging Characteristics

Imaging approach to leiomyosarcoma typically includes assessment of the primary tumor and a concurrent evaluation for metastases. There are, however, no pathognomonic imaging findings for leiomyosarcoma. Accurate differentiation of leiomyosarcoma from degenerative and cellular leiomyomas is a challenge due to overlap in MR morphology and enhancement characteristics [9]. Several recent studies have concluded that there are no 'objective' imaging characteristics to distinguish a benign from a malignant mesenchymal tumor in the uterus aside from the presence of metastatic or diffuse disease [3].

Ultrasound

The initial workup of a suspected uterine sarcoma should include a transvaginal ultrasound [6]. The uterine/endometrial vascularization can be assessed using transvaginal pulsed and color Doppler ultrasonography, which evaluates blood flow impedance of uterine, myometrial, and/or endometrial vessels [7]. Leiomyosarcomas often contain an irregular vessel distribution with low impedance to flow and high peak systolic velocities [4]. The ability of this technique to differentiate benign vs. malignant disease remains controversial, with early studies suggesting its utility yet subsequent studies not confirming these results [3].

Magnetic Resonance Imaging (MRI)

Magnetic resonance imaging (MRI) may play an important role in differentiating and determining proper management of leiomyomsarcomas [7]. Leiomyosarcomas often are seen as a mass distorting normal uterine anatomy, with or without regions of necrosis and hemorrhage [9]. These masses may enhance with gadolinium-DTPA [3]. Sarcomas within the uterus typically appear as a large infiltrating myometrial mass with heterogeneous hypointensity on T1-weighted imaging (T1WI) with foci of high signal and intermediate/high intensity on T2-weighted imaging (T2WI) [7, 9]. This is in contrast to benign leiomyoma with low-intensity on T2WI; however, degenerative or cellular leiomyoma can have increased T2WI signal intensity [7]. Other MRI findings that have been reported include low signal intensity reminiscent of leiomyoma, or a mass with focally infiltrative margins [4]. Other features that suggest a malignant process involve the presence of necrosis in cystic regions on T2WI and irregular margins with hyperintense regions on T1WI [9]. Typically, leiomyosarcomas have no evidence of calcification [4]. Thus in summary, leiomyomas with 'atypical' imaging features continue to pose challenges in differentiating leiomyoma from leiomyosarcomas as objective image analysis is not particularly sensitive [10].

Diffusion-Weighted Imaging (DWI)

Diffusion-weighted imaging (DWI) uses Brownian motion to define tissue characteristics; this technique creates an image based on the movement of water molecules within the tissue [7, 9]. This technique delineates malignant lesions as hyperintense regions. The apparent diffusion coefficient (ADC) can be determined using this technique, and tissues with a different viscosity or altered intracellular:extracellular water ratio can be identified. Malignant tumors typically have a decreased ADC [7]. The greatest sensitivity and specificity was obtained when this technique was combined with T2-weighted MRI [3]. The use of this modality is however limited, as there remains a considerable overlap between benign and malignant imaging features [9]. Lack of standardization, routine availability and technical expertise may be additional impediments in this regard.

Positron Emission Tomography (PET) Scan

In PET scans, the increased glucose metabolism by metabolic cells results in higher levels of fluoro-deoxyglucose (FDG) uptake which is detected and used to reconstruct an image that provides metabolic and anatomic information. This imaging modality is typically combined with a CT scan. PET-CT is a highly sensitive and specific modality for detecting recurrence and is therefore most suited as a surveillance monitoring tool to detect metastases or recurrences after an initial histological diagnosis has been confirmed [7]. However, the true sensitivity and specificity of this modality remains poorly understood [3]. Routine PET scans, therefore have no significant advantage in the current surveillance strategy of physical exams and conventional imaging such as CT or MRI.

Staging Workup

An initial chest x-ray is recommended, as up to 10% of leiomyosarcomas can present with 'silent' pulmonary metastases [11]. As uterine leiomyosarcomas are inherently aggressive neoplasms, computed tomography (CT) scanning of the chest, abdomen, and pelvis is warranted to evaluate for extra-pelvic spread [6].

Biopsy/Curettage Characteristics

As leiomyosarcomas arise in the myometrium, most cases are not diagnosed from endometrial sampling [7]. Endometrial curettage is only diagnostic in 30% of patients with uterine leiomyosarcoma [6].

Histopathological Characteristics

Leiomyosarcoma are normally solitary intramural masses not associated with leiomyomas [8]. On gross exam, uterine leiomyosarcomas may appear as large and irregular masses with necrosis and/or hemorrhage [9]. They usually have a poorly-defined border and may appear as large fleshy soft, gray/white lesions with areas of hemorrhage and necrosis in contrast to the whorled and fibrous appearance of a conventional leiomyoma. The myxoid subtypes may appear grossly different, with a gelatinous texture with free fluid exudation [8].

As there are no pathognomonic clinical or imaging features for the preoperative identification of leiomyosarcomas, accurate diagnosis typically relies on histopathological evaluation. Leiomyosarcomas are malignant mesenchymal tumors and as such are composed of cells exhibiting features of smooth muscle lineage. They are usually sufficiently differentiated to allow recognition of their smooth muscle origin [4]. These tumors demonstrate spindle cells in intersecting sharply demarcated fascicles with abundant eosinophilic cytoplasm and elongated hyperchromatic nuclei [2]. Abundant mitosis of >20 per 10high power fields (HPF) are typical [8]. Focal pleomorphism is common; however, extensive pleomorphism resembling an undifferentiated soft tissue sarcoma or clear cell areas may also be focally present [2, 8].

While traditionally the mitotic index has been used to differentiate malignant vs. benign, it is now well understood that tumors of a low mitotic index may exhibit malignant behavior [12]. In response, new criteria have been developed. A diagnosis of leiomyosarcoma can be made in the presence of two of the following three characteristics:

a) diffuse nuclear atypia,
b) increased mitotic rate of >10 per 10HPFs
c) coagulative tumor necrosis [2, 7].

Indicators of atypia include nuclear pleomorphism, nucleomegaly, nuclear membrane irregularity, hyperchromatism with prominent nuclei. Only mitotic figures identified by the presence of hairy chromatin extending from a central dense mass of chromosomes in the presence of discernible cytoplasm should be included in the mitotic count, as lymphocytes, mast cells, stripped nuclei, degenerated cells, or precipitated hematoxylin may mimic true mitotic figures, resulting in a falsely elevated mitotic count [5]. Additionally, endogenous and exogenous hormones may physiologically increase mitotic counts, and delayed fixation may decrease these counts [13]. Accurate calculation of the mitotic index is imperative as this factor is most strongly associated with tumor behavior and thus impacts patient prognosis [14].

Differentiation between true coagulative necrosis of leiomyosarcoma from the hyaline or ulcerative necrosis of uterine leiomyomas is paramount for accurate diagnosis [12]. Coagulative necrosis, also known as 'tumor cell necrosis' is characterized by the presence of an abrupt transition point from viable to necrotic cells, without the presence of an interposed granulation or fibrous zone. By contrast, hyaline necrosis, also termed 'infarct-type necrosis' contains a region of connective tissue, whether granulation or fibrous depending on the age of the infarct, that separates viable cells from necrotic cells. Finally, ulcerative necrosis is most common on the surface of a submucosal leiomyoma and contains inflammatory cells surrounding a foci of necrotic debris [15].

Two subtypes of leiomyosarcoma have been described: epithelioid and myxoid. Diagnostic criteria of these subtypes have a lower criteria diagnostic threshold. Diagnosis of epithelioid leiomyosarcoma requires the presence of >5 mitoses/10HPF with any degree of cytological atypia and/or tumor cell necrosis [5]. Epithelioid leiomyosarcoma characteristically contains abundant eosinophilic cytoplasm and may have a centrally placed nucleus; rarely they can contain rhabdoid cells, resembling primitive skeletal muscle precursors. The mitotic rate cannot be accurately assessed in the myxoid subtype of leiomyosarcoma which is composed of a hypocellular stroma with dispersed malignant cells

[8]. Criteria for malignancy in this subset of tumors includes either i) the presence of severe atypia with/without tumor cell necrosis and any mitotic index or ii) mitotic index >2/10HPF without tumor cell necrosis or atypia [5]. Infiltrative tumor margin may be a useful feature in diagnosing either epithelioid or myxoid leiomyosarcoma. Rare histopathologic characteristics of leiomyosarcomas have been reported that include osteoclast-like giant cells, xanthomatous change, or an oncocytic appearance due to the presence of abundant mitochondria [8].

The relationship between leiomyoma and leiomyosarcoma remains poorly defined, with many authors suggesting that these are separate entities rather than a continuum. On the other hand, other authors suggest that it may be challenging to differentiate malignant vs. benign lesions as there is a continuum from benign→borderline→high-grade leiomyosarcoma [2]. The latter hypothesis is not in current vogue. Regardless of the pathophysiology, accurate distinction between these two entities can be challenging, as there are no preoperative imaging characteristics or serum markers to reliably differentiate them [11]. Leiomyoma variants such as symplastic (atypical, bizarre, or pleomorphic), mitotically-active, and cellular leiomyomas may demonstrate nuclear atypia, high mitotic index, and high cellularity respectively. As such, these benign tumors may be misdiagnosed as leiomyosarcoma by the unwary [16].

Immunohistochemical Characteristics

Leiomyosarcomas are typically reactive for smooth muscle markers that include alpha smooth muscle actin, desmin, h-caldesmon, and histone deacetylase 8 (HDAC8); however, epithelioid/myxoid tumors may not express these markers [2, 5]. Uterine leiomyosarcomas typically express platelet derived growth factor receptor-alpha, Wilms' tumor gene 1, aromatase, and gonadotropin-releasing hormone receptor. Androgen receptor positivity is detected in 40% of uterine leiomyosarcomas [7]. Estrogen-receptor and progesterone-receptor markers are positive in up to 60% of cases [5]. These tumors usually have no expression of epidermal growth factor receptor and ERBB2 [7]. Although KIT expression has been occasionally documented, these findings alone are insufficient for identifying targets for treatment [4].

Overexpression of cell cycle proteins p16, p53, and Ki67 may additionally suggest a malignant process; however, they are not predictive of outcome [11, 17]. Increased expression of p16 with p53 and MIB1 has been shown to be highly suggestive of leiomyosarcoma rather than leiomyoma or STUMP [16]. Overexpression of p53 is detected in 25% of leiomyosarcomas and 7% of atypical leiomyomas, whereas its expression is less frequent in STUMPs and leiomyomas with bizarre nuclei, and is nonexistent in conventional leiomyomas [13]. The interpretation of the expression of cell cycle regulatory proteins in the diagnosis of leiomyosarcoma warrants caution as upregulation, though more common in leiomyosarcoma, is also present in atypical and cellular leiomyomas [13]. The marker MMP2 may be used to aid in differentiating leiomyosarcomas from leiomyomas as greater expression is associated with malignancy. Additionally, CD44v3 is not expressed in leiomyosarcoma yet is typically expressed in leiomyomas [8]. Fascin expression is identified in 90% of leiomyosarcomas and 50% of STUMPs but rarely in leiomyomas [5].

Diagnostic Pitfalls

Though the diagnosis of conventional leiomyoma is routine for the pathologist, there are many variants of these tumors that can be misinterpreted as leiomyomsarcoma or another type of uterine neoplasm for the unwary pathologist. The following section addresses some of the more common leiomyoma variants and unusual growth patterns seen in these smooth muscle tumors that can potentially lead to diagnostic confusion and error.

Leiomyoma Variants [8, 15, 18]

1. Mitotically Active Leiomyomas

Mitotically active leiomyomas smooth muscle tumors with no atypia, necrosis, or invasion of the vasculature/muscle. These benign tumors may have 15-20 mitoses/10HPF, rarely even >20mitoses/10HPF, yet will behave in a benign manner. Up to 15% have microscopic vascular invasion within the tumor confines. Mitotically-active leiomyomas are most common in the submucosa and thus are subject to trauma. These tumors are usually identified in reproductive-aged women, typically in the secretory phase of menstruation, or in the presence of pregnancy or exogenous hormone use.

2. Symplastic Leiomyomas

Symplastic leiomyomas often the most difficult to distinguish from leiomyosarcoma. Histopathological examination reveals nuclear atypia, with bizarre, grossly enlarged hyperchromatic nuclei. Chromatin may have a 'smudged' appearance, and the nuclei may contain cytoplasmic pseudoinclusions mimicking eosinophilic macronucleoli. Distribution of bizarre cells may be multifocal or diffuse. They typically have <10 mitoses/10HPF. A minority of symplastic leiomyomas may have hemorrhagic foci, hydropic change, and/or infarct-type necrosis. Features that may aid in differentiating symplastic leiomyomas from leiomyosarcoma may include multifocal rather than diffuse nuclear atypia, absence of tumor necrosis, and low mitotic count with no increased expression of MIB1/PCNA on immunohistochemistry.

3. Pseudosarcomatous Leiomyomas

Pseudosarcomatous leiomyomas may cause a diagnostic dilemma as they are difficult to distinguish from leiomyosarcomas. These tumors fit within the criteria of a true leiomyosarcoma, with nuclear atypia and coagulative necrosis, yet are only a benign variant of the conventional leiomyoma. Three key features distinguishing a pseduosarcomatous leiomyoma rather than a leiomyosarcoma have been proposed:

a) cellularity/pleomorphism heterogeneity with dense cytoplasm and less hyperchromatic nuclei,
b) intermingled regions of the conventional leiomyoma, and
c) the presence of intense estrogen and/or progesterone receptor staining [12].

4. Cellular Leiomyomas

Cellular leiomyomas are otherwise normal leiomyomas with a high degree of cellularity. This benign variant accounts for only <5% of all leiomyomas. Hemorrhage or infarct-type necrosis may be present; however, cellular leiomyomas do not have an elevated mitotic count. Dense cellularity, prominent vascularity, and irregular margins may cause diagnostic confusion. When well-circumscribed, they may appear similar to an endometrial stromal nodule; when their borders are irregular their histopathological appearance is reminiscent of low-grade endometrial stromal sarcoma. Features that may indicate a cellular leiomyoma rather than a stromal neoplasm include a fascicular growth pattern in the periphery, and the absence of foamy histiocytes.

5. Apoplectic Leiomyomas

Apoplectic leiomyomas are hormone-sensitive benign tumors that arise most commonly in women who are pregnant or on oral contraceptive therapy. Use of tamoxifen or clomiphene may precipitate rapid growth, causing clinical suspicion of a malignant process. Features of apoplectic leiomyoma may additionally be appreciated in leiomyomas treated with GnRH agonists prior to excision. Patients may present with the typical picture of abnormal uterine bleeding/pain, or as an acute abdomen secondary to leiomyoma rupture causing hemoperitoneum. These tumors, also called 'hemorrhagic cellular leiomyoma', may have increased mitotic counts up to 2-10/10HPF around foci of hemorrhage. On histopathological exam, regions of hemorrhage, edema, myxoid change, focal hypercellularity, nuclear pleomorphism and increased mitotic activity may be appreciated. Intimal myxoid change and fibrosis, medial hypertrophy, fibrinoid necrosis and thrombosis are potential vascular changes. The presence of 'red degeneration' (dusky red discoloration of the uterus) is characteristically seen during pregnancy.

6. Degenerative Leiomyoma

Degenerative leiomyoma may be a confounding diagnosis. This may include hemorrhage, hyalinization, hydropic/myxoid/mucinous/cystic degeneration, and true necrosis. Hyaline degeneration is common in leiomyomas, often with dystrophic calcification. This may cause compartmentalization of smooth muscle cells creating an epithelial-like appearance of an epithelioid leiomyoma. Hydropic degeneration, characterized by well-to-poorly circumscribed zones of edematous connective tissue, is often misinterpreted as myxoid degeneration [15]. Additional findings may include occasional fibroblasts, flocculent/granular eosinophilic proteinaceous material, dystrophic calcification, and numerous blood vessels. "Perinodular hydropic change" may be present, in which sparsely cellular hydropic connective tissue divides the leiomyoma into small nodules, potentially mimicking leiomyomatosis.

7. Myxoid Leiomyomas

Myxoid leiomyomas are tumors characterized by abundant acellular pale material rich in mucins. On gross examination, they have a soft gray jelly-like appearance. On histopathological evaluation stellate-shaped neoplastic cells are widely separated by extracellular material. These lesions are often indistinguishable from myxoma. In this context, the infiltrative borders of a myxoid leiomyosarcoma in contrast to well-circumscribed border of myxoid leiomyoma may be useful in distinguishing between these two neoplasms.

8. Leiomyoma with Heterologous Elements

Leiomyoma with heterologous elements the most common of which is lipoleiomyoma, have no additional clinical implications. Leiomyomas have been reported to contain mature bone, cartilage, skeletal muscle, or epithelial elements. Endometrial, endocervical, and tubal-type glands have also been reported within a leiomyoma.

9. Pyomyomas

Pyomyomas are the result of a bacterial infection within a leiomyoma and are characterized by a prominent number of inflammatory and hematopoietic cells. On gross evaluation, an abscess cavity within the tumor is appreciable.

Unusual Growth Patterns of Smooth Muscle Tumors [8, 15, 18]

1. Leiomyomatosis

Leiomyomatosis may be concerning to the clinician, as patients typically present with uterine enlargement. On microscopic examination, countless nodules composed of cytologically benign mitotically inactive smooth muscle cells are visualized. These nodules are often ill-defined. They may coalesce with adjacent nodules and the surrounding myometrium, and may contain clustered capillaries in a hyalinized stroma.

2. Cotyledonoid-Dissecting Leiomyomas

(Sternberg tumor) typically presents as a placenta-like mass extruding into the vascular channels. These tumors are often lobulated with irregular and indistinct margins, and may protrude into the broad ligament and/or pelvic cavity. While their growth pattern is aggressive and destructive, with a grossly sarcomatous appearance, these are benign lesions as there is no mitotic activity, atypia, or necrosis on histopathological evaluation. Micronodules of smooth muscle in a swirling pattern with marked vascularity and hydropic/hyaline degeneration may be present.

3. Intravascular Leiomyomatosis

Intravascular leiomyomatosis may appear concerning, as these tumors typically appear as smooth muscle masses that extend into the pelvic blood vessels, occasionally extending up to the inferior vena cava and the right side of the heart. Histopathology can reveal any of the morphological variants of uterine leiomyoma.

4. Benign Metastasizing Leiomyoma

Benign metastasizing leiomyoma may be iatrogenic, alleged to arise from fragments of a curetted or surgically removed leiomyoma that enter the lymphatics. They may also present as multiple pulmonary nodules [8]. Less common sites of involvement include the retroperitoneal and mediastinal lymph nodes, soft tissue, and bone. Histopathological examination of these tumors reveals no criteria for malignancy.

5. Parasitic Leiomyoma

Parasitic leiomyoma are otherwise unremarkable leiomyomas attached to the pelvic peritoneum, typically in a patient with uterine leiomyomas. They are thought to arise from subserosal pedunculated uterine leiomyomas that lose their attachment to the uterus.

Smooth Muscle Tumor of Unknown Malignant Potential (STUMP) [14, 16, 19]

The term 'smooth muscle tumor of unknown malignant potential' (STUMP) is reserved for tumors that neither confidently fit the category for a benign nor malignant lesion; it perhaps represents lesions found along the spectrum between leiomyoma and leiomyosarcoma. Consistent with this definition, on radiologic evaluation these tumors appear identical to leiomyomas or leiomyosarcomas. They are diagnosed when a tumor demonstrates one or more of the criteria of a smooth muscle malignancy but not all criteria necessary to diagnose leiomyosarcoma. They have been reported as subserosal, intramural, and submucosal lesions. There remains the risk, however, of the term "STUMP" becoming a 'dumping group' for the aforementioned leiomyoma variants. There continues to be limited knowledge regarding the unpredictable behavior of these tumors, and the most appropriate treatment for STUMP remains unknown. Studies have shown that most tumors classified as 'STUMP' behave in a benign fashion; however, these tumors are heterogenous in behavior and have the potential to recur and/or metastasize. The diagnosis of STUMP in a myomectomy or hysterectomy specimen remains a dilemma for clinicians regarding further management. STUMP therefore remains a diagnostic challenge to both clinicians and pathologists. It is proposed that patients with STUMP should at least be counseled regarding the potential for recurrence as leiomyosarcoma. Additionally, STUMP patients are recommended to have closer surveillance than the usual yearly examination and may benefit by consultation with a dedicated gynecologic oncologist [19].

Other Uterine Sarcomas [9]

An understanding of the differential diagnosis of uterine leiomyosarcoma necessitates an appreciation for the taxonomy of uterine sarcomas as it is from within the mesenchymal tumors of this group that uterine leiomyosarcoma must be distinguished. The World Health Organization classifies endometrial cancer into epithelioid, mesenchymal, and mixed. Pure mesenchymal tumors of the female genital tract include smooth muscle and endometrial stromal tumors. The smooth muscle tumor category is then further subdivided to include leiomyomas, leiomyosarcoma, and smooth muscle tumors of uncertain malignant potential (STUMP). The endometrial stromal tumors are then subdivided to endometrial stromal nodules, low-grade ESS, and undifferentiated endometrial sarcoma. Mixed epithelial and mesenchymal tumors include carcinosarcoma, adenosarcoma, carcinofibroma, adenofibroma, and adenomyoma. The accurate diagnosis of uterine leiomyosarcoma therefore necessitates exclusion of these other mesenchymal tumors. As previously discussed, the clinical presentation of uterine sarcomas is nonspecific; it therefore provides no clues of the underlying etiology. A brief summary of the radiological, and histopathology findings common to each of these mesenchymal tumors is available in Table 1 [3, 6, 8, 9, 10, 20].

Prognostic Features

While a number of patient and histopathologic tumor features have been proposed, no clear evidence is available to indicate the factors that are truly prognostic. Factors including age, menopause status, mitotic count, and adjuvant therapy have all been reported as potential prognostic factors. Poor prognosis has been documented in association with advanced stage, high grade and mitotic index, vascular space invasion, lack of primary surgery, older age group at presentation, and African-American race [3]. Clear tumor margins post-operatively are a positive prognostic factor for patients with leiomyosarcoma [6].

Leiomyosarcoma is staged using the 2009 FIGO system, with uterine sarcoma-specific criteria including tumor size and extension beyond the uterus; however, the predictive accuracy has not improved from the 1988 FIGO system, which was used for many years prior to the emergence of new guidelines. A normogram to predict postoperative 5-year survival has been developed, which takes into account tumor size, histological grade, uterine cervical involvement, regional & distant metastases, age at diagnosis, and mitotic index [21]. This normogram is reported to have better prognostic accuracy and individualized prediction of overall survival than the standard FIGO system [5]. Mitotic count is generally accepted to be the most important prognostic factor, and has been reported multiple times to significantly impact survival. The Gynecologic Oncology Group (GOG) found mitotic count to be the only factor to significantly affect progression-free survival in patients with early-stage leiomyosarcoma [1]. Similarly, a Norwegian study following 419 patients found on multivariate analysis that the number of mitoses is a significant independent prognostic factor [22]. In patients with early-stage disease, the size of the tumor and the number of mitoses are reported to impact survival; however, with late stage malignancy only the mitotic count is significant. Other authors have, however, disputed this claim and reported no correlation between prognosis and mitotic count [1]. Tumor size has also been reported to be an independent prognostic marker. Tumors $<$5cm have been associated with an improved 5-year crude survival of 64.0% versus 56.4% for tumors 5-10cm, and 29.3% for tumors greater than 10cm [22]. Combining mitotic rate and tumor size allows for patient to be stratified as low-risk (MI $\leq$10; tumor diameter $\leq$10cm), medium-risk (MI $\geq$10 or tumor diameter $>$10cm), and high-risk (MI$>$10 and tumor diameter $>$10cm), in which 'high-risk' patients have a 5.3-fold greater risk of death [6]. Tumor factors such as the type of border (pushing vs. infiltrative), the degree of nuclear pleomorphism, and the presence of vascular invasion are attributed as additional risk factors for early recurrence.

As the myometrium is a rich vascular organ, the aggressive behavior of uterine leiomyosarcomas is often credited to involvement of the vascular space resulting in early hematogenous metastases. These tumors will typically have a higher Ki67 expression and often a shortened survival [8]. The presence of metastatic/diffuse disease at presentation confers a poor prognosis, with few to no patients surviving 5 years post-diagnosis in the stage IV population compared with 51% 5-year-crude-survival in stage I [6]. Expression of a number of immunohistochemical proteins is prognostically significant, including overexpression of p53 and positive staining to bcl-2. P53 positive stage I-II tumors have a higher recurrence rate than the overall expected five-year recurrence rates which ranges from 45-73% [23]. Tumor related factors such as DNA ploidy and S-phase fraction (SPF) have been reported to have independent prognostic significance [24].

Treatment options for uterine leiomyosarcoma may be surgical or medical. As only ~3% of early stage uterine leiomyosarcomas present with lymphatic spread, lymphadenectomy is often not indicated as it has failed to be an independent prognostic factor for survival [4]. Many studies also suggest that lymph node metastases are usually only found in cases with extra-uterine disease associated with rapid progression of the sarcoma. The necessity of oophorectomy remains debatable. High grade, advanced stage disease, and oophorectomy are associated with significantly reduced disease-specific survival on multivariate analysis [23]. Oophorectomy is typically conducted due to the small risk of ovarian metastases and the potential for hormone-sensitive leiomyosarcoma. The standard treatment of leiomyosarcoma is, therefore, simple hysterectomy with oophorectomy and without lymphadenectomy [4]. In premenopausal women, an isolated hysterectomy may be considered to preserve fertility and endogenous estrogen. The value of adjuvant therapy for uterine leiomyosarcoma remains indeterminate. The rationale to eradicate micrometastases with adjuvant chemotherapy has not been validated in the postoperative management of uterine leiomyosarcoma, with several studies showing no proven survival benefit [4, 21]. Adjuvant radiotherapy, similarly, seems to have no real benefit in reducing local recurrence or improving overall survival in uterine leiomyosarcoma. For patients with advanced or recurrent disease, treatment options are limited to being palliative [4].

Conclusion

Uterine leiomyosarcoma is a rare, aggressive, lethal, malignant neoplasm. Despite advances in imaging techniques including the availability of new modalities, there remain no pathognomonic imaging characteristics that can provide a preoperative definitive diagnosis. The lack of serum markers further relegates the diagnosis of uterine leioymosarcoma solely to pathological evaluation. Though conventional leiomyoma is extremely common, there are many variants of these smooth muscle neoplasms with marked histomorphologic diversity that continue to cause diagnostic dilemma for the pathologist. Additionally, neoplasms such as STUMP continue to pose a challenge both for the clinician and the pathologist.

Though treatment is primarily surgical for uterine leiomyosarcomas, given the rarity of this lesion, guidelines for management remain largely ill defined and consensus-based rather than evidence-based. The role of adjuvant therapy – chemo or radiation – is undetermined and appears to confer no real survival benefit, as reported in the published literature. Despite the proposal of many clinical and tumor prognostic factors, the stage of the tumor is the best determinant for outcome in terms of recurrence and overall survival. Future multi-institutional research strategies with multidisciplinary teams of dedicated gynecological pathologists and gynecological oncologists are recommended to develop treatment algorithms for improved survival. Table 1 outlines the key pathology and radiology findings seen in mesenchymal and mixed tumors of the uterus. (Table cells highlighted with a grey background are benign neoplasms.)

Table 1. Differential Diagnosis (Pathology & Radiology) of benign vs. malignant uterine sarcomas [8, 9, 10, 20]

			Pathology	Radiology
Mesenchymal Tumors	Endometrial Stromal & Related Tumors	Endometrial stromal sarcoma	• Worm-like tumor plugs in myometrial vessels and lymphatics • Infiltrating margin • Densely cellular tumor • Vascular space invasion • Little atypia, mitosis, or myometrial infiltration	• Heterogenous intensity (CECT) • Bands low signal intensity • Tumor extension along vessels or ligaments • Isointense relative to myometrium on T1WI • Hyperintense on T2WI
		Undifferentiated endometrial sarcoma	• No resemblance to endometrial stroma • No evidence smooth muscle • Pleomorphic cells • High mitotic index • Marked cytological atypia	• Same as ESS on CECT & MRI • Vascular & lymphatic invasion
		Endometrial stromal nodule	• No myometrial/vascular invasion • Cells resemble proliferative phase of stromal cells	• Same as ESS on CECT & MRI
	Smooth Muscle Tumors	Leiomyosarcoma	• Cytological atypia • Tumor cell necrosis • Elevated mitotic index	• Hyperintense regions T1WI • Intermediate/High intensity on T2WI
		Leiomyoma	• Vary depending on subtype • 'atypical leiomyoma' → cytologic atypia	• Low signaling T1WI & T2WI
		STUMP	• Atypia or necrosis or high mitotic rate (doesn't satisfy criteria of leiomyosarcoma)	• Indistinguishable from leiomyosarcoma
Mixed Epithelial & Mesenchymal Tumors	Carcinosarcoma*		• Mixture epithelial malignancy (often adenocarcinoma) + stromal malignancy • +/- heterologous components: cartilage, fat, bone, rhabdoid, choriocarcinoma, melanocytic differentiation • High-grade stroma	• Hypo- to isointense to endometrium on T2WI • Enhances more than endometrial carcinoma
	Adenosarcoma		• Benign epithelial component + sarcomatous mesenchymal element (homologous or heterologous)	• Multi-septated cystic mass • Low signal intensity areas on T2WI

*-Recent updates seem to favor 'carcinosarcoma' as a de-differentiated/metaplastic variant of endometrial carcinoma [3, 6].

-The grey bars indicate "non-malignant lesions.

References

[1] Rauh-Hain JA, Oduyebo T, Diver EJ, Guseh SH, George S, Muto MG, del Carmen MG. Uterine leiomyosarcoma. An updated series. *Int J Gynecol Cancer.* 2013; 23: 1036-43.

[2] Serrano C, George S. Leiomyosarcoma. *Hematol Oncol Clin N Am.* 2013; 27: 957-74.

[3] Seddon BM, Davda R. Uterine sarcomas – recent progress and future challenges. *European Journal of Radiology.* 2011; 78: 30-40.

[4] Amant F, Coosemans A, Debiec-Rychter M, Timmerman D, Vergote I. Clinical management of uterine sarcomas. *Lancet Oncol.* 2009; 10: 1188-98.

[5] Chiang S, Oliva E. Recent developments in uterine mesenchymal neoplasms. *Histopathology.* 2013; 62: 124-37.

[6] Trope CG, Abeler VM, Kristensen GB. Diagnosis and treatment of sarcoma of the uterus. A review. *Acta Oncologica.* 2012; 51: 694-705.

[7] Wu TI, Yen TC, Lai CH. Clinical presentation and diagnosis of uterine sarcoma, including imaging. *Best Practice & Research Clinical Obstetrics and Gynaecology.* 2011; 25: 681-9.

[8] Brown L. Pathology of uterine malignancies. *Clinical Oncology.* 2008; 20: 433-47.

[9] Tirumani SH, Ojili V, Shanbhogue AKP, Fasih N, Ryan JG, Reinhold C. Current concepts in the imaging of uterine sarcoma. *Abdom Imaging.* 2013; 38: 397-411.

[10] Cornfeld D, Israel G, Martel M, Weinreb J, Schwartz P, McCarthy S. MRI appearance of mesenchymal tumors of the uterus. *European Journal of Radiology.* 2010; 74: 241-9.

[11] Sutton G. Uterine sarcomas 2013. *Gynecologic Oncology.* 2013; 130: 3-5.

[12] Watanabe K, Suzuki T. Uterine leiomyoma versus leiomyosarcoma: a new attempt at differential diagnosis based on their cellular characteristics. *Histopathology.* 2006; 48: 563-8.

[13] Mills AM, Ly A, Balzer BL, Hendrickson MR, Kempson RL, McKenney JK, Longacre TA. Cell cycle regulatory markers in uterine atypical leiomyoma and leiomyosarcoma. *Am J Surg Pathol.* 2013; 37: 634-42.

[14] Vilos GA, Marks J, Ettler HC, Vilos AG, Prefontaine M, Abu-Rafea B. Uterine smooth muscle tumors of uncertain malignant potential: diagnostic challenges and therapeutic dilemmas. Report of 2 cases and review of the literature. *The Journal of Minimally Invasive Gynecology.* 2012; 19(3): 288-95.

[15] Clement PB. The pathology of uterine smooth muscle tumors and mixed endometrial stromal-smooth muscle tumors: a selective review with emphasis on recent advances. *Int J Gynecol Pathol.* 2000; 19: 39-55.

[16] O'Neill CJ, McBride HA, Connolly LE, McCluggage WG. Uterine leiomyosarcomas are characterized by high p16, p53, and MIB1 expression in comparison with usual leiomyomas, leiomyoma variants and smooth muscle tumours of uncertain malignant potential. *Histopathology.* 2007; 50: 851-8.

[17] Chen L, Yang B. Immunohistochemical analysis of p16, p53 and Ki-67 expression in uterine smooth muscle tumors. *Int J Gynecol Pathol.* 2008; 27: 326-32.

[18] Wilkinson N, Rollason TP. Recent advances in the pathology of smooth muscle tumours of the uterus. *Histopathology.* 2001; 39: 331-41.

[19] Guntupalli SR, Ramirez PT, Anderson ML, Miliam MR, Bodurka DC, Malpica A. Uterine smooth muscle tumor of uncertain malignant potential: a retrospective analysis. *Gynecologic Oncology*. 2009; 113: 324-6.

[20] Szklaruk J, Tamm EP, Choi H, Varavithya V. MR imaging of common and uncommon large pelvic masses. *Radiographics*. 2003; 23(2): 403-24.

[21] Zivanovic O, Jacks LM, Iasonos A, Leitao M, Soslow RA, Veras E, Chi DS, Abu-Rustum NR, Barakat RR, Brennan MF, Hensley ML. A normogram to predict postresection 5-year overall survival for patients with uterine leiomyosarcoma. *Cancer*. 2012; 118: 660-9.

[22] Abeler VM, Royne O, Thoresen S, Danielsen HE, Nesland JM, Kristensen GB. Uterine sarcomas in Norway. A histopathological and prognostic survey of a total population from 1970 to 2000 including 419 patients. *Histopathology*. 2009; 54: 355-64.

[23] Wu TI, Chang TC, Hsueh S, Hsu KH, Chou HH, Huang HJ, Lai CH. Prognostic factors and impact of adjuvant chemotherapy for uterine leiomyosarcoma. *Gynecologic Oncology*. 2006; 100: 166-72.

[24] Blom R, Guerrieri C, Stal O, Malmstrom H, Simonsen E. Leiomyosarcoma of the uterus: a clinicopathologic, DNA flow cytometric, p53, and mdm-2 analysis of 49 cases. *Gynecologic Oncology*. 1998; 68: 54-61.

In: Leiomyosarcoma
Editor: Rosemary H. Leach
ISBN: 978-1-63117-940-2

Chapter 10

Clinical Manifestation and Imaging Diagnosis of Leiomyosarcoma

Ying Wang and Ri-sheng Yu
Department of Radiology, the Second Affiliated Hospital,
Zhejiang University School of Medicine, China

Abstract

Leiomyosarcoma (LMS), one of the most commonly diagnosed subtypes of sarcoma, is an aggressive malignancy of smooth muscle (SM) origin for which the basis of transformation and mechanisms of progression are mostly unknown. This tumor usually occurs in middle-aged or older adults. Given the variety of anatomical locations of SM tissues, LMS can arise in various regions of the body, and forms a significant percentage of retroperitoneal, vascular, extremity, and uterine sarcomas. Imaging studies often demonstrate LMS as a nonspecific soft tissue mass; the definitive diagnosis relies on histological examination. Following diagnosis of LMS, the first line of defense is surgical resection of the primary tumor, radiotherapy or chemotherapy is also needed due to common involvement of adjacent tissues and high recurrence rates. Although tumors from the various regions are histologically similar, they often have different clinical courses and chemotherapeutic responses. Clinically, LMS of cutaneous origin usually has a favorable outcome than of deep tissue origin, such as the frequent retroperitoneal tumors. This review delineates the risk factors, diagnosis and treatment of LMS in different sites; aim to better manage the care of those diagnosed with LMS.

Introduction

Leiomyosarcoma (LMS) is a mesenchymal tumor of ubiquitous origin, originating from smooth muscle cells, represents approximately 9% of all soft tissue sarcomas (including retroperitoneum) and is the third most frequently documented sarcoma after malignant fibrous histiocytoma and liposarcoma [1]. It usually occurs in middle-aged or older adults, and commonly arises from the retroperitoneum, alimentary tract, genitourinary tract, and soft tissues [2]. Metastases from LMS tend to be hematogenously spread with the liver and lung being the most frequent sites.

Risk Factors

LMS is a sarcoma associated with Epstein-Barr virus (EBV) [3]. The existing published data show that the cytogenetic and molecular genetic changes in LMS are complex, there are no consistent, recurrent aberrations demonstrated at the chromosomal level [4, 5]. A comprehensive review published in 2009 compiled the CGH studies to date and demonstrated that more than 20 chromosomes were affected, with regions encompassing over 2,200 genes [6]. Yang J [6] reported that the most frequent losses were detected in 10q and 13q, the regions where tumor suppressor genes PTEN and Rb reside and the most frequent gains were detected in 17p. In some reported studies these aberrations were found as frequently as in 50% (10q) and 78% (13q) of the patient samples analyzed [7]. These findings suggest that loss of PTEN and/or RB1 may contribute to initiation or progression of LMS. Studies showed that the extent of cytogenetic changes was associated with tumor size [6]. However, the underlying molecular which determinants driving soft tissue LMS inception, proliferation, and metastasis is little known about. With the advent of expression arrays, mRNA profiling provided further insight into the molecular classification of LMS [8, 9]. These initial studies demonstrated that on a molecular level independent LMS samples display a high degree of heterogeneity [8]. Subsequent to these publications, mRNA profiles have been used to categorize LMS samples based on the potential for metastasize [10], as well as to define 3 distinct subtypes based on a comprehensive genomic analysis [11]. Again, these studies highlight the complexity of this disease, and further define the molecular alterations in LMS tissues.

Imaging Features

Retroperitoneal LMS is often large and heterogeneous [12]. Masses demonstrate a central low density in keeping with hemorrhage, necrosis or cystic change on CT. LMS has a non-specific appearance on MRI, revealing a non-fatty mass. Moderate contrast enhancement is seen at the periphery of the large primary and metastatic lesions [13], whereas smaller lesions may be homogeneous [12]. Liver metastases are well defined with central necrosis. Calcification is uncommon but has been reported. Large deep lesions tend to be heterogeneous with areas of necrosis. Superficial lesions, which are usually smaller, may be homogeneous.

Tumors arising from large vessels, commonly the IVC, femoral vein or greater saphenous vein, are intraluminal, extraluminal or a combination of both. These lesions are well defined, may expand the vessel lumen and appear isointense to muscle on T1-weighted images (T1WI) and hyperintense on T2-weighted images (T2WI) [14].

LMS of bone is purely osteolytic with aggressive features such as endosteal scalloping, permeation, poor definition of margins and lack of sclerosis on conventional radiographs [15].

Lesions of the long bones involve the metaphysis, often with extension into the diaphysis or epiphysis. On MRI the tumor is clearly defined. It is isointense to muscle on T1WI, intermediate to hypointense to fat on spin-echo T2WI [15].

Treatment and Prognosis

Following diagnosis of LMS, the first line of defense is surgical resection of the primary tumor. Unfortunately, given the location and common involvement of adjacent tissues, wide margins of resection are not always possible, and recurrence rates are high. Patients may also undergo radiotherapy at this time, and chemotherapy is common in the case of systemic metastatic spread. But to date, in complete resection sarcoma, published studies show better local control of the disease but no survival benefit for adjuvant treatment with chemotherapy and radiotherapy [16, 17].

The prognosis for LMS is poor with an overall 5 year survival rate of 35%. Prognosis is worse for tumors greater than 5 cm and for those arising from the retroperitoneum [18]. LMS of deep tissue origin, such as the frequent retroperitoneal tumors, are highly aggressive, commonly recur after resection, and despite therapeutic attempts, have a 5-year survival rate of less than 50% [19], while LMS of cutaneous origin always has a favorable outcome [20].

Leiomyosarcoma of Different Sites

Retroperitoneum

Leiomyosarcoma of the inferior vena cava Retroperitoneal LMS is rare tumor of the mesenchymal cells, most often arising from the inferior vena cava. To date, only approximately 400 cases of LMS of the inferior vena cava have been reported in the literature [21]. LMS of the inferior vena cava is seen principally in adults with a striking preponderance for women (M: F ratio of 1:5) and the majority of patients present in their fifth to sixth decade. Laskin WB [22] advocated that the high incidence of retroperitoneal LMS and LMS of the inferior vena cava in the female population raises speculation that some cases may represent metastatic spread from a uterine primary. Kuyalat [23] found that 21% of females with LMS of the inferior vena cava reported in the literature had a history of surgery for another tumor, most commonly a uterine smooth muscle tumor, indirectly supports this possibility.

Retroperitoneal LMS of the inferior vena cava is slow growing, and at the time of diagnosis, it is often very large, making curative resection difficult [24]. Due to its extensive tumor growth, some patients will present with flank masses; however, most have nonspecific symptoms, and the tumor is discovered incidentally. Kulaylat [23] concluded that the diagnosis of LMS of the inferior vena cava was often delayed and stated that nearly 33% were diagnosed postmortem. Those who do have symptoms most commonly present with right-sided abdominal or flank pain. Patients may also present with lower extremity edema, which is more often secondary to deep vein thrombosis as opposed to complete or partial occlusion of the inferior vena cava by the tumor or thrombus. In addition, there have also been documented 16% to 25% cases of patients presenting with Budd–Chiari syndrome [25, 26].

The role of imaging in the management of LMS of the inferior vena cava is diagnosis (including biopsy), pre-operative planning, detection of recurrence and metastases. On ultrasound (US), these tumors appear to be heterogeneous as areas of necrosis are hypoechoic. Doppler flow studies can be used to evaluate the extent of IVC obstruction and to evaluate for thrombosis of the hepatic and renal veins [27]. On CT imaging, the tumors typically appear as heterogeneous masses with enhancement of the periphery [28]. Areas of hemorrhage and necrosis may be noted within the mass on CT. On MRI imaging, LMS has low signal intensity on T1WI, while demonstrate high signal intensity on T2WI [28]. Retroperitoneal LMS is more often diagnosed on CT or MRI.

As for treatment, a curative procedure for localized LMS of the inferior vena cava that is, a complete (local) or radical resection of the tumor, including involved viscera, provides the best hope for prolonged survival [29-31]. In patients who do not undergo surgical resection, survival is generally measured in months. In fact, Hollenbeck [24] claimed a 3-year overall survival rate of 76% for patients with LMS of the inferior vena cava managed in this manner, but a 0% survival for patients with incompletely excised tumors. A study on clinicopathologic analysis of 40 LMS of the inferior vena cava cases showed 5 closely associated clinicopathologic factors with prognosis: level III inferior vena cava and right atrial involvement by sarcoma, predominant intraluminal growth, a compromised liver, and residual postsurgical macroscopic disease, negatively impact on the clinical course of disease [22].

Alimentary Tract

Esophageal leiomyosarcoma Esophageal LMS is the most common of the pure mesenchymal tumors of the esophagus, accounting for less than 1% of all malignant esophageal tumors [32-34]. It is commonly located in the middle and lower thoracic esophagus because smooth muscle predominates in that area [35]. Esophageal LMS had, in the past, been classified as polypoid in 60% of cases and infiltrative in 40% [36]. As for the radiographic findings in LMS of the esophagus, Levine [37] reported that esophageal LMS had radiographic features similar to those of LMS found elsewhere in the GI tract. It is important to be aware of the limitations of endoscopy in diagnosing esophageal LMS. LMS has a slow and indolent clinical course, followed by late recurrence, and eventual death of patients from the disease. Hematogenous metastasis is the cause of most of the cases of tumor recurrence and death. Patients with polypoid and intramural tumors, tumors in an intrathoracic location, and well-differentiated tumors have a better prognosis than patients with infiltrating lesions, tumors in cervical locations, and poorly differentiated tumors [38, 39].

Gastric leiomyosarcoma Gastric LMS reported to account for 0.1-2% of all gastric malignancies [40]. The most common symptoms and signs of large tumors are abdominal pain, palpable mass and abdominal distension. None of these symptoms is specific to LMS. The disease most frequently occurs in the upper third of the gastric body, followed by the middle third and then the lower third [41]. For diagnosis of the disease, roentgenography, US, CT and angiography are effectively used, and angiography in particular enabled clarification of the vascularization of the tumors, by which it is often possible to determine the organ in which the tumors initially developed. Differential diagnoses can mainly be gastrointestinal stromal tumors (GISTs). GISTs are neoplasms that are believed to arise from the interstitial cells of Cajal, the c-kit-positive and so-called pacemaker cells of the gastrointestinal myenteric plexus. Diagnosis of GISTs frequently relies on positive immunoreactivity to c-kit, a property of these neoplasms that is observed in more than 95% of human GISTs [42]. GISTs can also be concurrently positive for SMA and S100 [43]. The lack of c-kit labeling in these neoplastic cells ruled out GISTs. LMS traditionally has cytoplasmic labeling for SMA, vimentin, laminin, desmin, and variably, S100.

There is universal acceptance in the literature that the treatment of choice is surgical excision. Most consider removal of the tumor together with a margin, by resection of the gastric wall or partial gastrectomy, as sufficient treatment. Prognosis in these tumors is dependent on histopathological grade, tumor size, and evidence of invasion of adjacent organs. Five year survival for patients with tumors of low grade malignancy is 81 % versus 32% for high grade tumors [44]. The median interval to recurrence is 24 months.

Small bowel leiomyosarcoma Small bowel LMS originates from smooth muscle cells within the muscularis mucosa or muscularis propria. It is the most common sarcoma that can develop in the small intestine [45]. It occurs most frequently in the jejunum, ileum, and duodenum, respectively [46]. The most common symptoms are ferriprive anemia and/or recurrent melena and surgical treatment remains the only effective treatment for small intestine LMS. It reported that 36% LMS had metastases. The location of the tumor, duration of symptoms, and age of the patient were not predictors for metastasis, but metastasis is more likely with a tumor size larger than 5 cm [47]. Small bowel LMS appears to metastasize hematogenously, especially to the liver (65% of metastases), other GI locations (15%), and the lungs (4%). Moreover, more than with other sarcomas, it does spread lymphogenously (13%) or via peritoneal route (18%) [48]. Since the small tumors are not likely to cause symptoms, a prolonged period can elapse before these slow-growing tumors are revealed [49]. At time of diagnosis, these tumors are mostly far-advanced and are frequently accompanied by complications, which deteriorate the prognosis [50]. In high-grade disease, the five-year survival rate is 5-20%, in contrast to 55% in low-grade disease [51, 52].

Rectal Leiomyosarcoma Rectal LMS is an uncommon malignancy accounting for less than 0.1% of all malignancies of the colon and rectum [53]. These tumors typically occur in the fifth and sixth decades of life and show a male predominance [54]. The presenting symptoms are rectal pain, constipation, rectal fullness, and diarrhea, although some patients may be asymptomatic [55]. According to the literature, most rectal LMS are identified as protruding masses during colonoscopic examination and are confirmed histologically [56-58]. However, if they are not detected by endoscopic examination, an accurate diagnosis may be difficult because their clinical presentation can mimic that of primary ovarian carcinoma. Radiological differentiation between LMS and leiomyomas is difficult, malignant potential can be missed on CT of MRI. In one series of 10 cases of colorectal LMS, 9 of 10 patients had lobulated tumor margins on CT or MRI [59]. Except in the case of 1 patient, the tumor appeared to be heterogeneous with varying degrees of internal necrosis. The spread of rectal LMS is mainly local or hematogenous, although lymphatic metastasis has been reported in some poorly differentiated tumors [59, 60]. The optimal treatment modality in patients with rectal LMS is controversial. Wide local excision and radical surgery, such as anterior resection or abdominoperineal resection, are commonly used. The overall prognosis is poor, with reported survival of 20-40% at 5 years and significant additional mortality reported during later years [61]. Tumor size and the degree of differentiation are known to be the most significant prognostic factors.

Hepatic leiomyosarcoma Primary hepatic LMS is a rare tumor, probably originating from smooth muscle cells of hepatic veins or bile duct [2]. There is no association with cirrhosis or other hepatic disorders [62]. However, there are an increasing number of reports of primary hepatic LMS in younger human immunodeficiency virus (HIV)-infected patients and immunosuppressed transplant patients [62, 63]. Grossly, primary hepatic LMS usually presents as a single large mass [64]. Clinically, the tumor has presented with hepatomegaly or an abdominal mass, commonly associated with pain and weight loss [62]. CT findings of primary hepatic LMS have been described as a large, well-defined, heterogeneous mass with internal and peripheral enhancement or cystic mass with an enhancing thick wall [2, 64]. MR imaging shows the tumor displays homogenous or heterogeneous hypointensity on T1WI and hyperintensity on T2WI with occasional observation of encapsulation [65]. The standard treatment for liver sarcomas is surgical resection followed by adjuvant chemotherapy however due to the rarity of the disease, there is very little data regarding optimal management and this remains empirical. Liver transplantation for primary hepatic sarcoma is controversial [66]. The efficacy of chemotherapy for LMS in general is unclear, In a retrospective study of first-line chemotherapy for unresectable or metastatic LMS from different primary sites the overall response rate was 18%; median progression-free survival and overall survival were 3.8 months and 9.7 months respectively [67]. The survival in most patients with primary sarcoma of the liver is poor. Complete resection of the primary tumor is only potentially curative treatment (R0 resection) for primary liver sarcoma. The largest case series of 22 primary hepatic sarcomas reported by Matthei found that no patient survived longer than 3 years after incomplete tumor resection; however, a long-term survival after curative surgery (R0 resection) for more than 10 years is possible [68].

Genitourinary Tract

Uterine leiomyosarcoma Uterine LMS accounts for approximately 1% of uterine cancer [69] with an estimated annual incidence of 0.64 per 100,000 women [70]. Uterine LMS may originate from the smooth muscle fibers of the uterus or its vessel smooth muscle, or come from the malignant transformation of leiomyomas; the latter accounts for 0.4-0.8% of the patients [71, 72]. Clinically, the most common presenting complaint is abnormal vaginal bleeding rather than pain or pelvic mass. Studies showed that ULMS have different clinical and genetic features from the other LMS [73-76]. Cho [73] found that Uterine LMS had specific gains and losses using the methods of genome wide array-based comparative genomic hybridization (array CGH) and fluorescence in situ hybridization (FISH). The regions of high-level gain were 7q36.3, 7q33-q35, 12q13-q15, and 12q23.3, while the regions of homozygous loss were 1p21.1, 2p22.2, 6p11.2, 9p21.1, 9p22.1, 14q32.33, and 14q32.33 qter. The regions with high-level gains included HMGIC, SAS, MDM2, and TIM1 genes. Wang [74] found that KIT is expressed in Uterine LMS, thus adjunctive diagnostic studies using c-kit may be useful in distinguishing LMS from benignl leiomyomas in uterine tumors that offer uncharacteristic features. Kowalewska [77] identified differential miRNA signatures the subtypes of uterine sarcomas.

US is the most common imaging modality in gynecology, but it cannot reliably confirm their degeneration nor differentiate leiomyomas from their malignant equivalent. CT can show uterine enlargement and deformation when leiomyomas are large enough and may show heterogeneous density when leiomyomas have degenerated. But CT is limited in both detection and characterization of leiomyomas, the only consistent finding in Uterine LMS on CT is the absence of calcifications. MRI has high soft tissue resolution and it has high value in locating and charactering a uterine mass. The increased signal intensity on T2WI, large patchs of hemorrhagic necrosis, irregular contour and poor circumscription might be the characteristics of Uterine LMS [78].

Uterine LMS is characterized by a propensity for early hematogenous spread, lymphatic spread is a rare event, and the overall prognosis is poor [79-81]. Surgical resection, including hysterectomy and bilateral salpingo-oophorectomy, is the recommended initial treatment strategy. A study on postresection 5-year overall survival for patients with Uterine LMS showed that the median overall survival for all patients was 3.75 years, the median follow-up for the surviving patients was 5.4 years, and the 5-year overall survival rate was 44.1% [82]. To date, no adjuvant treatment strategies have demonstrated a survival benefit for the patient with Uterine LMS. The benefits of chemotherapy are limited, though the combination of gemcitabine and docetaxel may be active in Uterine LMS [83], and radiotherapy can result in a lower rate of local recurrence but still has no effect on patients' overall survival [72].

Renal leiomyosarcomas Renal LMS is a rare tumor with only 0.12% of renal malignancies confirmed as LMS [84]. It may arise from the smooth muscle fibers of renal pelvis, renal capsule or renal vessel, last one is the most frequent. LMS of the kidney has preponderance in women, with a gradually incidence in the later period of life [85]. Grossly, the tumor has the appearance of a leiomyoma with a well-circumscribed margin and a whorled cut surface. It is frequently diagnosed on histological examination because it does not have any specific diagnostic features clinically and radiologically. The most common symptoms and signs are like those of renal cell carcinoma, namely pain, palpable mass, and hematuria, all of which are indicators of an extensive local disease. Neither US, CT nor MRI is able to differentiate between LMS and renal cell carcinomas [84].

Renal LMS has rapid growth and a high metastatic tendency, and show both local and distant recurrence. These characteristics lead to a very poor prognosis with a 5-year survival rate of 29-36%, and most patients die within 1 year of diagnosis [86]. Radical nephrectomy is the treatment of choice [87]. The major prognostic factor is total surgical resection, when it is completed, 5 years disease free survival could be of 60%. Although the role of lymphadenectomy in renal cancer remains controversial, given the extent of the tumor in the present case, this could have been done [88]. Besides surgical margins, major prognostic factors become histological grade, with 5 years disease-free survival of 90% for low grade tumors, and 30% for high grade tumor [87].

Surgery followed by chemotherapy and radiation has been advocated in the past with limited success [89, 90]. However, the possibility of treatment with KIT tyriosine kinase inhibitors such as sunitinib has been reported in phase II trial [91]. Radical operations, size <5 cm, low histologic grade, and negative lymph node metastasis are all associated with a better prognosis [92].

Nonvisceral Soft Tissue

LMS of soft tissues is a relatively uncommon malignant tumor that has the phenotypic features of smooth muscle differentiation and may occur anywhere in the body, especially in the extremities, trunk wall, and superficial parts of the head and neck region. It is generally thought to account for 5-10% of soft tissue sarcomas [4, 93-94]. In one study of 75 soft tissue LMS, 33% were noted to arise in extremity soft tissues. Several recent reports have indicated that a reliable and reproducible diagnosis of LMS is difficult without immunohistochemistry, but the available markers are not completely specific or sensitive [95, 96]. It is well known that an adequate surgical margin is the most important factor for local control. A study on nonvisceral soft tissue LMS in 225 Patients showed that the 5-year and 10-year overall survival rates were 64% and 46%, respectively [97]. The strongest risk factor related to death was the presence of metastases either at the time of primary diagnosis or subsequently, and tumor depth, tumor size, malignancy grade, and surgical margins are other important risk factors [97].

Superficial leiomyosarcoma Superficial LMS is rare, malignant smooth muscle neoplasm that arise in the dermis or subcutaneous tissue. It accounts for only 3% of all soft tissue sarcoma and is subdivided in two subtypes depending on its origin and location: subcutaneous and cutaneous types [21]. Subcutaneous LMS is by far the most common subtype. Primary cutaneous LMS accounts for only 2-3% of all superficial soft tissue sarcomas [98]. Generally, superficial LMS occurs as a solitary, slowly-enlarging lesion most commonly on the extensor surface of the proximal extremities, which coincide with the hair bearing areas. The lesions usually occur on the legs (50-75%) [21]. Well-known predisposing factors are precursor leiomyomas, trauma, radiation, chemicals and sunlight [99]. Cutaneous LMS originates from the arrector pili muscles or genital dartoric muscles, and presents as small, single or several intradermal nodules [99,100]. Sometimes it shows ulceration due to fixation to the epidermis. Subcutaneous LMS originates from the blood vessels of smooth muscles and presents as a larger movable mass in the subcutis without epidermal change. Overlying skin discoloration occurs more frequently in the cutaneous LMS than in the subcutaneous LMS [101]. In both types, spontaneous pain or tenderness was reported. Other common symptoms such as pruritus, bleeding, and a burning sensation were noted. Cutaneous LMS grows slowly and has a better prognosis than subcutaneous LMS. The metastatic potential is 5-10% for the cutaneous form compared with 30-60% for the subcutaneous form [101]. Superficial LMS expresses vimentin and smooth muscle actin in 100% of cases; however, desmin expression is seen in only about 60% of cases. CK and S-100 stains may sparsely be positive.

Treatment of superficial LMS consists mainly of wide local excision including a 2-5 cm excision margin with a depth including the subcutaneous tissue [102]. Chemotherapy may only be considered for preoperative tumor volume reduction, but is not therapeutic. Moreover, radiotherapy is contraindicated due to the causative factor itself [102]. Recently, Mohs micrographic surgery has been utilized for the removal of various sarcomas, especially superficial LMS [103]. Jensen [104] identified several poor prognostic factors, namely tumor size ≥5 cm, acral location, deep localization with fascia involvement and high histological grade. Cutaneous LMS has fewer incidences of local recurrence (30-50%) and negligible potential for distant metastases (0-10%). In contrast, subcutaneous LMS may develop local recurrence in about 40-60% and distant metastasis in 20-60% of patients [105].

Other Sites

Pulmonary leiomyosarcoma Pulmonary LMS is a mesenchymal tumor that appears to originate from smooth muscle cells of the bronchial wall or a vessel wall, and accounts for less than 0.5% of all malignant pulmonary tumors [106]. Pulmonary LMS can be classified by type as intraluminal, intrapulmonary, or pulmonary vascular [107]. The intrapulmonary type is the most common. The pulmonary vascular type grows along the vascular wall and occurs in the pulmonary artery, where it may cause stenosis or obstruction [108]. Clinically, patients with pulmonary LMS may present with symptoms similar to those seen in other primary pulmonary tumors, including fever, cough, hemoptysis, sputum production, dyspnea and chest pain, or they may be asymptomatic [109].

It is difficult to differentiate pulmonary LMS from lung cancer, pulmonary tuberculosis, mediastinal tumor, pulmonary artery sarcoma, and pulmonary artery stenosis. Radiographically, pulmonary LMS appears as a sharply defined, heterogeneous density that is smooth in contour with calcification in areas of presumed ischemic tissue damage. When a chest radiograph shows a solitary oval or round, well-circumscribed, calcified, and heterogeneous nodule or mass, pulmonary LMS should be considered along with other types of lung cancer and pulmonary tuberculosis. Pulmonary LMS is usually located in the periphery of the lung, but may be central and adherent to hilar structures.

Applicable therapeutic methods include surgical resection, which, if complete, is usually curative for small and well differentiated sarcomas [110]. Radical surgical extirpation is generally the optimal treatment [110]. Poorly differentiated and non-resectable tumors can be treated with palliative radiotherapy or chemotherapy. Median survival is 48 months, and the 5-year survival rate ranges between 38% and 48% [111]. Other therapeutic methods include radiotherapy and adjuvant chemotherapy, but the results are not very satisfactory. Factors for a poor prognosis have been described: tumor size (over 4-5 cm), the degree of histological malignancy, endobronchial invasion and the impossibility of performing complete resection [112].

Leiomyosarcoma of bone Primary LMS of bone is exceedingly rare, accounting for less than 0.7% of all primary malignant bone tumors [113]. To date, around 90 cases have been described [114]. Most patients cite pain as their primary complaint. Swelling is also a common presenting symptom. About 20% cases present with pathologic fracture. Similar to the more common primary sarcomas of bone, LMS most often involves the appendicular skeleton.

Plain radiographs characteristically show a solitary osteolytic lesion with a permeative appearance, indistinct margins, irregular cortical erosion, and minimal to no sclerosis or periosteal reaction. In the long bones, most cases are metaphyseal, with occasional extension into the diaphysis or epiphysis. Although intralesional calcifications are not considered typical radiographic features of LMS of bone or soft tissue, a recent study demonstrated that nearly 20% of these tumors may contain areas of calcification, mimicking more commonly mineralized neoplasms such as osteosarcoma [115]. CT scans typically show an intramedullary lesion with associated cortical destruction and extension into the surrounding soft tissues. These findings can also be demonstrated by MRI, in which the lesion is usually hypointense or isointense relative to skeletal muscle on T1WI and hyperintense on T2WI. The radiographic characteristics of histologically low-grade LMS of bone may be slightly different. The lesional margins are usually more distinct and may often be delimited by a surrounding rim of sclerotic bone, thereby mimicking benign tumors such as nonossifying fibroma or giant cell tumor of bone.

Surgical excision with wide margins remains the gold standard for curative management, amputation usually being reserved for tumors surrounding the neurovascular bundle, or with extensive soft tissue involvement. Many of the case series published have reflected that prognosis is based on the stage of diagnosis: with Enneking stages 1b or 2a cases achieving 100% survival, stage 2b tumors having a 60% survival at 5 years and 43% survival at 10 and 15 years [114].

References

[1] O'Sullivan PJ, Harris AC, Munk PL. Radiological imaging features of non-uterine leiomyosarcoma. *Br. J. Radiol.* 2008, 81: 73-81.

[2] Ferrozzi F, Bova D, Zangrandi A, Garlaschi G. Primary liver leiomyosarcoma: CT appearance. *Abdom Imaging.* 1996, 21:157-160.

[3] Takacs M, Segesdi J, Banati F, et al., The importance of epigenetic alterations in the development of epstein-barr virus-related lymphomas. *Mediterr J. Hematol. Infect Dis.* 2009, 1: 2009012.

[4] Evans HL, Shipley J. In: Pathology and genetics of tumours of soft tissue and bone. Fletcher DCM, Unni KK, Mertens F, editor. Lyon, IARC Press; 2002. *Leiomyosarcoma;* pp. 131-134.

[5] Wang R, Lu YJ, Fisher C, Bridge JA, Shipley J. Characterization of chromosome aberrations associated with soft-tissue leiomyosarcomas by twenty-four-color karyotyping and comparative genomic hybridization analysis, *Genes Chromosomes Cancer.* 2001, 31: 54-64.

[6] Yang J, Du X, Chen K, et al., Genetic aberrations in soft tissue leiomyosarcoma. *Cancer letters.* 2009, 275: 1-9.

[7] Otaño-Joos M, Mechtersheimer G, Ohl S, et al., Detection of chromosomal imbalances in leiomyosarcoma by comparative genomic hybridization and interphase cytogenetics. *Cytogenet Cell Genet.* 2000, 90: 86-92.

[8] Skubitz KM, Skubitz AP. Differential gene expression in leiomyosarcoma. *Cancer.* 2003, 98: 1029-1038.

[9] Nielsen TO, West RB, Linn SC, et al., Molecular characterisation of soft tissue tumours: a gene expression study. *Lancet.* 2002, 359: 1301-1307.

[10] Lee EK, Lee MJ, Abdelmohsen K, et al., miR-130 suppresses adipogenesis by inhibiting peroxisome proliferator-activated receptor gamma expression. *Mol. Cell Biol.* 2011, 31: 626-638.

[11] Beck A, Lee CH, Witten D, et al., Discovery of molecular subtypes in leiomyosarcoma through integrative molecular profiling. *Oncogene.* 2010, 29: 845-899.

[12] Lane RH, Stephens DH, Reiman HM. Primary retroperitoneal neoplasms: CT findings in 90 cases with clinical and pathologic correlation. *AJR Am. J. Roentgenol.* 1989, 152: 83-89.

[13] Munk PL, Lee MJ, Poon PY, Goddard KJ, Knowling MA, Hassell PR. Computed tomography of retroperitoneal and mesenteric sarcomas: a pictoral essay. *Can. Assoc. Radiol. J.* 1996, 47:335-341.

[14] Kransdorf MJ, Murphy MD. Imaging of soft tissue tumors. Philadelphia, PA: WB Saunders, 1997: 221-226.

[15] Sundaram M, Akduman I, White LM, McDonald DJ, Kandel R, Janney C. Primary leiomyosarcoma of bone. *AJR Am. J. Roentgenol.* 1999, 172:771-776.

[16] Pervaiz N, Colterjohn N, Farrokhyar F, et al., A systematic meta-analysis of randomized controlled trials of adjuvant chemotherapy for localized resectable softtissue sarcoma. *Cancer.* 2008, 113:573-581.

[17] Mahmood T, Agresta S, Vigil CE, et al., Phase II study of sunitinib malate, a multitargeted tyrosin kinase inhibitor in patients with relapsed or refractory soft tissue sarcomas. Focus on three prevalent histologies: leiomyosarcoma, liposarcoma and malignant fibrous histiocytoma. *Int. J. Cancer.* 2011, 129:1963-1969.

[18] Wile AG, Evans HL, Romsdahl MM. Leiomyosarcoma of soft tissue: a clinicopathologic study. *Cancer.* 1981, 48:1022-1032.

[19] Bonvalot S, Rivoire M, Castaing M, et al., Primary retroperitoneal sarcomas: a multivariate analysis of surgical factors associated with local control. *J. Clin. Oncol.* 2009, 27: 31-38.

[20] Svarvar C, Böhling T, Berlin O, et al., Clinical course of nonvisceral soft tissue leiomyosarcoma in 225 patients from the Scandinavian Sarcoma Group. *Cancer.* 2007, 109: 282-291.

[21] Lee HM, Jeong DS, Park PW, Kim WS, Sung K, Lee YT. Surgical treatment for an invasive leiomyosarcoma of the inferior vena cava. *Korean J. Thorac. Cardiovasc. Surg.* 2013, 46:373-376.

[22] Laskin WB, Fanburg-Smith JC, et al., Leiomyosarcoma of the inferior vena cava: clinicopathologic study of 40 cases. *Am. J. Surg. Pathol.* 2010, 34:873-881.

[23] Kulaylat MN, Karakousis CP, Doerr RJ, et al., Leiomyosarcoma of the inferior vena cava: a clinicopathologic review and report of three cases. *J. Surg. Oncol.* 1997, 65: 205-217.

[24] Hollenbeck ST, Grobmyer SR, Kent KC, et al., Surgical treatment and outcomes of patients with primary inferior vena cava leiomyosarcoma. *J. Am. Coll Surg.* 2003, 197:575-579.

[25] Hilliard NJ, Heslin MJ, Castro CY. Leiomyosarcoma of the inferior vena cava. Three case reports and review of the literature. *Annals Diagn Pathol.* 2005, 9:259-266.

[26] Mingoli A, Cavallaro A, Sapienza P, et al., International registry of inferior vena cava leiomyosarcoma: analysis of a world series on 218 patients. *Anticancer Res.* 1996, 16:3201-3205.

[27] Bieliūniene E, Kavaliauskiene G, Mitraite D, et al., Leiomyosarcoma of the inferior vena cava. *Medicina* (Kaunas). 2010, 46: 200-203.

[28] Ganeshalingam S, Rajeswaran G, Jones RL, et al., Leiomyosarcomas of the inferior vena cava: diagnostic features on cross-sectional imaging. *Clin Radiol.* 2011, 66:50-56.

[29] Barbara ZD, Brigitte S, Girma T, Sharon W, Surgical Management of Retroperitoneal Leiomyosarcoma Arising from the Inferior Vena Cava. *J. Gastrointest Surg.* 2013, 17: 2166-2171.

[30] Cho SW, Marsh JW, Geller DA, et al., Surgical management of leiomyosarcoma of the inferior vena cava. *J. Gastrointest Surg*. 2008, 12:2141-2148.

[31] Ito H, Hornick JL, Bertagnolli MM, et al., Leiomyosarcoma of the inferior vena cava: survival after aggressive management. *Annals Surg. Oncol.* 2007, 14:3534-3541.

[32] Jang SS, Kim WT, Ko BS, et al., A case of rapidly progressing leiomyosarcoma combined with squamous cell carcinoma in the esophagus. *World J. Gastroenterol.* 2013, 19: 5385-5388.

[33] Almeida JM. Leiomyosarcoma of the esophagus. *Chest.* 1982, 81:761-763.

[34] Galandiuk S, Hermann RE, Cosgrove DM, Gassman JJ. Cancer of the esophagus. The Cleveland Clinic experience. *Ann. Surg*. 1986, 203:101-108.

[35] Zhang BH, Zhang HT, Wang YG. Esophageal leiomyosarcoma: clinical analysis and surgical treatment of 12 cases. *Dis. Esophagus*. 2012:Epub ahead of print

[36] Lokesh V, Naveen T, Pawar YS. Spindle cell sarcoma of esophagus: a rare case presentation. *J. Cancer Res. Ther*. 2010, 6:100-101.

[37] Levine MS, Buck JL, Pantongrag-Brown L, Buetow PC, Hallman JR, Sobin LH. Leiomyosarcoma of the esophagus: Radiographic findings in 10 patients. *AJR Am. J. Roentgenol*. 1996, 167:27-32.

[38] Koga H, Iida M, Suekane H, et al., Rapidly growing esophageal leiomyosarcoma: case report and review of the literature. *Abdom Imaging*. 1995, 20:15-19.

[39] Rocco G, Trastek VF, Deschamps C, Allen MS, Miller DL, Pairolero PC. Leiomyosarcoma of the esophagus: results of surgical treatment. *Ann. Thorac. Surg*. 1998, 66:894-896.

[40] Ito Y, Takagi K, Tomita T, et al., A case report of gastric leiomyosarcoma showing pedunculated extragastric development. *Prog. Dig Endosc*. 1996, 49:198-199. (in Japanese).

[41] Skandalakis JE, Gray SW, Shepard D. Smooth muscle tumors of the stomach. *Int. Abstr. Surg*. 1960, 110:209-226.

[42] Miettinen M, Lasota J. Gastrointestinal stromal tumors: review on morphology, molecular pathology, prognosis, and differential diagnosis. *Arch. Pathol. Lab Med.* 2006,130:1466-1478.

[43] Head KW, Cullen JM, Dubielzig RR, et al., Histological classifications of tumors of the intestines of domestic animals. In: Histological classification of tumors of the alimentary system of domestic animals, ed. Schulman FY, 2003, 2nd series, vol. X, pp. 87–110. Armed Forces Institute of Pathology, Washington, DC.

[44] Tsianos GB, Argiropoulos-Rakas CA, Karkanias GG. Hemoperitoneum secondary to exogastric leiomyosarcoma: a case report. *Hepatogastroenterology*. 1995, 42:885-887.

[45] Bilimoria KY, Bentrem DJ, Wayne JD, et al., Small bowel cancer in the United States. *Ann Surg*, 2009, 249: 63-71.

[46] Akwari OE, Dozois RR, Weiland LH, Beahrs OH. Leiomyosarcoma of the small and large bowel. *Cancer.* 1978, 42: 1375-1384.

[47] Blanchard DK, Budde JM, Hatch GF 3rd, et al., Tumors of the small intestine. *World J. Surg*. 2000, 24: 421-429.

[48] Skandalakis JE, Gray SW, Skandalakis LJ. Metastasis of malignant smooth muscle tumors of the gastrointestinal tract: pattern and process. *J. Med. Assoc. Ga.* 1991, 80: 701-709.

[49] Gill SS, Heuman DM, Mihas AA. Small intestinal neoplasms. *J. Clin. Gastroenterol.* 2001, 33: 267-282.

[50] North JH, Pack MS. Malignant tumors of the small intestine: a review of 144 cases. *Am. Surg.* 2000, 66: 46-51.

[51] Edge SB, Byrd DR, Compton CC, et al., AJCC (American Joint Committee on Cancer) Cancer Staging Manual. 7th ed. New York: Springer, 2010; 285.

[52] Licht JD, Weissmann LB, Antman K. Gastrointestinal sarcomas. *Semin. Oncol.* 1988, 15: 181-188.

[53] Minsky BD, Cohen AM, Hajdu SI. Conservative management of anal leiomyosarcoma. *Cancer.* 1991, 6:1640-1643.

[54] Kahlifa AA, Bong WL, Rao VK, Williams MJ. Leiomyosarcoma of the rectum. Report of a case and review of the literature. *Dis. Colon Rectum.* 1986, 6:427-432.

[55] Meijer S, Peretz T, Gaynor JJ, Tan C, Hajdu SI, Brennan MF. Primary colorectal sarcoma. A retrospective review and prognostic factor study of 50 consecutive patients. *Arc Surg.* 1990, 6:1163-1168.

[56] Basu I, Lemonas P. Leiomyosarcoma of the rectum following pelvic irradiation: a difficult histological diagnosis. *Ann. R. Coll. Surg. Engl.* 2012, 6:44-45.

[57] Hsieh TH, Clark BD, Iswara K. Rectal Leiomyosarcoma: an unusual rectal malignancy mimicking fecal impaction in a 19-year-old man. *Clin. Gastroenterol. Hepatol.* 2009, 6: 18.

[58] Zbar AP, Sokolowsky N, Sandiford N, Prussia PR. Leiomyosarcoma of the rectum. A report of two cases and review of the literature. *West Indian Med. J.* 2004, 6:122-125.

[59] Lee SH, Ha HK, Byun JY, et al., Radiological features of leiomyomatous tumors of the colon and rectum. *J. Comput. Assist. Tomogr.* 2000, 6:407-412.

[60] Ouh YT, Hong JH, Min KJ, So KA, Lee JK. Leiomyosarcoma of the rectum mimicking primary ovarian carcinoma: a case report. *J. Ovarian Res.* 2013, 6:27.

[61] Hatch KF, Blanchard DK, Hatch GF, et al., Tumors of the rectum and anal canal. *World J. Surg.*. 2000, 6: 437-443.

[62] Gates LK Jr, Cameron AJ, Nagorney DM, Goellner JR, Farley DR. Primary leiomyosarcoma of the liver mimicking liver abscess. *Am. Gastroenterol.* 1995, 90:649-652.

[63] Brichard B, Smets F, Sokal E, et al., Unusual evolution of an Epstein-Barr virus-associated leiomyosarcoma occurring after liver transplantation. *Pediatr Transplant.* 2001, 5:365-369.

[64] Soyer P, Bluemke DA, Riopel M, Hruban RH, Fishman EK. Hepatic leiomyosarcomas: CT features with pathologic correlation. *Eur. J. Radiol.* 1995, 19:177-182.

[65] Yu RS, Chen Y, Jiang B, Wang LH, Xu XF. Primary hepatic sarcomas: CT findings. *Eur. Radiol.* 2008, 18: 2196-2205.

[66] Husted TL, Neff G, Thomas MJ, et al., Liver transplantation for primary or metastatic sarcoma to the liver. *Am. J. Transpl.* 2006, 6:392-397.

[67] Oosten AW, Seynaeve C, Schmitz PI, et al., Outcomes of first-line chemotherapy in patients with advanced or metastatic leiomyosarcoma of uterine and non-uterine origin. *Sarcoma.* 2009, 2009:348910.

[68] Matthaei H, Krieg A, Schmelzle M, et al., Long-term survival after surgery for primary hepatic sarcoma in adults. *Arch. Surg.* 2009, 144:339-344.

[69] Norris HJ, Zaloudek CJ. In Mesenchymal tumors of the uterus. In Pathology of the female genital tract. Secondth editionth edition. Edited by Blaustein A. New York: Springer; 1982:352.

[70] Harlow BL, Weis NS, Lofton S: The epidemiology of sarcoma of the uterus. *J. Natl. Cancer Inst*. 1986, 76:399.

[71] Baird DD, Garrett TA, Laughlin SK, Davis B, Semelka RC, Peddada SD. Short-term change in growth of uterine leiomyoma: tumor growth spurts. *Fertil Steril*. 2011, 95: 242-246.

[72] Amant F, Coosemans A, Debiec-Rychter M, Timmerman D, Vergote I. Clinical management of uterine sarcomas. *Lancet Oncol*. 2009; 10: 1188-1198.

[73] Cho YL, Bae S, Koo MS, et al., Array comparative genomic hybridization analysis of uterine leiomyosarcom. *Gynecol. Oncol*. 2005, 99: 545-551.

[74] Wang L, Felix JC, Lee JL, et al., The proto-oncogene c-kit is expressed in leiomyosarcomas of the uterus. *Gynecol. Oncol*. 2003, 90:402-406.

[75] Ylisaukko-oja SK, Kiuru M, Lehtonen HJ, et al., Analysis of fumarate hydratase mutations in a population-based series of early onset uterine leiomyosarcoma patients. *Int. J. Cancer*. 2006, 119:283-287.

[76] Lehtonen HJ, Kiuru M, Ylisaukko-Oja SK, et al., Increased risk of cancer in patients with fumarate hydratase germline mutation. *J. Med. Genet*. 2006, 43:523-526.

[77] Kowalewska M, Bakula-Zalewska E, Chechlinska M, et al., microRNAs in uterinesarcomas and mixed epithelial-mesenchymal uterine tumors: a preliminary report. *Tumour Biol*. 2013, 34:2153-2160.

[78] Zhang HJ, Zhan FH, Li YJ, Sun HR, Bai RJ, Gao S. Fluorodeoxyglucose positron emission tomography/computed tomography and magnetic resonance imaging of uterine leiomyosarcomas: 2 cases report. *Chin. Med. J*. (Engl). 2011, 124:2237-2240.

[79] Ueda SM, Kapp DS, Cheung MK, et al., Trends in demographic and clinical characteristics in women diagnosed with corpus cancer and their potential impact on the increasing number of deaths. *Am. J. Obstet Gynecol*. 2008, 198:218.

[80] Zivanovic O, Leitao MM, Iasonos A, et al., Stage-specific outcomes of patients with uterine leiomyosarcoma: a comparison of the International Federation of Gynecology and Obstetrics and American Joint Committee on Cancer staging systems. *J. Clin. Oncol*. 2009, 27:2066-2072.

[81] Leitao MM, Sonoda Y, Brennan MF, Barakat RR, Chi DS. Incidence of lymph node and ovarian metastases in leiomyosarcoma of the uterus. *Gynecol. Oncol*. 2003, 91:209-212.

[82] Zivanovic O, Jacks LM, Iasonos A, et al., A nomogram to predict postresection 5-year overall survival for patients with uterine leiomyosarcoma. *Cancer*. 2012, 118:660-669.

[83] Hensley ML, Ishill N, Soslow R, et al., Adjuvant gemcitabine plus docetaxel for completely resected stages I-IV high grade uterine leiomyosarcoma Results of a prospective study. *Gynecol. Oncol*. 2009, 112:563-567.

[84] Dhawan S, Chopra P, Dhawan S. Primary renal leiomyosarcoma: a diagnostic challenge. *Urology Annals*. 2012, 4:48-50.

[85] Niceta P, Lavengood RW Jr, Fernandes M, Tozzo PJ. Leiomyosarcoma of kidney. Review of the literature. *Urology*. 1974, 3:270-277.

[86] Dominici A, Mondani N, Nesi G, Travaglini F, Di Cello V, Rizzo M. Cystic leiomyosarcoma of the kidney. *Urol. Int*. 2000, 65:229-231.

[87] Miettinen M, Fetsch JF. Evaluation of biological potential of smooth muscle tumours. *Histopathology.* 2006, 48:97-105.

[88] Montgomery JS, Leibovich BC. Lymph node excision for renal cancer. *J. Urol.* 2013,189: 419-421.

[89] Miller JS, Zhou M, Brimo F, Guo CC, Epstein JI. Primary leiomyosarcoma of the kidney: a clinicopathologic study of 27 cases. *Am. J. Surg. Pathol.* 2010, 34:238-242.

[90] Ellouze S, Abid N, Kossentini M, et al., Leiomyosarcoma of the kidney. *Clinical Genitourinary Cancer.* 2011, 9:68-69.

[91] Mahmood T, Agresta S, Vigil CE, et al., Phase II study of sunitinib malate, a multitargeted tyrosin kinase inhibitor in patients with relapsed or refractory soft tissue sarcomas. Focus on three prevalent histologies: leiomyosarcoma, liposarcoma and malignant fibrous histiocytoma. *Int. J. Cancer.* 2011, 129:1963-1969.

[92] Raut CP, Pisters PW. Retroperitoneal sarcomas: combined-modality treatment aproaches. *J. Surg. Oncol.* 2006, 94:81-87.

[93] Weiss SW, Goldblum JR. Enzinger and Weiss's Soft Tissue Tumours. 5. St. Louis Mosby; 2008. *Leiomyosarcoma;* pp. 545–564.

[94] Hashimoto H, Daimaru Y, Tsuneyoshi M, Enjoji M. Leiomyosarcoma of the external soft tissue. *Cancer.* 1986, 57:2077-2088.

[95] Daugaard S. Current soft-tissue sarcoma classifications. *Eur. J. Cancer.* 2004, 40:543-548.

[96] Fields JP, Helwig EB. Leiomyosarcoma of the skin and subcutaneous tissue. *Cancer.* 1981,47:156-169.

[97] Coindre JM. Immunohistochemistry in the diagnosis of soft tissue tumours. *Histopathology.* 2003, 43:1-16.

[98] Torres T, Oliveira A, Sanches M, Selores M. Superficial cutaneous leiomyosarcoma of the face: report of three cases. *J. Dermatol.* 2011, 38:373-376.

[99] Lin JY, Tsai RY. Subcutaneous leiomyosarcoma on the face. *Dermatol Surg.* 1999, 25:489-491.

[100] De Giorgi V, Sestini S, Massi D, Papi F, Alfaioli B, Lotti T. Superficial cutaneous leiomyosarcoma: a rare, misleading tumor. *Am. J. Clin. Dermatol.* 2008, 9:185-187.

[101] Blaise G, Nikkels AF, Quatresooz P, Hermanns-Lê T, Piérard GE. Childhood cutaneous leiomyosarcoma. *Pediatr. Dermatol.* 2009, 26:477-479.

[102] Choy C, Cooper A, Kossard S. Primary cutaneous diffuse leiomyosarcoma with desmoplasia. *Australas J. Dermatol.* 2006, 47:291-295.

[103] Tsutsumida A, Yoshida T, Yamamoto Y, Itoh T, Minakawa H, Sugihara T. Management of superficial leiomyosarcoma: a retrospective study of 10 cases. *Plast Reconstr Surg.* 2005, 116:8-12.

[104] Jensen ML, Jensen OM, Michalski W, Nielsen OS, Keller J. Intradermal and subcutaneous leiomyosarcoma: A clinicopathological and immunohistochemical study of 41 cases. *J. Cutan Pathol.* 1996, 23:458-463.

[105] Holst VA, Junkins-Hopkins JM, Elenitsas R. Cutaneous smooth muscle neoplasms: clinical features, histologic findings, and treatment options. *J. Am. Acad. Dermatol.* 2002, 46:477-490.

[106] Pui MH, Yu SP, Chen JD. Primary intrathoracic malignant fibrous histiocytoma and angiosarcoma. *Australas Radiol.* 1999;43:3-6.

[107] Yu H, Ren H, Miao Q, Cui Q, Zhang Z, Xu L. Pulmonary leiomyosarcoma--report of three cases. *Chin. Med. Sci. J.* 1996, 11:191-194.

[108] Pain JA, Sayer RE. Primary leiomyosarcoma of the pulmonary artery. *Eur. J. Respir. Dis.* 1984, 65:139-143.

[109] Petrov DB, Vlassov VI, Kalaydjiev GT, et al., Primary pulmonary sarcomas and carcinosarcomas--postoperative results and comparative survival analysis. *Eur. J. Cardiothorac Surg.* 2003, 23:461-466.

[110] Luthra M, Khan H, Suhail MF, Avadhani V. Primary pulmonary leiomyosarcoma -- a case report. *Arch Bronconeumol.* 2012, 48:476-478.

[111] Jakubcová T, Jakubec P. Primary pulmonary sarcomas. *Klin. Onkol.* 2009, 22:139-153.

[112] Porte HL, Metois DG, Leroy X, Conti M, Gosselin B, Wurtz A. Surgical treatment of primary sarcoma of the lung. *Eur. J. Cardiothorac. Surg.* 2000;18(2):136-42.

[113] Frings A, Leithner A, Liegl-Atzwanger B. Leiomyosarcoma of bone: a case report. *Case Rep. Med.* 2011, 2011:980257.

[114] Brewer P, Sumathi V, Grimer RJ, et al., Primary leiomyosarcoma of bone: analysis of prognosis. *Sarcoma.* 2012, 2012:636849.

[115] Bush CH, Reith JD, Spanier SS. Mineralization in musculoskeletal leiomyosarcoma: radiologic-pathologic correlation. *AJR Am. J. Roentgenol.* 2003. 180:109-113.

In: Leiomyosarcoma
Editor: Rosemary H. Leach
ISBN: 978-1-63117-940-2

Chapter 11

Gastrointestinal Leiomyosarcoma (GI-LMS) and GI Stromal Tumor (GIST)

Kensuke Adachi, M.D., Ph.D. [1,*] *and Kazuaki Enatsu, M.D., Ph.D.* [2]
[1]Department of Surgery;
[2]Department of Pathology; Tokyo Metropolitan Tama Medical Center, Japan

Abstract

The vast majority of mesenchymal neoplasms of the gastrointestinal (GI) tract are currently identified as GI stromal tumors (GISTs). According to the World Health Organization's classification of the tumors of the digestive system 2010, primary GI leiomyosarcoma (GI-LMS) in the post-GIST era is so rare that there are no significant data on clinicopathological features of this tumor. Because of different treatment options available, it is crucial to distinguish the GI-LMS from the GIST accurately, on the basis of histological criteria combined with smooth muscle antigens as well as GIST-specific molecular markers. In this review, we summarize immunohistochemical diagnosis, prognostic factors as well as clinical management of the GI-LMS and the GIST.

Keywords: Gastrointestinal leiomyosarcoma, gastrointestinal stromal tumor, GIST

Introduction

It is only recently that the gastrointestinal stromal tumor (GIST) has been recognized as the most frequent mesenchymal neoplasm of the gastrointestinal (GI) tract [1]. GI mesenchymal neoplasms now include the broad spectrum of both malignant and benign non-epithelial tumors which comprise neoplasms of leiomyogenic, neurogenic, and other stromal origins [1-3]. However, in the pre-GIST era, i.e., prior to the advent of KIT (c-kit, CD117)

* Correspondence: Kensuke Adachi MD, PhD, Address: 2-8-29, Musashidai, Fuchu, Tokyo, 183-8524, Japan, TEL: +81-42-323-5111, FAX: +81-42-323-9209, E-mail: kensuke_adachi@tmhp.jp.

staining, it was difficult to classify GI mesenchymal tumors on the basis of histological criteria because they usually possess incompletely differentiated features [3], i.e., they often lack fully differentiated characteristics of smooth muscle or neural cells [4].

KIT immunochemistry allowed a detailed clinicopathological study of the GIST [5]. Although the GI leiomyosarcoma (GI-LMS) grossly and histologically resembles the GIST, the GI-LMS has definite features of smooth muscle differentiation [6-10]. Moreover, GI-LMSs are always negative for KIT staining with absent gene mutations of KIT, whereas most GISTs are positive for KIT with gene mutations. In the pre-GIST era, most GI mesenchymal tumors labelled as the GI-LMS were actually GISTs [6-9]. The so-called GI leiomyoblastoma had been previously recognized as an epilelioid GI mesenchymal tumor [11,12], while the GI autonomic nerve tumor (GANT) characterized by a neuroendocrine phenotype had been classified as a distinct entity on the basis of electron microscopic findings [13,14]. However, KIT immunochemistry eventually concluded that the former was identical to an epithelioid GIST, and the latter to another variant of the GIST [15].

Consequently, the primary GI-LMS has become strikingly less common than the GIST. Given the aforementioned features, the GI-LMS is now seen as entirely distinct from the GIST; however, clinicopathological and immunohistochemical features of the GI-LMS have yet to be elucidated in the post-GIST era.

Case Report

In January, 2012, a 74-year-old man presented to our hospital with a huge, palpable liver tumor. A T2-weighted axial MRI demonstrated a heterogeneous tumor in the hepatic right lobe (*Figure 1A*). The patient had a history of a total gastrectomy for the bulky gastric submucosal tumor (SMT) > 10 cm in size (*Figure 1C*), in February, 1993 (in the pre-GIST era). The cut surface of the gastric tumor was yellowish-gray (*Figure 1D*). This case was provisionally diagnosed as a gastric LMS because of marked proliferation of spindle cells without expression of S-100 protein (*Figure 2A*). Despite the large size of the gastric tumor, pathology could not detect any necrotic area of the specimen at all. In addition, the mitotic rate showed <1 mitosis/50 high-power fields (HPFs).

A hepatic right anterior sectionectomy was carried out. The cut surfaces of the hepatic lesion were shown in *Figure 1B*. Microscopy of the specimen revealed spindle cells arranged in an interlacing fascicular growth-pattern reminiscent of the features observed in the prior gastric LMS (*Figure 2B*). Further examination of KIT yielded positive staining in both tumors (*Figure 2C, 2D*), although CD 34 staining was only reactive for the gastric lesion (*Figure 2E, 2F*). The Ki-67 score of the hepatic lesion was about 5% whereas that of the primary disease indicated <1% (*Figure 2G, 2H*). Genetic analysis in each lesion revealed the same in-flame deletions involving exon 11 of KIT at codon 558–559.

These findings led unequivocally to the correct diagnosis as a "true" liver metastasis from a prior gastric GIST (spindle cell type). It was made remarkable by the fact that it occurred 19 years after primary surgery. The patient regained his health with no indication of recurrence 2 years after his hepatectomy despite receiving no postoperative adjuvant chemotherapy.

Risk factors of recurrence including tumor size and location, and mitotic rates have been well-established in the GIST [16]; however, the present case constitutes an exception, showing that the GIST sometimes gives rise to 'delayed metastases' even though there may be no evidence for tumor necrosis, aneuploidy, or cellular pleomorphism in the primary lesion.

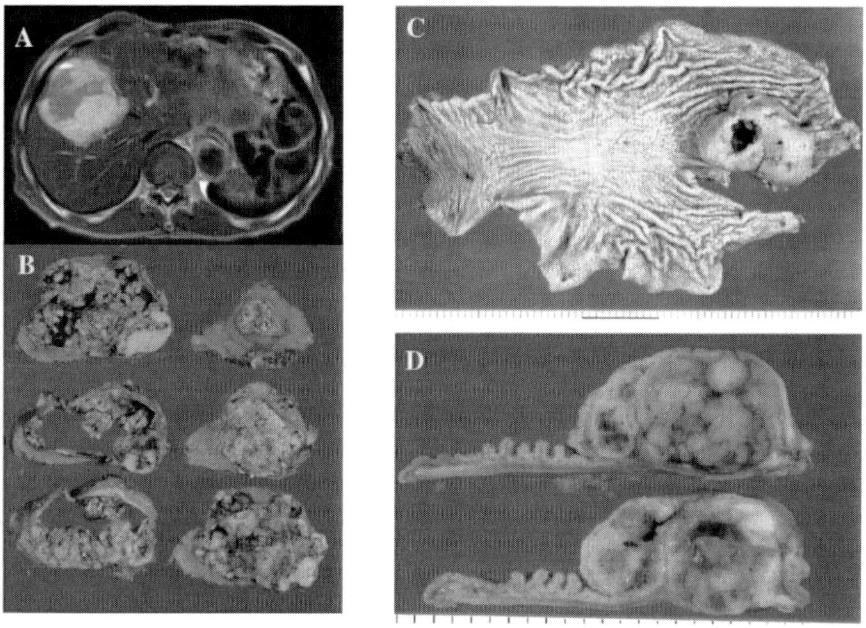

Figure 1. Clinical features of both hepatic and gastric lesions. A: A T-2 weighing MRI revealed a heterogenous tumor in the hepatic right lobe. B: Cut surfaces of the hepatic lesion. C: The gastric lesion 19 years before hepatectomy. D: The cut surface of the gastric lesion.

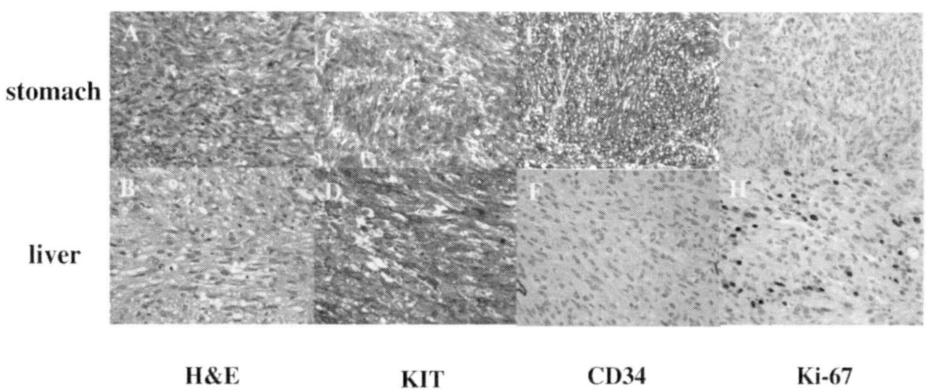

Figure 2. Immunohistochemical studies on each lesion. A & B: hematoxylin & eosin stain, C & D: KIT stain, E & F: CD34 stain, G & H: Ki-67 stain.

Clinical Features

The accurate incidence of GI-LMS and GIST is difficult to determine because only recently have these tumors been recognized as distinct entities. The GIST is a common type of sarcoma with an annual incidence of 10-15 cases per million, whereas the GI-LMS is extremely rare with 1-2% of GIST incidence [17-19]. Although most of these tumors are sporadic neoplasms and occur in adults over the age of 40, they can also occur in children, adolescence, and younger adults. GISTs can also occur in association with hereditary syndromes including Carney's triad (gastric GIST, extra-adrenal paraganglioma, and pulmonary chondroma), and von Recklinghausen disease (neurofibromatosis) [20-23].

A number of etiologic factors have been implicated in soft-tissue LMS. LMS is known to be closely associated with TP53 carriers [24] and commonly arises in immunocompromised hosts including human immunodeficiency virus (HIV)-infected [25], or Ebstein-Barr virus (EBV)-infected patients [26-28], post- transplant patients [27], and children with congenital immunodeficiency [28-30]. A few cases of the GI-LMS reportedly have a history of radiotherapy, or retinoblastoma as well [30]. The molecular and genetic pathomechanisms of GI-LMSs require further investigation.

The clinical behavior of both GI-LMSs and GISTs varies considerably among patients and depends upon tumor size, tumor location, extent of disease, and site of involvement [9]. Small tumors are asymptomatic and are detected incidentally during abdominal exploration, or endoscopic and radiologic examination. Like other sarcomas, both types of tumors initially tend to displace adjoining structures without invading them, and then reach large proportions before producing symptoms due to mass or invasive effects. On endoscopy, they appear similar to SMTs. They often manifest as exophytic tumors with protrusion into the bowel lumen. GI-LMSs occur preferentially in the small and large intestine, whereas gastric tumors are extremely rare [31-33]. In contrast, approximately 50-60% of GISTs occur in the stomach, followed by the small intestine (30-40%), the colon and rectum (5%), and the esophagus (5%) [6]. These features also suggest the GI-LMS is distinct from the GIST [31].

Most recurrences of operable GISTs and GI-LMSs take place within the first 5 years after surgery [34]. Approximately 50% of the patients with both primary diseases who undergo curative resection will survive 5 years; however, the natural course of each disease is unpredictable. GIST can occasionally recur later, as in the case described above, sometimes 20 years after surgery. Similarly, the low grade GI-LMS carries the risk of malignant behavior despite its mitotic activity. Recurrence of the GIST tends to involve the liver and peritoneal lining, whereas the lymph nodes, lung, and bone are infrequent metastatic sites, and generally become involved only in the late stages of the disease [31]. Like the GIST, the GI-LMS rarely spreads to regional lymph nodes and instead normally metastasizes to the liver and the lung [32,33].

Molecular Basis of GIST

The GIST attracted widespread interest because the principal pathological genetic mutations were identified as gain-of-function mutations in the KIT proto-oncogene (a tyrosine kinase receptor proto-oncogene), the resulting expression of KIT protein in most cases of GIST [5]. Moreover, molecularly- targeted, tyrosine kinase inhibitors against these defects have been developed and revolutionized the treatment of the GIST [34,35]. Because of the excellent response of GISTs to this specific treatment with a tyrosin kinase inhibitor such as imatinib methylate, differentiating clearly between the GIST and the GI-LMS is of paramount importance. Imatinib selectively inhibits specific tyrosine kinases, including KIT, and the platelet-derived growth factor receptor-alpha (PDGFA). Initially, imatinib was developed as a PDGFRA inhibitor and was first introduced clinically into the treatment of chronic myelogenous leukemia (CML). CML is characterized by a balanced translocation between chromosomes 9 and 22, resulting in Philadelphia chromosomal products (BCR-ABL fusion protein), which are also targeted by imatinib [36].

The KIT proto-oncogene encodes the KIT protein [5], which belongs to the group of transmembrane glycoproteins. It is expressed in the interstitial cells of Cajal, from which the GIST is believed to derive, hematopoietic cells, mast cells, and germ cells [37,38]. Binding of the KIT ligand induces dimerization and autophosphorylation of KIT. These processes initiate a cascade of intracellular signaling involved in tumorigenesis, proliferation, and differentiation [39-41]. A gain-of-function mutation often occurs in KIT, resulting in ligand-independent or constitutive activation of its tyrosine kinase function. KIT mutation is usually somatic and occurs in up to 90% of GISTs. The most frequent sites of mutation are in exon 11 (70%) or exon 9 (10%), whereas exons 13 or 17 are rarely involved [42]. Although activating KIT mutations have been reported in a number of other malignant tumors such as mastocytoma, germ cell tumors, acute myeloid leukemia, and neuroblastoma, in contrast to the GIST, KIT activation is unlikely to play a pathogenetic role in these tumors [43-49].

Approximately 3% of all GISTs harbor an activating mutation in PDGFA gene [47]. The sites of mutation are found in exon 12 and 18 [40-42]. Less than 5% of GISTs do not have a detectable mutation in either KIT or PDGFRA. At the chromosomal level, several abnormalities have been found in the GIST, including early loss of chromosomes 14p and 22q [49], suggesting that chromosomal derangements may constitute an additional mechanism for tumor progression.

Histopathological Diagnosis

Microscopically, the GI-LMS consists of long, spindle-shaped cells having eosinophilic fibrillary cytoplasm and ovioid or cigar-shaped nuclei with a blunt end. High mitotic activity with tumor necrosis is present. Its histological appearance is similar to that of the GIST, and may have been a source of confusion before the use of KIT immune staining became standard in case of a spindle cell morphology. The GIST generally has scant stroma and uniform cytology with eosinophilic fibrillary cytoplasm and nuclei containing fine chromatin and inconspicuous nucleoli as well [5-9].

The GI-LMS originates from smooth muscle cells within the muscularis mucosa or propria. Its benign counterpart, GI-leiomyoma, arises in smooth muscle cells as well [32]. Because of the unlikelihood of any malignant transformation in its pathogenesis, the GI-LMS may be derived de novo. The GI-LMS shows smooth muscle actin (SMA) and desmin reactivity, whereas it lacks expression of KIT and CD 34, as well as mutations of KIT and PDGRFA genes, which are the definitive characteristics of the GIST [32,33].

Histologically, GISTs can be classified into 3 subgroups, namely, the spindle cell type (70%), the epithelioid type (20%), and the mixed type (10%) which contains both features [31]. The spindle cell GIST shows uniform fusiform cells in intersecting fascicles or whorls, whereas the epithelioid GIST typically includes round cells in a nested pattern. The latter tends to show less intense KIT expression than the former [30]. The GIST is believed to be originated from the interstitial cell of Cajal, an intestinal pace maker cell or its stem cell-like precursor [37,38]. This cell acts as a regulator of intestinal motility within the GI autonomic nervous system [49].

Immunohistochemically, GISTs are almost always immunopositive for KIT (94%), while about 60-70% of GISTs are positive for CD34 [50]. KIT overexpression is a feature of KIT gene mutations although PDGFRA mutations and other unknown mechanisms also may result in KIT expression even in the absence of KIT mutations [50,51]. Sometimes, the GIST may lack the characteristics of smooth muscle cells, and instead show features of neural cells. Approximately 30-40% of GISTs are positive for SMA and 5% are also reactive to the S-100 protein. Because the GIST rarely expresses desmin, it is relatively well-confined to smooth muscle tumors with a spindle cellular morphology [51]. However, it is important to note that desmin is also expressed in the epithelioid or KIT-negative GIST [43,44].

Distinguishing the GIST from the GI-LMS has been facilitated by immunohistochemical detection of KIT, CD34, and the specific markers of smooth muscle differentiation mentioned above [33,34]. Importantly, KIT immunoreactivity is not exclusive to the GIST because mastocytoma, melanoma, angiosarcoma, Ewing's sarcoma, and GI neuroendocrine tumor may also express KIT [52]. However, these KIT-expressing neoplasms often lack pathological gene mutations in the KIT gene and may not be responsive to treatment of a tyrosine kinase inhibitor. Thus, the overall expression pattern is crucial in distinguishing the GI-LMS from the GIST [31].

KIT-negative GIST poses a diagnostic dilemma. It usually presents in the gastric region, showing an epithelioid phenotype without desmin reactivity, and commonly harboring PDGFRA mutations [32]. PDGFRA mutations, KIT mutations in exon 9 or 11, pediatric-type GISTs, or treatment with tyrosine kinase inhibitors including imatinib may bring about loss or attenuation of KIT expression [51,52]. DOG1.1, a mouse monoclonal antibody, was recently reported to have superior sensitivity and specificity compared with KIT and CD34 and to possess an additional advantage of detecting KIT-negative GIST by enabling a cytoplasmic and membranous immune staining exclusively of the GIST cells and native interstitial cells of Cajal. Furthermore, unlike KIT, DOG1.1 is negative in mast cells [53]. However, DOG1.1-negative exceptional cases with contradictory or ambiguous findings may require further molecular genetic analysis [32]. Therefore, for an unequivocal diagnosis of GI-LMS in the post-GIST era, a tumor should possess the histological features of LMS combined with the definitive profile including immunohistochemical positivity for SMA and desmin, and negativity for KIT, CD34, and DOG1.1 (*Table 1*).

Prognostic Factors and Clinical Management

GI-LMS

The World Health Organization (WHO) and the American Joint Committee on Cancer (AJCC) in conjunction with the College of American Pathologists, now recommend that sarcomas be graded according to the French Federation Nationale des Centres de Lutte Contre le Cancer (FNCLCC) or National Cancer Institute (NCI) grading systems [54-56].

Table 1. Comparison of GI-LMS and GIST

	GI-LMS	GIST
Cell of origin	**Smooth muscle**	**Interstitial cell of Cajar**
Cellular markers		
KIT	-	+
CD34	-	+
DOG1.1	-	+
SMA	+	-
desmin	+	-

The FNCLCC histological grading system evaluates 3 tumor parameters: (a) the degree of tumor differentiation, (b) number of mitotic figures per 10 high power fields (HPFs), and (c) quantity of tumor necrosis. These figures are then totaled to produce an overall histological grade (*Table 2*). The cut-off for mitotic counts in the FNCLCC system is 10 or 20 mitoses per 10 HPFs, equivalent to 50 or 100 per 50 HPFs.

Table 2. FNCLCC grading system: definition of parameters

(a) Tumor differentiation

Score 1: sarcomas closely resembling normal adult mesenchymal tissue (e.g., low grade leiomyosarcoma).

Score 2: sarcomas for which histological typing is certain (e.g., myxoid liposarcoma).

Score 3: embryonal and undifferentiated sarcomas, sarcomas of doubtful type, synovial sarcomas, osteosarcomas, PNET.[1]

(b) Mitotic count

Score 1: 0-9 mitoses per 10 HPF[2]

Score 2: 10-19 mitoses per 10 HPF

Score 3: ≧20 mitoses per 10 HPF

(c) Tumor necrosis

Score 0: no necrosis

Score 1: <50% tumor necrosis

Score 2: ≧50% tumor necrosis

Histological grade

Grade 1: total score 2, 3

Grade 2: total score 4, 5

Grade 3: total score 6, 7, 8

[1] PNET: primitive neuroectodermal tumor.

[2] A high power field (HPF) measures 0.1734 mm^2.

The NCI grading system uses the histologic diagnosis combined with (1) degree of cellularity, (2) cellular pleomorphism, and (3) mitotic activity. This grading system also identifies the importance of the degree of necrosis. In addition, the International Union against Cancer (UICC)/AJCC staging system for soft tissue sarcoma assesses the tumor size (cut-off, 5 cm) as well as the depth of tumor (T), lymph node metastasis (N), and distant metastasis (M), and employs a histological grading system similar to that used in the FNCLCC system.

According to the previous reports, more than 50 cases of GI-LMS have been described in the post-GIST era [6,9,32,33]. The histopathological features of these tumors have been well documented; however, most reported cases suffered for lack of information from accurate grading. Although survival analysis is hindered by small case numbers and limited survival data available, tumor size may emerge as an important prognostic factor; i.e., tumor size < 5 cm was correlated significantly with a more favorable prognosis, while, unlike cases of the GIST, mitotic counts and primary tumor site were unrelated to prognosis [33].

Because most GI-LMSs have a number of mitoses irrespective of biological behavior, mitotic count may not be of prognostic value, e.g., a tumor with two mitoses per 50 HPFs has a much lower risk for recurrence than a tumor with 12 mitoses per 50 HPFs, whereas it makes very little difference whether a tumor has 50 or 100 mitoses per 50 HPFs, the cut-off for mitotic counts in the FNCLCC system. Despite the paucity of GI-LMSs, the FNCLCC and AJCC systems might be applicable to the GI-LMS because the GI-LMS differs from the GIST and possess clinicopathologic features that may more closely parallel soft-tissue or vascular LMS rather than other GI stromal neoplasms. A risk stratification of the GI-LMS based on the tumor depth (e.g., submucosa or above versus muscularis propria or beyond) might be of prognostic value; however, the risk indicators for adverse outcomes in cases of the GI-LMS have yet to be clarified.

Reportedly, GI-LMSs may be more sensitive to conventional chemotherapeutic agents including doxorubicin and ifosfamide than GISTs [31]. However, unlike for the GIST, at present, there is no specific molecular therapy for the GI-LMS. Because of the different treatment options available, distinguishing these tumors is crucial. The ability to distinguish the GI-LMS from the GIST accurately will enable identification of clinical symptomology, and outcomes of the GI-LMS. Accurate staging of the GI-LMS in the future can help steer surgeons, oncologists, and pathologists toward appropriate management based on risk-stratified categorization of the GI-LMS.

GIST

GIST has varying malignancy potential. Micro-GISTs, with a diameter of less than 1 cm, occur in approximately 30% of the middle-aged and elderly general population [17-19]. Micro-GISTs seldom have malignancy potential, even though most of them harbor an activating mutation in KIT or PDGFRA, which are considered the key drivers of GIST molecular pathogenesis [57,58]. Large GISTs and GISTs with high mitotic indices have formidable recurrence activity, with metastases typically in the liver and peritoneal cavity [59]. The GIST most commonly arises in the stomach and gastric GISTs have a more favorable outcome of than those from the small intestinal, colorectal, or esophageal origin [34,59].

Complete surgical resection is the mainstay for treatment of GISTs. When the GIST adheres to the adjoining structures, an en bloc resection may be indicated. Because the GIST is soft and fragile, surgery without meticulous procedures may bring about tumor rupture, which may increase the risk of peritoneal recurrence. Lymphadenectomy generally is not indicated unless the regional lymph nodes are involved because GIST rarely metastasizes there. Although imatinib has become the first-line treatment of metastatic GIST, extended surgery may be considered first in case of the primary GIST with a synchronous metastatic disease, if possible [31].

Imatinib can induce a partial tumor response in 45% of patients and stable disease in approximately 30% [60]. Remarkably, the 2-year survival of patients with metastatic disease is now reported to be approximately 70% [60]. By contrast, before the introduction of imatinib, the median survival after surgical resection of recurrent GIST was only 15 months [61]. Although imatinib is very efficacious against GISTs, this agent rarely induces a complete remission. The median time to disease progression with imatinib therapy is 2 years. Some patients with metastatic GIST who have focal resistance to imatinib may benefit from resection [62]. The resection of metastatic GISTs in conjunction with imatinib therapy may prove to be a potent therapeutic strategy. A multimodal approach involving resection of resistant clones may benefit some patients; however, in patients with metastatic GISTs with multifocal resistance, surgery is generally not indicated.

Multifocal resistance to imatinib should be treated with another targeted agent such as sunitinib which has activity against KIT and PDGFRA as well as the vascular endothelial cell growth factor (VEGF) and fms-related tyrosine kinase 3 (Flt3) receptors. Sunitinib may have activity against GISTs harboring secondary KIT mutations which confer resistance to imatinib [63]. Conventional forms of adjuvant therapy play a limited role in the management of patients with a metastatic GIST. The efficacy of systemic chemotherapy with the currently available agents is unknown. The response rate of the GIST to conventional chemotherapy is reportedly 5%. In contrast, the GI-LMS shows a more favorable response to conventional chemotherapy due probably to the lower expression of multi-drug resistant (MDR) proteins than seen in the GIST [4,31].

Unfortunately, resistance to these tyrosine kinase inhibitors is an emerging clinical problem. Detailed study of the mechanisms of resistance is in progress and will hopefully provide insight into creating strategies to circumvent this dilemma. Through a better understanding of the biology of the GIST, the rationale for an effective combination of surgical and molecular therapy has been developed and serves as a paradigm for the treatment of other solid tumors for which newer targeted therapies are being developed [31].

As mentioned above, metastatic GISTs are often lethal despite treatment with tyrosine kinase inhibitors. Estimates of the risk of recurrence are crucial in the management of operable GIST [54]. Adjuvant imatinib has been reported to increase the time to GIST recurrence, and patients with a high risk of recurrence have longer survival with 3 years of adjuvant imatinib therapy than with 1 year [34].

Currently, almost all patients with GIST, even those with a complete resection, are given imatinib because the recent National Comprehensive Cancer Network and European Society for Medical Oncology guideline suggest use of imatinib for patients with intermediate-risk to high-risk GIST [64]. However, this practice increases the risk for adverse effects and the cost for patients and health-care systems. Although adjuvant imatinib is generally well tolerated, most patients suffer some adverse effects including fatigue, edema, skin rash, diarrhea, and abdominal pain.

Since many patients with the GIST can be cured by surgery alone and might not benefit greatly from adjuvant treatment, risk stratification is necessary in the management of operable

GIST [65]. It is crucial to predict accurately the risk of recurrence for each patient, and to identify unequivocally those who would benefit from adjuvant imatinib therapy [66]. A few risk-stratification schemes including the National Institutes of Health (NIH) consensus classification, the modified NIH consensus criteria, and the Armed Forces Institute of Pathology (AFIP) criteria are available for operable GIST.

In the NIH consensus classification [50], tumors are stratified into four risk groups based on two factors—size and mitosis count (very low risk: size <2.0 cm and mitosis count <5 per 50 HPFs; low risk: size 2.0–4.9 cm and mitosis count <5 per 50 HPFs; intermediate risk: size ≦5.0 cm and mitosis count 6–10 per 50 HPFs, or size 5.0–10.0 cm and mitosis count <5 per 50 HPFs; high risk: size >5.0 cm and mitosis count >5 per 50 HPFs, or size >10.0 cm with any mitosis count, or mitosis count >10 per 50 HPFs irrespective of size). The modified NIH classification differs from the NIH consensus classification by considering ruptured GIST as a high-risk tumor irrespective of other features, and by including in the high-risk category small (≦5.0 cm), non-gastric tumors with frequent mitoses (>5 per 50 HPFs), and intermediate size (5.1–10.0 cm) non-gastric tumors with few mitoses (5 per 50 HPFs)[59]. The AFIP classification stratifies tumors with few mitoses (<5 per 50 HPFs) into four categories based on size (group 1: <2.0 cm; group 2: 2.1–5.0 cm; group 3a: 5.1–10.0 cm; group 3b: >10.0 cm) and tumors with frequent mitoses (>5 per 50 HPFs) into four groups (group 4: <2.0 cm; group 5: 2.1–5.0 cm; group 6a: 5.1–10.0 cm; group 6b: >10.0 cm)[58]. The AFIP classification takes into account tumor site (gastric, duodenal, jejunal and ileal, or rectal) as well. Reportedly, the modified NIH classification is the best criteria to identify a single high-risk group for consideration of adjuvant therapy [34, 65,66].

Tumor rupture, whether spontaneous or surgical, was thought to be associated with a high risk of peritoneal recurrence, and is currently identified as an independent prognostic parameter [34,65,66]. Although some mutations, such as deletions involving KIT exon 11 at codons 557–558, are associated with unfavorable prognosis, they are not yet considered to be independent risk factors [59]. Reportedly, GIST patients who were identified as having an intermediate risk of recurrence showed a clinical course similar to that of the low-risk group; in other words, only the high-risk patients would likely benefit from adjuvant imatinib therapy [34]. The subset of high-risk patients who are likely to benefit from adjuvant therapy should be considered separately from those who will do just as well without it. This personalized approach will ultimately reduce costs and side effects in patients who can be adequately treated by surgery alone, and allow focus on high-risk patients who need more intensive treatment [34,67].

Conclusion

Prior to the advent of KIT immunochemistry, most GI stromal neoplasms which had been labeled as GI-LMSs were actually identical to GISTs. The GIST is the most frequent GI-mesenchymal neoplasm, while the GI-LMS is extremely rare. The distinction between the GIST and the GI-LMS has been facilitated by immunohistochemical detection of KIT as well as specific markers of smooth muscle differentiation. Further investigation using modern diagnostic criteria are needed to define the biology of the GI-LMS in the post-GIST era.

References

[1] Yamaguchi U, Hasegawa T, Masuda T, et al.: Differential diagnosis of gastrointestinal stromal tumor and other spindle cell tumors in the gastrointestinal tract based on immunohistochemical analysis. *Virchows Arch.* 2004; 445:142–150.

[2] Howe JR, Karnell LH, Scott-Conner C: Small bowel sarcoma:Analysis of survival from the National Cancer Data Base. *Ann. Surg. Oncol.* 2001; 8:496–508.

[3] Suster S: Gastrointestinal stromal tumors. *Semin. Diagn. Pathol.* 1996; 13: 297–313.

[4] Plaat BE, Hollema H, Molenaar WM, et al.: Soft tissue leiomyosarcomas and malignant gastrointestinal stromal tumors: Differences in clinical outcome and expression of multidrug resistance proteins. *J. Clin. Oncol.* 2000; 18: 3211–3220.

[5] Hirota S, Isozaki K, Moriyama Y, et al.: Gain-of-function mutations of c-kit in human gastrointestinal stromal tumors. *Science* 1998; 279: 577–580.

[6] Miettinen M, Furlong M, Sarlomo-Rikala M, et al.: Gastrointestinal stromal tumors, intramural leiomyomas, and leiomyosarcomas in the rectum and anus: A clinicopathologic, immunohistochemical, and molecular genetic study of 144 cases. Am *J. Surg. Pathol.* 2001; 25: 1121–1133.

[7] Miettinen M, Kopczynski J, Makhlouf HR, et al.: Gastrointestinal stromal tumors, intramural leiomyomas, and leiomyosarcomas in the duodenum: A clinicopathologic, immunohistochemical, and molecular genetic study of 167 cases. *Am. J. Surg. Pathol.* 2003; 27: 625–641.

[8] Miettinen M, Lasota J: Gastrointestinal stromal tumors-Definition, clinical, histological, immunohistochemical, and molecular genetic features and differential diagnosis. *Virchows Arch.* 2001; 438: 1–12.

[9] Miettinen M, Sarlomo-Rikala M, Sobin LH, et al.: Gastrointestinal stromal tumors and leiomyosarcomas in the colon: A clinicopathologic, immunohistochemical, and molecular genetic study of 44 cases. *Am. J. Surg. Pathol.* 2000; 24: 1339–1352.

[10] Lee YT: Leiomyosarcoma of the gastro-intestinal tract: General pattern of metastasis and recurrence. *Cancer Treat. Rev.* 1983; 10: 91–101.

[11] Stout AP. Bizarre smooth muscle tumors of the stomach. *Cancer* 1962; 15:400-9.

[12] Mazur MT, Clark HB. Gastric stromal tumors: reappraisal of histogenesis. *Am. J. Surg. Pathol.* 1983; 7: 507-19.

[13] Herrera GA, Pinto De Morales H, Grizzle WE, et al. Malignant small bowel neoplasm of enteric plexus derivation (plexosarcoma): light and electron microscopic study confirming the origin of the neoplasm. *Dig. Dis. Sci.* 1984; 29: 275-84.

[14] Walker P, Dvorak AM. Gastrointestinal autonomic nerve (GAN) tumor: ultrastructural evidence for a newly recognized entity. *Arch. Pathol. Lab. Med.* 1986; 110: 309-16.

[15] Lee JR, Joshi V, Griffin JW, Lasota J, et al. Gastrointestinal autonomic nerve tumor: immunohistochemical and molecular identity with gastrointestinal stromal tumor. *Am. J. Surg. Patho.* 2001; 25: 979-987.

[16] Adachi K, Hashimoto T, Enatsu K. A liver metastasis 19 years after primary surgery discloses the correct diagnosis. *Digest. Liver Dis.* 2013; 45: e8.

[17] Nilsson B, Bumming P, Meis-Kindblom JM, et al. Gastrointestinal stromal tumors: the incidence, prevalence, clinical course, and prognostication in the preimatinib mesylate era—a population-based study in western Sweden. *Cancer* 2005; 103: 821–29.

[18] Mucciarini C, Rossi G, Bertolini F, et al. Incidence and clinicopathologic features of gastrointestinal stromal tumors: a population-based study. *BMC Cancer* 2007; 7: 230.

[19] Tryggvason G, Gislason H, Magnusson MK, Jonasson JG. Gastrointestinal stromal tumors in Iceland, 1990–2003: the Icelandic GIST study, a population based incidence and pathologic risk stratification study. *Int. J. Cancer* 2005; 117: 289–93.

[20] DeMatteo RP, Lewis JJ, Leung D, et al.: Two hundred gastrointestinal stromal tumors: Recurrence patterns and prognostic factors for survival. Ann Surg 2000; 231: 51–58.

[21] Nishida T, Hirota S, Taniguchi M, et al.: Familial gastrointestinal stromal tumours with germline mutation of the KIT gene. *Nat. Genet* 1998; 19: 323–324.

[22] Chompret A, Kannengiesser C, Barrois M, et al.: PDGFRA germline mutation in a family with multiple cases of gastrointestinal stromal tumor. *Gastroenterology* 2004; 126: 318–321.

[23] Gold JS, Dematteo RP: Combined surgical and molecular therapy: The gastrointestinal stromal tumor model. *Ann. Surg*. 2006; 244: 176–184.

[24] Ognjanovic S, Olivier M, Bergemann TL, Hainaut P. Sarcomas in TP53 germline mutation carriers. A review of the IARC TP53 database. *Cancer* 2012; 118: 1387-96.

[25] McClain KL, Leach CT, Jenson HB, et al. Association of Epstein-Barr virus with leiomyosarcomas in children with AIDS. *N. Engl. J. Med.* 1995; 332: 12.

[26] Tetzlaff MT, Nosek C, Kovarik CL. Epstein-Barr virus–associated leiomyosarcoma with cutaneous involvement in an African child with human immunodeficiency virus: a case report and review of the literature. *J. Cutan. Pathol.* 2011; 38: 731-9.

[27] Nur S, Rosenblum WD, Katta UD, Islam H, Brown K, Ramaswamy G. Epstein-Barr virus–associated multifocal leiomyosarcomas arising in a cardiac transplant recipient: autopsy case report and review of the literature. *J. Heart Lung Transplant.* 2007; 26: 944-52.

[28] Reyes C, Abuzaitoun O, De Jong A, Hanson C, Langston C. Epstein-Barr virus associated smooth muscle tumors in ataxia telangiectasia: a case report and review. *Hum. Pathol.* 2002; 33: 133.

[29] Deyrup AT, Lee VK, Hill CE, et al. Epstein-Barr virus–associated smooth muscle tumors are distinctive mesenchymal tumors reflecting multiple infection events: a clinicopathologic and molecular analysis of 29 tumors from 19 patients. *Am. J. Surg. Pathol.* 2006; 30:75.

[30] Pauser U, Grimm H. Intramucosal leiomyosarcoma of the stomach following hereditary retinoblastoma in childhood—a case report and review of the literature. *World J. Surg. Oncol. 2008*; 6: 131.

[31] Katz S, DeMatteo RP. Gastrointestinal stromal tumors and leiomyosarcoma. *J. Surg. Oncol.* 2008; 97: 350-359.

[32] Aggarwal G, Sharma S, Zheng M, et al. Primary leimyosarcoma of the gastrointestinal tract in the postgastrointestinal stromal tumor era. *Ann. Diagn. Pathol.* 2012;16: 532-40.

[33] Yamamoto H, Tobo T, Setsu N, et al. Clinicopathological features of primary leiomyosarcoma of the gastrointestinal tract following recognition of gastrointestinal stromal tumours. *Histopathology* 2013; 61: 194-207.

[34] Joensuu H, Vehtari A, Riihimaki J, et al. Risk of recurrence of gastrointestinal stromal tumour after surgery: an analysis of pooled population-based cohorts. *Lancet Oncol.* 2011; 13: 265-274.

[35] Heinrich MC, Griffith DJ, Druker BJ, et al.: Inhibition of c-kit receptor tyrosine kinase activity by STI 571, a selective tyrosine kinase inhibitor. *Blood* 2000; 96:925–932.

[36] Druker BJ, Talpaz M, Resta DJ, et al.: Efficacy and safety of a specific inhibitor of the BCR-ABL tyrosine kinase in chronic myeloid leukemia. *N. Engl. J. Med.* 2001; 344: 1031–1037.

[37] Kindblom LG, Remotti HE, Aldenborg F, et al.: Gastrointestinal pacemaker cell tumor (GIPACT): Gastrointestinal stromal tumors show phenotypic characteristics of the interstitial cells of Cajal. *Am. J. Pathol.* 1998; 152:1259–1269.

[38] Sanders KM: A case for interstitial cells of Cajal as pacemakers and mediators of neurotransmission in the gastrointestinal tract. Gastroenterology 1996; 111:492–515.

[39] Sommer G, Agosti V, Ehlers I, et al.: Gastrointestinal stromal tumors in a mouse model by targeted mutation of the Kit receptor tyrosine kinase. *Proc. Natl. Acad. Sci. USA* 2003; 100:6706–6711.

[40] Rubin BP, Singer S, Tsao C, et al.: KIT activation is a ubiquitous feature of gastrointestinal stromal tumors. *Cancer Res.* 2001; 61: 8118–8121.

[41] Lux ML, Rubin BP, Biase TL, et al.: KIT extracellular and kinase domain mutations in gastrointestinal stromal tumors. *Am. J. Pathol.* 2000; 156: 791–795.

[42] Antonescu CR, Sommer G, Sarran L, et al.: Association of KIT exon 9 mutations with nongastric primary site and aggressive behavior: KIT mutation analysis and clinical correlates of 120 gastrointestinal stromal tumors. *Clin. Cancer Res.* 2003; 9: 3329–3337.

[43] Tsujimura T, Morimoto M, Hashimoto K, et al.: Constitutive activation of c-kit in FMA3 murine mastocytoma cells caused by deletion of seven amino acids at the juxtamembrane domain. *Blood* 1996; 87:273–283.

[44] Tian Q, Frierson HF Jr, Krystal GW, et al.: Activating c-kit gene mutations in human germ cell tumors. *Am. J. Pathol.* 1999; 154: 1643–1647.

[45] Kanakura Y, Ikeda H, Kitayama H, et al.: Expression, function and activation of the proto-oncogene c-kit product in human leukemia cells. *Leuk Lymphoma* 1993; 10:35–41.

[46] Cohen PS, Chan JP, Lipkunskaya M, et al.: Expression of stem cell factor and c-kit in human neuroblastoma. The Children's Cancer Group. *Blood* 1994; 84:3465–3472.

[47] Heinrich MC, Corless CL, Duensing A, et al.: PDGFRA activating mutations in gastrointestinal stromal tumors. *Science* 2003; 299:708–710.

[48] Ma CK, Amin MB, Kintanar E, et al.: Immunohistologic characterization of gastrointestinal stromal tumors: A study of 82 cases compared with 11 cases of leiomyomas. *Mod. Pathol.* 1993; 6:139–144.

[49] Breiner JA, Meis-Kindblom J, Kindblom LG, et al.: Loss of 14q and 22q in gastrointestinal stromal tumors (pacemaker cell tumors). *Cancer Genet. Cytogenet.* 2000; 120:111–116.

[50] Fletcher CD, Berman JJ, Corless C, et al.: Diagnosis of gastrointestinal stromal tumors: A consensus approach. *Hum. Pathol.* 2002; 33:459–465.

[51] Heinrich M, Corless C, Blanke C, et al. Molecular correlates of imatinib resistance in gastrointestinal stromal tumors. *J. Clin. Oncol.* 2006; 24:4764-4774.

[52] Miettinen M, Sobin LH, Sarlomo-Rikala M: Immunohistochemical spectrum of GISTs at different sites and their differential diagnosis with a reference to CD117 (KIT). *Mod. Pathol.* 2000; 13: 1134–1142.

[53] Liegl B, Hornick JL, Corless CL, et al. Monoclonal antibody DOG1.1 shows higher sensitivity than KIT in the diagnosis of gastrointestinal stromal tumors, including unusual subtypes. *Am. J. Surg. Pathol.* 2009; 33:437-446.

[54] Fletcher DM, Unni KK, Mertens F. World Health Organization classification of tumours: pathology and genetics of tumours of soft tissue and bone. Lyon, France: IARC Press; 2002.

[55] Edge SB, Byrd DR, Compton CC, et al. AJCC cancer staging handbook. Chicago, Illinois: *Springer*; 2010.

[56] Costa J, Wesley RA, Glatstein E, Rosenberg SA. The grading of soft tissue sarcomas. Results of a clinicohistopathologic correlation in a series of 163 cases. *Cancer* 1984; 53:530-41.

[57] Eisenberg BL, Trent JC. Adjuvant and neoadjuvant imatinib therapy: current role in the management of gastrointestinal stromal tumors. *Int. J. Cancer* 2011; 129: 2533–42.

[58] Miettinen M, Lasota J. Gastrointestinal stromal tumors: pathology and prognosis at different sites. *Semin. Diagn. Pathol.* 2006; 23: 70–83.

[59] Joensuu H. Risk stratification of patients diagnosed with gastrointestinal stromal tumor. *Hum. Pathol.* 2008; 39: 1411–19.

[60] van Oosterom AT, Judson I, Verweij J, et al.: Safety and efficacy of imatinib (STI571) in metastatic gastrointestinal stromal tumours: A phase I study. *Lancet* 2001; 358:1421–1423.

[61] Demetri GD, von Mehren M, Blanke CD, et al.: Efficacy and safety of imatinib mesylate in advanced gastrointestinal stromal tumors. *N. Engl. J. Med.* 2002; 347:472–480.

[62] Verweij J, Casali PG, Zalcberg J, et al.: Progression-free survival in gastrointestinal stromal tumours with high-dose imatinib: Randomised trial. *Lancet* 2004; 364:1127–1134.

[63] Prenen H, Cools J, Mentens N, et al.: Efficacy of the kinase inhibitor SU11248 against gastrointestinal stromal tumor mutants refractory to imatinib mesylate. *Clin. Cancer Res.* 2006; 12:2622–2627.

[64] Eisenberg BL, Trent JC. Adjuvant and neoadjuvant imatinib therapy: current role in the management of gastrointestinal stromal tumors. *Int. J. Cancer* 2011; 129: 2533–42.

[65] Rutkowski P, Bylina E, Wozniak A, et al. Validation of the Joensuu risk criteria for primary resectable gastrointestinal stromal tumour—the impact of tumour rupture on patient outcomes. *Eur. J. Surg. Oncol.* 2011; 37: 890–96.

[66] Rutkowski P, Nowecki ZI, Michej W, et al. Risk criteria and prognostic factors for predicting recurrences after resection of primary gastrointestinal stromal tumor. *Ann. Surg. Oncol.* 2007; 14: 2018–27.

[67] Duensing A. Closing in on accurate risk prediction and disease management for patients with operable GIST. *Lancet Oncol.* 2012; 13:220-221.

In: Leiomyosarcoma
Editor: Rosemary H. Leach

ISBN: 978-1-63117-940-2

Chapter 12

Primary Ovarian Leiomyosarcoma: A Very Rare Entity

Georgios Androutsopoulos[1*], Emmanouil Terzakis[2] and Georgios Decavalas[1]

[1]Department of Obstetrics and Gynecology, University of Patras, Medical School, Rion, Greece

[2]nd Department of Gynecology, St. Savvas Anticancer-Oncologic Hospital, Athens, Greece

Abstract

Primary ovarian sarcoma is a very rare tumor, accounting 1% of all ovarian malignancies. The most common histologic subtypes are: mixed mullerian tumor, stromal cell sarcoma and fibrosarcoma.

Primary ovarian leiomyosarcoma is an extremely rare histologic subtype of ovarian sarcomas. Until now, about 66 cases have been reported in English literature. Among them, 43 were primary ovarian leiomyosarcoma without heterologous elements and 23 were primary ovarian leiomyosarcoma with heterologous elements.

It is usually occurs in postmenopausal women, although sometimes younger women may be affected. The mean age at diagnosis is 52 years (range 12-84 years).

The precise histogenesis of primary ovarian leiomyosarcoma is relative unknown. It is probably originates from smooth muscle present in the walls of the blood vessels in the cortical stroma, in the corpus luteum, in the ovarian ligaments at their point of attachment to the ovary, in remnants of Wolffian ducts and in totipotential cells of ovarian mesenchyme.

Most patients with primary ovarian leiomyosarcoma usually have nonspecific symptoms and signs. Also they have pressure symptoms on adjacent organs.

* Corresponding author: Georgios Androutsopoulos MD, Lecturer, Department of Obstetrics & Gynecology, Nikolaou Apostoli 21, Patras, 26332, Greece, Tel: +306974088092, Email: androutsopoulosgeorgios @hotmail.com.

Primary ovarian leiomyosarcoma is typically present as a solitary, large, lobular, soft, fleshy, solid mass with hemorrhage and cystic degeneration. It is usually unilateral and may reach more than 10 cm in diameter.

The diagnostic criteria for primary ovarian leiomyosarcoma are: hypercellularity, nuclear atypia, pleomorphism, coagulative necrosis and high mitotic activity.

Immunohistochemical staining for primary ovarian leiomyosarcoma is generally positive for muscle specific actin, SMA, desmin, vimentin, p53 and proliferation markers and negative for cytokeratins and S-100.

Due to the rarity of primary ovarian leiomyosarcoma, it is very difficult to determine the optimal therapy. Surgery is the baseline therapy and complete resection should be attempted whenever possible. Postoperative adjuvant radiotherapy is used for local disease control. Postoperative adjuvant chemotherapy is used in patients with locally advanced or metastatic disease.

The prognosis of primary ovarian leiomyosarcoma is generally unfavorable, depending on mitotic activity and stage at diagnosis. Most patients die with extended local disease and multiple distant metastases.

1. Introduction

Primary ovarian sarcoma (POS) is a very rare tumor, accounting 1% of all ovarian malignancies. [1-3] According to the source of origin, POS classified into: teratoid, mesenchymal and mullerian. [1,3,4]

The most common histologic subtypes of POS are: mixed mullerian tumor, stromal cell sarcoma and fibrosarcoma.[1,3,4] Other less common histologic subtypes of POS are: leiomyosarcoma, neurofibrosarcoma, rhabdomyosarcoma, chondrosarcoma, angiosarcoma and liposarcoma. [1,3,4]

It is obvious that primary ovarian leiomyosarcoma (POLMS) is an extremely rare histologic subtype of POS. [4,5]

2. Epidemiology

POLMS most commonly occurs in postmenopausal women. [5,6] However, sometimes younger women may be affected. [5,7-9] The mean age at diagnosis is 52 years (range 12-84 years). [5,7,10-13] Only 10% of patients are younger than 30 years. [5,10]

Until now, 66 cases of POLMS have been reported in English literature. [5,10,11,14,15] Among them, 43 cases were POLMS without heterologous elements and 23 cases were POLMS with heterologous elements. [7,10,14-16]

3. Pathogenesis

The precise pathogenesis of POLMS is relative unknown. [10]

It is probably originates from smooth muscle present in the walls of the blood vessels in the cortical stroma, in the corpus luteum, in the ovarian ligaments (at their point of attachment to the ovary), in remnants of Wolffian ducts and in totipotential cells of ovarian mesenchyme.

[5,10,13,16-22]. Moreover it can probably originates from smooth muscle metaplasia of endometriotic stroma or smooth muscle present in mature cystic teratomas and in the walls of mucinous cystic tumors. [5,10,21,23-26]

Malignant transformation of an ovarian leiomyoma and migration of a uterine leiomyoma are very rare mechanisms of pathogenesis. [7,10,27,28]

4. Symptoms & Signs

The most common presenting symptoms and signs are: abdominal/pelvic pain, abdominal/pelvic mass and abdominal bloating. [5,11,14,28]

Many patients have pressure symptoms on adjacent organs (bladder, bowel and ureter). [5,28]

5. Pathology

POLMS is typically present as a large, solitary, lobular, soft, fleshy, solid mass. [5,14,27] It is usually unilateral. [5,7,14,18,27] Tumor size may reach more than 10 cm (range 4-30 cm). [5,7,14,18,27] Moreover, tumor has areas with hemorrhage, cystic degeneration and necrosis. [5,10,14,27]

The diagnostic criteria for POLMS are: hypercellularity, nuclear atypia, pleomorphism, coagulative necrosis and high mitotic activity (>5 mitotic figures per 10 high-power fields). [5,10,14,27,29]

Immunohistochemical staining for POLMS is generally positive for muscle specific actin, SMA, desmin, vimentin, p53 and proliferation markers and negative for cytokeratins and S-100. [6,10,13,18,27]

Mitotic activity and stage have a direct correlation with the malignant potential and aggressiveness of POLMS. [13,16,30]

6. Treatment

Due to the rarity of POLMS, it is very difficult to determine the optimal therapy. [16]

6.1. Surgery

Surgery is the baseline therapy, for most patients with POLMS. [7,14,15,28] The extent of surgery ranges from conservative (fertility-sparing surgery) to radical (systematic surgical staging). [5,7-10]

Systematic surgical staging includes: total hysterectomy, bilateral salpingo-oophorectomy, omentectomy, pelvic and para-aortic lymphadenectomy and complete resection of all disease. [7,11,12,14,16,28,31]

6.2. Postoperative Adjuvant Radiotherapy

Postoperative adjuvant radiotherapy is used for local disease control. [14,28]

Especially in patients with disease confined to the ovary, the role of postoperative adjuvant radiotherapy remains controversial. [6,7,14-16,28,31,32]

6.3. Postoperative Adjuvant Chemotherapy

Postoperative adjuvant chemotherapy is used in patients with locally advanced or metastatic disease [7,14,28]. Various chemotherapeutic protocols including cisplatin have been applied. [7,16,29]

It seems that postoperative adjuvant chemotherapy has only modest effect in progression free survival and overall survival. [5,7]

Especially in patients with disease confined to the ovary, the role of postoperative adjuvant chemotherapy remains controversial. [6,7,9,14-16,28,31,32]

7. Disease Recurrence

The mean time of disease recurrence in patients with POLMS, is 19 months. [5,7]

The most common sites of disease recurrence, are: abdomen and pelvis. [5,10] Other less common sites of disease recurrence, are: lung, bone, liver, mediastinum, brain and preauricular lymph node. [5,10]

8. Prognosis

The prognosis of patients with POLMS is generally unfavorable. [5-7,16] The most important prognostic factors are: mitotic activity and stage at diagnosis. [5,6,10,13,14,16]

Most patients with POLMS recur within 19 months after initial diagnosis. [5,7,14] Moreover, most patients with POLMS die within 23 months after initial diagnosis. [5,7,14] They usually die with extended local disease and multiple distant metastases. [28]

Additional studies are needed in order to understand more about nature, clinical behavior and treatment of POLMS. [11]

References

[1] Sood, A; Sorosky, J; Gelder, M; Buller, R; Anderson, B; Wilkinson, E; et al. Primary ovarian sarcoma: analysis of prognostic variables and the role of surgical cytoreduction. *Cancer*, 1998, 82(9), 1731-7.

[2] Anderson, B; Turner, DA; Benda, J. Ovarian sarcoma. *Gynecol Oncol*, 1987, 26(2), 183-92.

[3] Sahin, A; Benda, J. An immunohistochemical study of primary ovarian sarcoma. An evaluation of nine tumors. *Int J Gynecol Pathol*, 1988, 7(3), 268-79.

[4] Azoury, R; Woodruff, J. Primary ovarian sarcomas. Report of 43 cases from the Emil Novak Ovarian Tumor Registry. *Obstet Gynecol*, 1971, 37(6), 920-41.

[5] Lerwill, M; Sung, R; Oliva, E; Prat, J; Young, R. Smooth muscle tumors of the ovary: a clinicopathologic study of 54 cases emphasizing prognostic criteria, histologic variants, and differential diagnosis. *Am J Surg Pathol*, 2004, 28(11), 1436-51.

[6] Friedman, H; Mazur, M. Primary ovarian leiomyosarcoma. An immunohistochemical and ultrastructural study. *Arch Pathol Lab Med*, 1991, 115(9), 941-5.

[7] Monk, B; Nieberg, R; Berek, J. Primary leiomyosarcoma of the ovary in a perimenarchal female. *Gynecol Oncol*, 1993, 48(3), 389-93.

[8] O'Sullivan, S; Das Narla, L; Ferraro, E. Primary ovarian leiomyosarcoma in an adolescent following radiation for medulloblastoma. *Pediatr Radiol*, 1998, 28(6), 468-70.

[9] Seracchioli, R; Colombo, F; Bagnoli, A; Trengia, V; Venturoli, S. Primary ovarian leiomyosarcoma as a new component in the nevoid basal cell carcinoma syndrome: a case report. *Am J Obstet Gynecol*, 2003, 188(4), 1093-5.

[10] Taskin, S; Taskin, E; Uzum, N; Ataoglu, O; Ortac, F. Primary ovarian leiomyosarcoma: a review of the clinical and immunohistochemical features of the rare tumor. *Obstet Gynecol Surv*, 2007, 62(7), 480-6.

[11] Zygouris, D; Androutsopoulos, G; Grigoriadis, C; Arnogiannaki, N; Terzakis, E. Primary ovarian leiomyosarcoma. *Eur J Gynaecol Oncol*, 2012, 33(3), 331-3.

[12] Inoue, J; Gomibuchi, H; Minoura, S. A case of a primary ovarian leiomyosarcoma. *J Obstet Gynaecol Res*, 2000, 26(6), 401-7.

[13] Nasu, M; Inoue, J; Matsui, M; Minoura, S; Matsubara, O. Ovarian leiomyosarcoma: an autopsy case report. *Pathol Int*, 2000, 50(2), 162-5.

[14] Arslan, O; Sumer, C; Cihangiroglu, G; Kanat-Pektas, M; Gungor, T. A rare tumor of the female genital tract: primary ovarian leiomyosarcoma. *Arch Gynecol Obstet*, 2011, 283(Suppl 1), 83-5.

[15] Goodall, E; Madhuri, T; Manuel, S. The management dilemma of leiomyosarcoma of the ovary. *World Journal of Oncology*, 2011, 2(5), 265-66.

[16] Rasmussen, C; Skilling, J; Sorosky, J; Lager, D; Buller, R. Stage IIIC ovarian leiomyosarcoma in a premenopausal woman with multiple recurrences: prolonged survival with surgical therapy. *Gynecol Oncol*, 1997, 66(3), 519-25.

[17] Nicotina, P; Antico, F; Caruso, C; Triolo, O. Primary ovarian leiomyosarcoma. Proliferation rate and survival. *Eur J Gynaecol Oncol*, 2004, 25(4), 515-6.

[18] Balaton, A; Vaury, P; Imbert, M; Mussy, M. Primary leiomyosarcoma of the ovary: a histological and immunocytochemical study. *Gynecol Oncol*, 1987, 28(1), 116-20.

[19] Doss, B; Wanek, S; Jacques, S; Qureshi, F; Ramirez, N; Lawrence, W. Ovarian smooth muscle metaplasia: an uncommon and possibly underrecognized entity. *Int J Gynecol Pathol*, 1999, 18(1), 58-62.

[20] Santini, D; Ceccarelli, C; Leone, O; Pasquinelli, G; Piana, S; Marabini, A; et al. Smooth muscle differentiation in normal human ovaries, ovarian stromal hyperplasia and ovarian granulosa-stromal cells tumors. *Mod Pathol*, 1995, 8(1), 25-30.

[21] Scully, R. Smooth-muscle differentiation in genital tract disorders. *Arch Pathol Lab Med*, 1981, 105(10), 505-7.

[22] Okamura, H; Virutamasen, P; Wright, K; Wallach, E. Ovarian smooth muscle in the human being, rabbit, and cat. Histochemical and electron microscopic study. *Am J Obstet Gynecol*, 1972, 112(2), 183-91.

[23] Fukunaga, M. Smooth muscle metaplasia in ovarian endometriosis. *Histopathology*, 2000, 36(4), 348-52.

[24] Hameed, A; Ying, A; Keyhani-Rofagha, S; Xie, D; Copeland, L. Ovarian mucinous cystadenoma associated with mural leiomyomatous nodule and massive ovarian edema. *Gynecol Oncol*, 1997, 67(2), 226-9.

[25] Kelley, R; Scully, R. Cancer developing in dermoid cysts of the ovary. A report of 8 cases, including a carcinoid and a leiomyosarcoma. *Cancer*, 1961, 14, 989-1000.

[26] Nichols, G; Mills, S; Ulbright, T; Czernobilsky, B; Roth, L. Spindle cell mural nodules in cystic ovarian mucinous tumors. A clinicopathologic and immunohistochemical study of five cases. *Am J Surg Pathol*, 1991, 15(11), 1055-62.

[27] Bouie, S; Cracchiolo, B; Heller, D. Epithelioid leiomyosarcoma of the ovary. *Gynecol Oncol*, 2005, 97(2), 697-9.

[28] Dixit, S; Singhal, S; Baboo, H; Vyas, R; Neema, J; Murthy, R; et al. Leiomyosarcoma of the ovary. *J Postgrad Med*, 1993, 39(3), 151-3.

[29] Bodner, K; Bodner-Adler, B; Czerwenka, K; Hudelist, G; Kimberger, O; Leodolter, S; et al. Bcl-2 expression in a primary leiomyosarcoma of the ovary: a case report. *Wien Klin Wochenschr*, 2003, 115(5-6), 191-5.

[30] O'Reilly, P; Raab, S; Niemann, T; Rodgers, J; Robinson, R. p53, proliferating cell nuclear antigen, and Ki-67 expression in extrauterine leiomyosarcomas. *Mod Pathol*, 1997, 10(2), 91-7.

[31] Dobbs, S; Brown, L; Hollingworth, J; Ireland, D. Surgical treatment of recurrent primary ovarian leiomyosarcoma. A case report. *Eur J Gynaecol Oncol*, 1999, 20(3), 172-3.

[32] Rampaul, R; Barrow, S; Naraynsingh, V. A primary ovarian leiomyosarcoma with micro-invasive features (stage I): is surgical excision enough? *Gynecol Oncol*, 1999, 73(3), 464.

In: Leiomyosarcoma
Editor: Rosemary H. Leach

ISBN: 978-1-63117-940-2

Chapter 13

Leiomyosarcoma in the Female Genital Tract: Risk Factors, Diagnosis and Treatment Options

Joo-Hyun Nam*, M.D., Ph.D. and Jeong-Yeol Park, M.D., Ph.D.
Department of Obstetrics and Gynecology,
University of Ulsan College of Medicine,
Asan Medical Center, Seoul, Korea

Abstract

Leiomyosarcoma, a malignant tumor that arises from mesenchymal tissues, is the most common soft-tissue sarcoma. Although rarely found in the female genital tract, leiomyosarcoma is the most malignant tumor that can occur in the female genital tract.

Although leiomyosarcomacan occur anywhere through the female genital tract (including the uterine body, uterine cervix, ovary, salpinx, vagina and vulva), it is most commonly found in the uterine body. Uterine leiomyosarcoma is the most common uterine sarcoma, with an incidence of uterine leiomyosarcoma of 0.64 per 100,000 women. It is the single largest site-specific group of leiomyosarcoma. Given the rarity of leiomyosarcoma in the female genital tract, the causes and risk factors are not well known.

The pretreatment diagnosis of leiomyosarcoma in the female genital tract is challenging because most cases are diagnosed after inadvertent surgery for presumed fibroids.

Surgery is the only curable treatment for leiomyosaroma, with rates of cure of other treatment modalities (including radiation therapy, chemotheprapy, and targeted therapy) remaining uncertain.

This review summarizes the most recent findings regarding the risk factors, diagnosis, and treatment options for leiomyosarcoma in the female genital tract.

* Corresponding Author: Joo-Hyun Nam, M.D., Ph.D. Department of Obstetrics and Gynecology, University of Ulsan College of Medicine, Asan Medical Center, Seoul, Korea.

Introduction

Leiomyosarcoma—a malignant tumor that arises from mesenchymal tissues—is the most common soft-tissue sarcoma. Although leiomyosarcoma rarely occurs in the female genital tract, it is the most malignant tumor that can occur in any part of this region—including the uterine body, uterine cervix, ovary, salpinx, vagina and vulva. Of these sites, the uterine body is the most common for this cancer. Given the rarity of leiomyosarcoma in the female genital tract, the causes and risk factors are not well known and pretreatment diagnosis is challenging because most cases are diagnosed after inadvertent surgery for presumed fibroids. The standard management of leiomyosarcoma in the female genital tract is also not yet well established. This review provides an up-to-date summary of findings regarding the risk factors, diagnosis, and treatment options for leiomyosarcoma in the female genital tract.

Body of Review

Leiomyosarcoma of the Uterine Corpus

1) Incidence and Risk Factors

Uterine sarcoma is a rare and aggressive type of uterine malignant neoplasm that comprises only 3% to 9% of all sarcomas. [1, 2] Uterine leiomyosarcomas are smooth-muscle tumors that comprise a subset of sarcomas that accounts for approximately 1% of uterine malignancies with an incidence of 0.64 per 10,000 women. [3, 4] Uterine leiomyosarcomas occur in women between the ages of 40–60 years. Fewer than 1% of benign uterine leiomyomas convert to a sarcomatous condition. [5, 6] Uterine leiomyosarcoma is most frequently observed in women in their 60s, and increasing age is a risk factor [7]. Use of tamoxifen for longer than five years is believed to make a small contribution to the risk for leiomyosarcoma. [8-10] Amongst female breast cancer patients who receive tamoxifen therapy, 17 of every10,000 develop uterine leiomyosarcoma. [10-13] The observation that 0.5% of uterine leiomyosarcoma patients have a history of pelvic radiation therapy suggests that this might also be a risk factor. [14]

2) Diagnosis

Vaginal bleeding, pelvic pain or pressure, and abdominopelvic mass are not specific presenting symptoms for differentiating uterine leiomyosarcoma from benign conditions. Imaging studies are usually not useful in differentiating between uterine leiomyosarcoma and benign tumor types, such as leiomyoma or adenomyosis. [15, 16] Notwithstanding reports that levels of tumor markers are elevated in uterine sarcomas, [17-19] the diagnostic value of CA-125 and other tumor markers for uterine leiomyosarcoma requires further investigation. Many cases are diagnosed as uterine leiomyosarcoma when there is a rapid growth either on examination or imaging over a short period of time, although most of these cases are still diagnosed as a benign tumor. [20] Postmenopausal women without hormonal replacement therapy who display tumor growth also show an increased risk of uterine leiomyosarcoma. [21] Thorough pelvic and abdominal examination including groin and supraclavicular nodes should be performed. Image analyses using MRI, CT, or PET/CT are helpful when identifying distant metastases, such as to the lungs or lymphatic system, when these are suspected. [22] Endometrial biopsy should be performed when symptoms suggest or findings indicate uterine malignancies; nonetheless, the sensitivity of endometrial biopsy ranges from 38% to 62%. [23-26]. The majority of uterine leiomyosarcomas are diagnosed incidentally after myomectomy or hysterectomy. [27] Mitotic index, the location of coagulative necrosis dissected from tumor, and cellular atypia are the three most important mainstays of diagnosing uterine leiomyosarcoma pathologically. [28, 29] Uterine leiomyosarcomas has characteristics of hypercellularity, severe nuclear atypia, and a mitotic rate of over 10 per 10 high power fields (Figure 1). [30, 31]

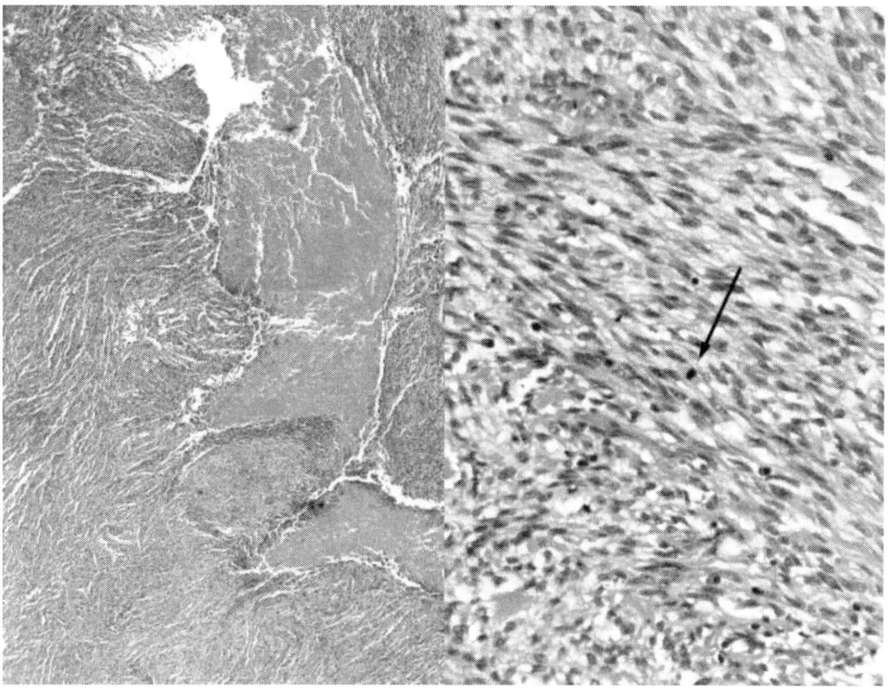

Figure 1. Uterine leiomyosarcoma showing hypercellularity, severe nuclear atypia, and a mitotic rate of over 10 per 10 high power fields (arrow). (Left: H&A, ×40; Right: H&A, ×200).

3) Treatment Options

Surgery

Surgical management is the first treatment modality in most cases of uterine leiomyosarcoma. [32, 33] The only chance for a cure in affected patients is complete surgical resection of the uterus-confined lesion. [32, 33] The stage of uterine leiomyosarcoma is determined surgically according to the International Federation of Gynecology and Obstetrics (FIGO) which was revised in 2009 (Table 1). [34]

The standard surgical procedure for the treatment of uterine leiomyosarcoma is simple hysterectomy. Bilateral salpingo-oophorectomy is recommended only for postmenopausal women. Unless there are ovarian metastatic lesions, bilateral salpingo-oophorectomy is not recommended for premenopausal women. The incidence of occult ovarian metastasis in normal appearing ovaries is low, and ranges between 3.4% and 3.9%. [35-37]. Preservation of the ovaries does not compromise the survival of patients with uterine leiomyosarcoma. [6, 36, 38-40]

Table 1. International Federation of Gynecology and Obstetrics (FIGO) staging system for uterine leiomyosarcoma (revised in 2009)

Stage	Definition
I	Tumor limited to uterus
IA	≤ 5 cm
IB	> 5 cm
II	Tumor extends to the pelvis
IIA	Adnexal involvement
IIB	Tumor extends to extrauterine pelvic tissue
III	Tumor invades abdominal tissues (not just protruding into the abdomen).
IIIA	One site
IIIB	> One site
IIIC	Metastasis to pelvic and/or para-aortic lymph nodes
IV IVA	Tumor invades bladder and/or rectum
IVB	Distant metastasis

Reference: Prat J. FIGO staging for uterine sarcomas. *Int J Gynaecol Obstet*. 2009;104: 177-178.

Surgical staging procedures—including lymphadenectomy, peritoneal biopsy, omentectomy, and peritoneal washing cytology—are controversial and are usually not recommended for the surgical management of early-stage uterine leiomyosarcoma. [32, 33] The incidence of occult lymph node metastasis is low (between 0% and 3.7%), and lymph node metastasis is commonly associated with peritoneal spread of the disease. [6, 35, 40-42] Accordingly, lymphadenectomy is indicated only in the event of peritoneal seeding or lymph node enlargement. [6, 39]

The goal of surgery in patients with extra-uterine spread of uterine leiomyosarcoma should be complete debulking of the disease. [32, 33] Given the frequency of hematogenous metastasis as the origin of uterine leiomyosarcoma, lung metastasis is not uncommon. Some studies report that the resection of isolated lung metastasis is associated with prolonged survival. [43-45] Given that the preoperative differential diagnosis of leiomyosarcoma and leiomyoma is nearly impossible, many cases of leiomyosarcomaare diagnosed after surgery for a presumed uterine leiomyoma. [46, 47] Hence, and notwithstanding the extremely low incidence of uterine leiomyosarcoma in patients undergoing surgery for presumed leiomyoma, many patients with uterine leiomyosarcoma experience inadvertent morcellation of uterine leiomyosarcoma. Recent reports have suggested that this has an adverse impact on the prognosis of uterine leiomyosarcoma. [21, 48, 49] Therefore, meticulous excision of uterine leiomyosarcoma without tumor injury is as important as a complete excision of these lesions.

Radiation Therapy, Chemotherapy, and Targeted Therapy

Treatment modalities other than surgical excision (including radiation therapy, chemotherapy, and targeted therapy) cannot achieve complete remission. [32, 33] These modalities are thus rarely selected as the primary treatment for uterine leiomyosarcoma but are used as an adjuvant therapy after surgical management. [32, 33] Radiation therapy has frequently been used as an adjuvant therapy after surgical excision of uterine leiomyosarcoma. However, the role of radiation therapy is controversial and only a few studies have suggested that it can improve local control rates. [50] Most studies suggest that radiation therapy does not improve local control rate orsurvival [51] In addition, a role for adjuvant radiation therapy in uterine leiomyosarcoma was not evident in a recent large-scale prospective randomized controlled trial. [52]

Doxorubicin and ifosfamide have been regarded as the most active chemotherapeutic agents for uterine leiomyosarcoma. The response rates to these agents are about 20% for doxorubicin, and between 20% and 30% for a combination of doxorubicin and ifosfamide. [53] However, recent clinical trials for the treatment of uterine leiomyosarcoma showed a higher response rate with a combination of gemcitabine and docetaxel. [47, 48] The response rate of this regimen was about 36% as a first-line treatment and about 27% as a second-line treatment for uterine leiomyosarcoma. [54, 55] A more recently tested regimen with a combination of gemcitamin and docetaxel followed by treatment with doxorubicin alone also showed promise in a phase-II study. However, the survival benefit of adjuvant chemotherapy for uterine leiomyosarcoma has not yet been confirmed and a clinical trial in this regard is ongoing.

Given the limited roles of radiation therapy, chemotherapy, or a combination of both in the management of uterine leiomyosarcoma, many targeted agents have been investigated as potential therapeutic regimens for this disease. These include VEGF-trap, [56] sunitinib, [57] pazopanib, [58] and bevacizumab (with doxorubicin) [59]. Although none of these agents was found to have the potential to cure uterine leiomyosarcoma, some do delay the progression of disease. A clinical trial to evaluate the therapeutic potential of adding bevacizumab to a combination of gemcitabine and docetaxel is underway.

Leiomyosarcoma of the Uterine Cervix

Leiomyosarcoma of the cervix is very uncommon, and constitutes less than 1% of all cervical malignancies. [60] Given its rarity, no large experimental study of leiomyosarcoma of the cervix has been undertaken to date. Most of the available data on these lesions are derived from case reports and small case series. [61]

Diagnostic tools for leiomyosarcoma of the cervix are almost identical to those for uterine leiomyosarcoma.

Tumor stage, grade, and mitotic count—which are the best prognostic indicators in patients with uterine leiomyosarcoma—are all associated with a reduced likelihood of survival. [62] Other factorsi ncluding tumor size, age, and menopausal status are suggested to predict the outcome. [30, 40,62] Older age, postmenopausal status, and larger tumor size (>5 cm) appear to be significantly associated with a reduced likelihood of survival. [40] If leiomyosarcoma was confined to the cervix, TAH-BSO should be warranted. Given that leiomyosarcoma rarely disseminates to lymph nodes, the value of routine lymphadenectomy has been questioned. [61] Several studies suggest that postoperative adjuvant pelvic irradiation tends to improve loco-regional control. [40, 62, 63] The impact of chemotherapy in cervical leiomyosarcomas is difficult to assess. Most patients can be candidates for chemotherapy because of its tendency to metastasize hematogenously. Doxorubicin and ifosfamide can be used as a first-line chemotherapy regimen for advanced leiomyosarcoma patients. Doxorubicin and ifosfamide show the largest response rates, as high as 30.3%. [53] Combined-modality treatments—including surgery, radiotherapy, and chemotherapy—should be considered in advanced-stage patients to achieve better survival.

Leiomyosarcoma of the Vagina

Carcinomas of the vagina are also rare, and account for only between2% and 3% of gynecologic malignancies. Approximately 3% of vaginal cancers are sarcomas, and approximately65% of sarcomas are leiomyosarcomas. [64-66] The vagina is the most common site of metastasis or direct extension from tumors originating in other genital sites (such as the cervix or endometrium) or from extragenital sites (including the rectum and bladder) [66]. About half of the patients with invasive cancer display abnormal vaginal bleeding, frequently after coitus or vaginal douching. Patients frequently report vaginal discharge, a palpable mass, dyspareunia, or pain in the perineum or pelvis. [66]

In general, surgery for leiomyosarcoma of the vagina is crucial for the treatment of high-risk, short- and long-term morbidity. However, a negative resection margin is very important. An insufficiently wide local excision might result in positive or close margins that require additional multimodality treatment of leiomyosarcoma. [66] Surgical intervention is possible as a primary treatment, but ensuring tumor-free resection margins is extremely important. Every effort should be made to never cut through the tumor, and it is very important to prevent spillage. [67] Although resection of lymph nodes is controversial, this should be considered when metastasis to the lymph nodes is suspected. The role of radiation therapy is controversial. Brachytherapy may be preferred over external-beam radiotherapy for smaller tissue volumes to minimize the effects on healthy tissue. Brachy therapy can also be regarded as an alternative to surgery when hysterectomy or colpectomy is required. [68, 69] For patients with localized disease, the role of adjuvant chemotherapy is even more poorly defined than that of radiation therapy; nonetheless, adjuvant chemotherapy has been considered owing to the high risk for distant relapse. [67] Ifosphamid, cisplatin, etoposide, gemcitabine, paclitaxel, and doxorubicin have shown modest-to-minimal response rates in advanced and recurrent leiomyosarcoma. [70] A combination of doxorubicin and ifosfamide is the most popular regimen. Supplementation of docetaxel therapy with gemcitabine has also shown effectiveness, particularly with leiomyosarcomas of uterine origin. [54]

Leiomyosarcoma of the Vulva

Leiomyosarcomas comprise only 1% of all types of vulvar cancer, and are the most common sarcoma of the vulva. They are believed to arise from the smooth muscles within the walls of blood vessels, as well as in round ligaments, erectile tissue, and erector-pili muscles.

[71] Painless palpable masses are the most common symptoms of leiomyosarcomas of the vulva. These masses are commonly misdiagnosed as benign lesion-like bartholin cysts. [72, 73] A vulvar smooth muscle tumor should be considered a sarcoma when at least three of the following four features are present: i) tumor diameter of 5 cm or greater, ii) infiltrating margin, iii) 5 or more mitoses per 10 hpf, and iv) grade-2 to -3 cytologicatypia. [73] Radical local excision is the primary treatment for leiomyosarcomas of the vulva, and lymphatic metastases are uncommon. Adjuvant treatment might be considered if surgical margins are involved.

Leiomyosarcoma of the Ovary

Primary ovarian leiomyosarcoma, an uncommon ovarian tumor that comprises less than 1% of all ovarian neoplasias, is usually diagnosed in postmenopausal women. The origin, etiology, clinical behavior, and proper treatment ovarian leiomyosarcoma remain unknown [74]. The prognosis is typically very poor, and depends on the tumor stage and mitotic activity within the tumor [75]. Recurrence reportedly occurs within a year after surgery, and cancer related death usually occurs within 2 years. [76, 77] Staging and treatment traditionally follow those of epithelial carcinoma of the ovary. Radical surgical excision is a mainstay of treatment, but the extent of surgery remains contentious. The expected benefits and optimal modality of adjuvant therapy are also uncertain.

Leiomyosarcoma of the Fallopian Tube

Leiomyosarcoma of the fallopian tube is an extremely rare tumor, with only a few reports in the literature. Presenting symptoms are usually ambiguous. Patients in the available literature complained of lower abdominal pain and pelvic pressure. Transvaginal sonography, CT, and MRI can be used to diagnose malignant fallopian tube tumors, but the identification of leiomyosarcoma is difficult [78, 79]. Surgery followed by adjuvant chemotherapy can be a reasonable treatment option. Successful treatment was reported in a 39-year-old woman with leiomyosarcoma confined to the right fallopian tube; in this case, there was no evidence of disease for 2 years after surgical resection followed by adjuvant doxorubicin and cisplatin chemotherapy [80].

References

[1] Nordal RR, Thoresen SO. Uterine sarcomas in Norway 1956-1992: incidence, survival and mortality. *Eur. J. Cancer*. 1997;33: 907-911.

[2] Trope CG, Abeler VM, Kristensen GB. Diagnosis and treatment of sarcoma of the uterus. A review. *Acta. Oncol*. 2012;51: 694-705.

[3] Zaloudek CJ, Norris HJ. Adenofibroma and adenosarcoma of the uterus: a clinicopathologic study of 35 cases. *Cancer*. 1981;48: 354-366.

[4] Harlow BL, Weiss NS, Lofton S. The epidemiology of sarcomas of the uterus. *J. Natl. Cancer Inst.* 1986;76: 399-402.

[5] Dinh TA, Oliva EA, Fuller AF, Jr., Lee H, Goodman A. The treatment of uterine leiomyosarcoma. Results from a 10-year experience (1990-1999) at the Massachusetts General Hospital. *Gynecol. Oncol.* 2004;92: 648-652.

[6] Giuntoli RL, 2nd, Metzinger DS, DiMarco CS, et al. Retrospective review of 208 patients with leiomyosarcoma of the uterus: prognostic indicators, surgical management, and adjuvant therapy. *Gynecol. Oncol.* 2003;89: 460-469.

[7] Norris HJ, Taylor HB. Mesenchymal tumors of the uterus. I. A clinical and pathological study of 53 endometrial stromal tumors. *Cancer.* 1966;19: 755-766.

[8] Mourits MJ, De Vries EG, Willemse PH, Ten Hoor KA, Hollema H, Van der Zee AG. Tamoxifen treatment and gynecologic side effects: a review. *Obstet. Gynecol.* 2001;97: 855-866.

[9] Yildirim Y, Inal MM, Sanci M, et al. Development of uterine sarcoma after tamoxifen treatment for breast cancer: report of four cases. *Int. J. Gynecol. Cancer.* 2005;15: 1239-1242.

[10] Wysowski DK, Honig SF, Beitz J. Uterine sarcoma associated with tamoxifen use. *N. Engl. J. Med.* 2002;346: 1832-1833.

[11] Wickerham DL, Fisher B, Wolmark N, et al. Association of tamoxifen and uterine sarcoma. *J. Clin. Oncol.* 2002;20: 2758-2760.

[12] Moinfar F, Azodi M, Tavassoli FA. Uterine sarcomas. *Pathology.* 2007;39: 55-71.

[13] ACOG committee opinion. No. 336: Tamoxifen and uterine cancer. *Obstet Gynecol.* 2006;107: 1475-1478.

[14] Fang Z, Matsumoto S, Ae K, et al. Postradiation soft tissue sarcoma: a multiinstitutional analysis of 14 cases in Japan. *J. Orthop. Sci.* 2004;9: 242-246.

[15] Rha SE, Byun JY, Jung SE, et al. CT and MRI of uterine sarcomas and their mimickers. *AJR Am. J. Roentgenol.* 2003;181: 1369-1374.

[16] Kitajima K, Murakami K, Kaji Y, Sugimura K. Spectrum of FDG PET/CT findings of uterine tumors. *AJR Am. J. Roentgenol.* 2010;195: 737-743.

[17] Goto A, Takeuchi S, Sugimura K, Maruo T. Usefulness of Gd-DTPA contrast-enhanced dynamic MRI and serum determination of LDH and its isozymes in the differential diagnosis of leiomyosarcoma from degenerated leiomyoma of the uterus. *Int. J. Gynecol. Cancer.* 2002;12: 354-361.

[18] Huang GS, Chiu LG, Gebb JS, et al. Serum CA125 predicts extrauterine disease and survival in uterine carcinosarcoma. *Gynecol. Oncol.* 2007;107: 513-517.

[19] Hoskins PJ, Le N. Preoperative tumor markers at diagnosis in women with malignant mixed mullerian tumors/carcinosarcoma of the uterus. *Int. J. Gynecol. Cancer.* 2008;18: 1200-1201.

[20] Parker WH, Fu YS, Berek JS. Uterine sarcoma in patients operated on for presumed leiomyoma and rapidly growing leiomyoma. *Obstet. Gynecol.* 1994;83: 414-418.

[21] Perri T, Korach J, Sadetzki S, Oberman B, Fridman E, Ben-Baruch G. Uterine leiomyosarcoma: does the primary surgical procedure matter? *Int. J. Gynecol. Cancer.* 2009;19: 257-260.

[22] Shah SH, Jagannathan JP, Krajewski K, O'Regan KN, George S, Ramaiya NH. Uterine sarcomas: then and now. *AJR Am. J. Roentgenol.* 2012;199: 213-223.

[23] Sagae S, Yamashita K, Ishioka S, et al. Preoperative diagnosis and treatment results in 106 patients with uterine sarcoma in Hokkaido, Japan. *Oncology.* 2004;67: 33-39.
[24] Jin Y, Pan L, Wang X, et al. Clinical characteristics of endometrial stromal sarcoma from an academic medical hospital in China. *Int. J. Gynecol. Cancer.* 2010;20: 1535-1539.
[25] Bansal N, Herzog TJ, Burke W, Cohen CJ, Wright JD. The utility of preoperative endometrial sampling for the detection of uterine sarcomas. *Gynecol. Oncol.* 2008;110: 43-48.
[26] Leibsohn S, d'Ablaing G, Mishell DR, Jr., Schlaerth JB. Leiomyosarcoma in a series of hysterectomies performed for presumed uterine leiomyomas. *Am. J. Obstet Gynecol.* 1990;162: 968-974; discussion 974-966.
[27] D'Angelo E, Prat J. Uterine sarcomas: a review. Gynecol Oncol. 2010;116: 131-139.
[28] Bell SW, Kempson RL, Hendrickson MR. Problematic uterine smooth muscle neoplasms. A clinicopathologic study of 213 cases. *Am. J. Surg. Pathol.* 1994;18: 535-558.
[29] Quade BJ, Wang TY, Sornberger K, Dal Cin P, Mutter GL, Morton CC. Molecular pathogenesis of uterine smooth muscle tumors from transcriptional profiling. *Genes. Chromosomes Cancer.* 2004;40: 97-108.
[30] Evans HL, Chawla SP, Simpson C, Finn KP. Smooth muscle neoplasms of the uterus other than ordinary leiomyoma. A study of 46 cases, with emphasis on diagnostic criteria and prognostic factors. *Cancer.* 1988;62: 2239-2247.
[31] Perrone T, Dehner LP. Prognostically favorable "mitotically active" smooth-muscle tumors of the uterus. A clinicopathologic study of ten cases. *Am. J. Surg. Pathol.* 1988;12: 1-8.
[32] Nam JH. Surgical treatment of uterine sarcoma. *Best Pract. Res. Clin. Obstet. Gynaecol.* 2011;25: 751-760.
[33] Nam JH, Park JY. Update on treatment of uterine sarcoma. *Curr. Opin. Obstet. Gynecol.* 2010;22: 36-42.
[34] Prat J. FIGO staging for uterine sarcomas. *Int. J. Gynaecol. Obstet.* 2009;104: 177-178.
[35] Leitao MM, Sonoda Y, Brennan MF, Barakat RR, Chi DS. Incidence of lymph node and ovarian metastases in leiomyosarcoma of the uterus. *Gynecol. Oncol.* 2003;91: 209-212.
[36] Gard GB, Mulvany NJ, Quinn MA. Management of uterine leiomyosarcoma in Australia. *Aust. N. Z. J. Obstet. Gynaecol.* 1999;39: 93-98.
[37] Bokhman JV, Yakovleva IA, Urmanchejeva AF. Treatment of patients with sarcoma of the uterus. *Eur. J. Gynaecol. Oncol.* 1990;11: 225-231.
[38] Berchuck A, Rubin SC, Hoskins WJ, Saigo PE, Pierce VK, Lewis JL, Jr. Treatment of uterine leiomyosarcoma. *Obstet. Gynecol.* 1988;71: 845-850.
[39] Van Dinh T, Woodruff JD. Leiomyosarcoma of the uterus. *Am. J. Obstet. Gynecol.* 1982;144: 817-823.
[40] Gadducci A, Landoni F, Sartori E, et al. Uterine leiomyosarcoma: analysis of treatment failures and survival. *Gynecol. Oncol.* 1996;62: 25-32.
[41] Park JY, Kim DY, Suh DS, et al. Prognostic factors and treatment outcomes of patients with uterine sarcoma: analysis of 127 patients at a single institution, 1989-2007. *J. Cancer Res. Clin. Oncol.* 2008;134: 1277-1287.

[42] Ayhan A, Tuncer ZS, Tanir M, Yuce K, Ayhan A. Uterine sarcoma: the Hacettepe hospital experience of 88 consecutive patients. *Eur. J. Gynaecol. Oncol.* 1997;18: 146-148.

[43] Levenback C, Rubin SC, McCormack PM, Hoskins WJ, Atkinson EN, Lewis JL, Jr. Resection of pulmonary metastases from uterine sarcomas. *Gynecol. Oncol.* 1992;45: 202-205.

[44] Weiser MR, Downey RJ, Leung DH, Brennan MF. Repeat resection of pulmonary metastases in patients with soft-tissue sarcoma. *J. Am. Coll Surg.* 2000;191: 184-190; discussion 190-181.

[45] Leitao MM, Brennan MF, Hensley M, et al. Surgical resection of pulmonary and extrapulmonary recurrences of uterine leiomyosarcoma. *Gynecol. Oncol.* 2002;87: 287-294.

[46] Kido A, Togashi K, Koyama T, Yamaoka T, Fujiwara T, Fujii S. Diffusely enlarged uterus: evaluation with MR imaging. *Radiographics.* 2003;23: 1423-1439.

[47] Fukunishi H, Funaki K, Ikuma K, et al. Unsuspected uterine leiomyosarcoma: magnetic resonance imaging findings before and after focused ultrasound surgery. *Int. J. Gynecol. Cancer.* 2007;17: 724-728.

[48] Morice P, Rodriguez A, Rey A, et al. Prognostic value of initial surgical procedure for patients with uterine sarcoma: analysis of 123 patients. *Eur. J. Gynaecol. Oncol.* 2003;24: 237-240.

[49] Park JY, Park SK, Kim DY, et al. The impact of tumor morcellation during surgery on the prognosis of patients with apparently early uterine leiomyosarcoma. *Gynecol. Oncol.* 2011;122: 255-259.

[50] Sampath S, Schultheiss TE, Ryu JK, Wong JY. The role of adjuvant radiation in uterine sarcomas. *Int. J. Radiat. Oncol. Biol. Phys.* 2010;76: 728-734.

[51] Wright JD, Seshan VE, Shah M, et al. The role of radiation in improving survival for early-stage carcinosarcoma and leiomyosarcoma. *Am. J. Obstet. Gynecol.* 2008;199: 536 e531-538.

[52] Reed NS, Mangioni C, Malmstrom H, et al. Phase III randomised study to evaluate the role of adjuvant pelvic radiotherapy in the treatment of uterine sarcomas stages I and II: an European Organisation for Research and Treatment of Cancer Gynaecological Cancer Group Study (protocol 55874). *Eur. J. Cancer.* 2008;44: 808-818.

[53] Sutton G, Blessing JA, Malfetano JH. Ifosfamide and doxorubicin in the treatment of advanced leiomyosarcomas of the uterus: a Gynecologic Oncology Group study. *Gynecol. Oncol.* 1996;62: 226-229.

[54] Hensley ML, Blessing JA, Mannel R, Rose PG. Fixed-dose rate gemcitabine plus docetaxel as first-line therapy for metastatic uterine leiomyosarcoma: a Gynecologic Oncology Group phase II trial. *Gynecol. Oncol.* 2008;109: 329-334.

[55] Hensley ML, Blessing JA, Degeest K, Abulafia O, Rose PG, Homesley HD. Fixed-dose rate gemcitabine plus docetaxel as second-line therapy for metastatic uterine leiomyosarcoma: a Gynecologic Oncology Group phase II study. *Gynecol. Oncol.* 2008;109: 323-328.

[56] Mackay HJ, Buckanovich RJ, Hirte H, et al. A phase II study single agent of aflibercept (VEGF Trap) in patients with recurrent or metastatic gynecologic carcinosarcomas and uterine leiomyosarcoma. A trial of the Princess Margaret Hospital, Chicago and California Cancer Phase II Consortia. *Gynecol. Oncol.* 2012;125: 136-140.

[57] Hensley ML, Sill MW, Scribner DR, Jr., et al. Sunitinib malate in the treatment of recurrent or persistent uterine leiomyosarcoma: a Gynecologic Oncology Group phase II study. *Gynecol. Oncol.* 2009;115: 460-465.

[58] Sleijfer S, Ray-Coquard I, Papai Z, et al. Pazopanib, a multikinase angiogenesis inhibitor, in patients with relapsed or refractory advanced soft tissue sarcoma: a phase II study from the European organisation for research and treatment of cancer-soft tissue and bone sarcoma group (EORTC study 62043). *J. Clin. Oncol.* 2009;27: 3126-3132.

[59] D'Adamo DR, Anderson SE, Albritton K, et al. Phase II study of doxorubicin and bevacizumab for patients with metastatic soft-tissue sarcomas. *J. Clin. Oncol.* 2005;23: 7135-7142.

[60] Fadare O. Uncommon sarcomas of the uterine cervix: a review of selected entities. *Diagn. Pathol.* 2006;1: 30.

[61] Khosla D, Gupta R, Srinivasan R, Patel FD, Rajwanshi A. Sarcomas of uterine cervix: clinicopathological features, treatment, and outcome. *Int. J. Gynecol. Cancer.* 2012;22: 1026-1030.

[62] Larson B, Silfversward C, Nilsson B, Pettersson F. Prognostic factors in uterine leiomyosarcoma. A clinical and histopathological study of 143 cases. The Radiumhemmet series 1936-1981. *Acta. Oncol.* 1990;29: 185-191.

[63] Major FJ, Blessing JA, Silverberg SG, et al. Prognostic factors in early-stage uterine sarcoma. A Gynecologic Oncology Group study. *Cancer.* 1993;71: 1702-1709.

[64] Copeland LJ, Gershenson DM, Saul PB, Sneige N, Stringer CA, Edwards CL. Sarcoma botryoides of the female genital tract. *Obstet. Gynecol.* 1985;66: 262-266.

[65] Martelli H, Oberlin O, Rey A, et al. Conservative treatment for girls with nonmetastatic rhabdomyosarcoma of the genital tract: A report from the Study Committee of the International Society of Pediatric Oncology. *J. Clin. Oncol.* 1999;17: 2117-2122.

[66] Peters WA, 3rd, Kumar NB, Andersen WA, Morley GW. Primary sarcoma of the adult vagina: a clinicopathologic study. *Obstet. Gynecol.* 1985;65: 699-704.

[67] Della Badia C, Karini H. Endometrial stromal sarcoma diagnosed after uterine morcellation in laparoscopic supracervical hysterectomy. J. Minim. *Invasive Gynecol.* 2010;17: 791-793.

[68] Magne N, Haie-Meder C. Brachytherapy for genital-tract rhabdomyosarcomas in girls: technical aspects, reports, and perspectives. *Lancet Oncol.* 2007;8: 725-729.

[69] Magne N, Oberlin O, Martelli H, Gerbaulet A, Chassagne D, Haie-Meder C. Vulval and vaginal rhabdomyosarcoma in children: update and reappraisal of Institut Gustave Roussy brachytherapy experience. *Int. J. Radiat. Oncol. Biol. Phys.* 2008;72: 878-883.

[70] Sutton G, Blessing J, Hanjani P, Kramer P. Phase II evaluation of liposomal doxorubicin (Doxil) in recurrent or advanced leiomyosarcoma of the uterus: a Gynecologic Oncology Group study. *Gynecol. Oncol.* 2005;96: 749-752.

[71] Lösch A, Joura EA, Stani J, Breitenecker G, Lahodny J. Leiomyosarcoma of the vulva. A case report. *The Journal of reproductive medicine.* 2001;46: 609-612.

[72] Jones IS, Crandon A, Sanday K. Vulvar sarcomas: A 25 plus-year experience from Queensland. *Open Journal of Obstetrics and Gynecology.* 2013;3: 37.

[73] Nielsen GP, Rosenberg AE, Koerner FC, Young RH, Scully RE. Smooth-muscle tumors of the vulva: a clinicopathological study of 25 cases and review of the literature. The *American journal of surgical pathology.* 1996;20: 779-793.

[74] Taskn S, Taskn EA, Üzüm N, Ataoglu Ö, Ortaç F. Primary ovarian leiomyosarcoma: a review of the clinical and immunohistochemical features of the rare tumor. *Obstetrical & gynecological survey*. 2007;62: 480-486.

[75] Lerwill MF, Sung R, Oliva E, Prat J, Young RH. Smooth muscle tumors of the ovary: a clinicopathologic study of 54 cases emphasizing prognostic criteria, histologic variants, and differential diagnosis. *The American journal of surgical pathology*. 2004;28: 1436-1451.

[76] Shakfeh SM, Woodruff DJ. Primary ovarian sarcomas: report of 46 cases and review of the literature. *Obstetrical & gynecological survey*. 1987;42: 331-349.

[77] Bouie SM, Cracchiolo B, Heller D. Epithelioid leiomyosarcoma of the ovary. *Gynecol. Oncol.* 2005;97: 697-699.

[78] Slanetz PJ, Whitman GJ, Halpern EF, Hall DA, McCarthy KA, Simeone JF. Imaging of fallopian tube tumors. *AJR. American journal of roentgenology*. 1997;169: 1321-1324.

[79] Tsili A, Tsampoulas C, Charisiadi A, et al. Adnexal masses: accuracy of detection and differentiation with multidetector computed tomography. *Gynecol. Oncol.* 2008;110: 22-31.

[80] Jacoby AF, Fuller Jr AF, Thor AD, Muntz HG. Primary leiomyosarcoma of the fallopian tube. *Gynecol. Oncol.* 1993;51: 404-407.

Index

A

D

E

F

G

H

I

J

K

L

M

N

O

P

Q

R

S

T

U

V

W

X

Y